THE PHYSICS OF
MEDICAL RADIOGRAPHY

February 3, 1896: the first case of x-rays being employed
for medical diagnosis in America. Dr. Edwin B. Frost,
physicist and astronomer (left), and his brother, Dr. Gilman
D. Frost, physician, x-raying a broken arm. The place:
Physics Laboratory in Reed Hall at Dartmouth College,
Hanover, New Hampshire. (Courtesy of Hitchcock Clinic,
Hanover, N.H.)

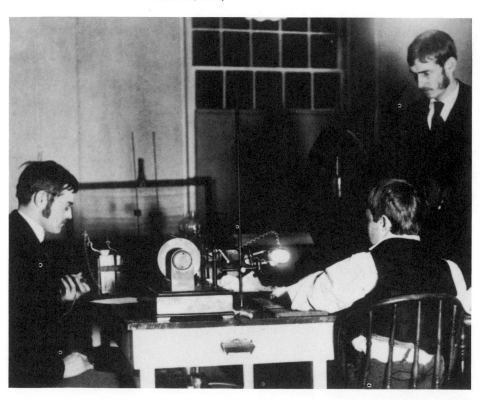

▲▼▲ **ADDISON-WESLEY PUBLISHING COMPANY**

THE PHYSICS OF
MEDICAL RADIOGRAPHY

ARTHUR RIDGWAY
British Columbia Institute of Technology

WALTER THUMM
British Columbia Institute of Technology

Reading, Massachusetts • Menlo Park, California • London • Don Mills, Ontario

To Brenda R. and Eileen T.

Preface

In Chapter 1 there is a summary of the "working rules," to explain the plan we had in mind when we wrote the book, and how the book should be used; this summary is addressed chiefly to the student. Here in the preface, however, we are addressing ourselves primarily to the instructor in medical radiography.

This text had its origins in a series of courses in medical radiography given over a period of years at the British Columbia Institute of Technology. Each course—of which physics naturally formed an important part—lasted five months. These courses made up the main didactic part of the student technician's two-year training program. The remainder of the student's instruction, chiefly practice, was undertaken in a number of affiliated hospital training schools.

This book was written to fill the need for a physics text aimed at the student diagnostic x-ray technician. We hope that our friends and colleagues elsewhere who have experienced the same difficulties we have in finding a text at a suitable level will find this text useful, and that our book will place physics in a perspective that is consistent with the present trend in the training of x-ray technicians.

We believe that health technology, and specifically medical radiography, is an emerging profession, and thus we welcome criticism and comment on this text. Only by such exchanges can those teaching in the health technologies ultimately develop a comprehensive library of texts in the basic sciences and special subjects at a level that is appropriate for tomorrow's health technologist.

The book is intended as a textbook, as opposed to a reference book; a text from which a course in physics for student x-ray technicians can be directly derived. For this reason, we have trimmed it to its present form instead of cramming into it everything which might possibly relate to the subject. At the same time, we have avoided giving the student the impression that physics for him, or her, stops here. There is something peculiarly final and limiting about a text if it gives no indication of the wider world that, after all, begins mere inches outside its covers. So we have included occasional clues to the existence of other horizons, in the hope that the student will read further on his own.

This statement is not to be construed as meaning that we have been completely rigorous in our presentation. We admit that we have not been able to resolve the dilemma of presenting physics at a relatively elementary level: to be as accurate and rigorous as possible in the light of present knowledge and thereby lose the student, or to make the presentation pedagogically tenable and hence somewhat less scientific. But we have tried to resolve the dilemma to the extent that we frequently cite the limitations of our presentation and, as stated above, indicate the existence of further horizons.

Physics in medical radiography has tended to be a dead-end subject; it is not as directly applied in the diagnostic x-ray department as it would be in radiotherapy. For this reason, we believe it is all the more important to make the student aware especially of the principles of physics during the didactic part of his training. If this is done, the medical radiographer will more readily be able to accommodate to whatever changes may come along in the future. Consequently, this is a physics text first and foremost. It does not include such topics as radiography, photography, apparatus, or any other subjects of medical radiography, except as they arise incidental to the physics. Other texts, which deal separately with these subjects, are now becoming available. On the other hand, we *have* illustrated the various physical principles by drawing on examples from medicine and in particular from medical radiography. Throughout the book we have encouraged the student to ask the question, "How does this topic relate to medical radiography?"

The lectures on which this text is based covered 60 hours, but excluded the last chapter and some of the detail in Chapter 8. The 60 hours included lectures, three two-hour written examinations, and two reviews. Concurrently with the lectures, the students at the British Columbia Institute of Technology spent 40 hours in laboratory experiments to reinforce the material presented in the classroom, and especially to relate the physics they were learning to the x-ray department. During the second half of the physics course these students also made a separate but related study of x-ray apparatus.

The prerequisite for entrance to the British Columbia Institute of Technology and the medical radiography program is secondary school graduation in an academic stream, the same as for university entrance. However, few of the members of the classes had had previous instruction in physics.

Since this text is primarily predicated on the student background described above, the first six chapters are concerned with relevant elementary physics. Nevertheless these chapters, as we mentioned earlier, contain many references which relate the physics to medical radiography and therefore provide a new perspective of this material for the student who has some knowledge of physics. For this reason, we feel that the book may also find use in programs for students who have had a general course in elementary physics either in secondary school or first-year college, or both. In fact, we have on a number of occasions gone deliberately further afield to provide material of interest and significance to those who enter x-ray work with such a background. *We feel that the instructor, when he selects the material he wishes to use, may readily omit those topics which he considers either too elementary or too advanced for his students, without, in most cases, doing significant damage to the continuity.* By and large, the syllabus followed is that of the Canadian Society of Radiological Technicians, which syllabus is very similar to that of the American Society of Radiologic Technologists and the British Society of Radiographers.

As a general rule, we have used conventional current direction and mks units, conforming to common practice in physics, electrical engineering, and electronics. In the realm of radiation physics we have employed the terminology of the 1962 recommendations of the ICRU.

The bibliographies at the end of each chapter are annotated for the convenience of instructor and student.

Acknowledgments

We want to acknowledge our indebtedness to the many colleagues, students, and friends whose comments and advice have helped us in the preparation of this text. Like the authors of any technical book we are, of course, also indebted to previous writers on our topic and allied ones.

Among our colleagues from the British Columbia Institute of Technology, those who provided particularly helpful comments were Miss P. M. Rogers of the Department of Medical Radiography; M. S. Bishop, Broadcast Communications Technology; D. Breckner, Computer Center; Dr. B. A. Bürgel, Dr. A. B. L. Whittles, and D. E. Thom of the Department of Physics. Mr. Thom deserves special thanks for his careful proofreading of the work at each stage of its development, as well as for his permission to use some of his notes on significant figures. For several of the photographs we are indebted to Mr. R. J. Smith of the Department of Medical Radiography.

Further afield, we owe thanks to Dr. R. H. Barrett of the Department of Anesthesiology, Hitchcock Clinic, Hanover, N.H., for much valuable, and little-known, information on early x-ray work at Dartmouth College; to Dr. A. Beiser, for permission to use much of the preliminary mathematics from his books, *Modern Technical Physics* and *The Mainstream of Physics* (Addison-Wesley, 1966), in our Appendix A; to Dr. D. E. Tilley of the Department of Physics, Le Collège Militaire Royal de Saint-Jean, Quebec, for invaluable comment on much of the basic physics, as well as on certain pedagogical aspects; and to Dr. Jacob Spira, of the Department of Radiology, Department of Health and Hospitals, Boston, Mass., for helpful constructive criticism on level and content.

For details of x-ray equipment, we acknowledge the cooperation of the General Electric Company and Picker X-Ray Engineering, Ltd.

Our thanks also go to E. C. Roper, principal of the B.C. Institute of Technology at the time the book was conceived and the main writing done, and to S. T. Richards, head of the Department of Health Technology, for the encouragement they gave us on our project.

We are also grateful to the members of the editorial staff of Addison-Wesley, who saw the book through its various stages in a most efficient manner.

Last, but by no means least, our thanks go to our wives for constructive ideas and for bearing with us during the hectic days of writing. In particular: Brenda Ridgway for much handwritten labor, clerical chores, and proofreading; Eileen Thumm for typing the draft and the manuscript, with a valuable assist from Mrs. Helen Cartmill.

We, however, assume full responsibility for any errors, including those which may be construed as having arisen from quoting other works out of context. In committing the book to print we fully realize that such a work is never finished, but merely abandoned.

North Vancouver, B.C.   A. R.
August 1968   W. T.

Contents

CHAPTER 1

The Structure of Matter

Any summary of the achievements of mankind is bound to be unfair to many people who made significant contributions. Nevertheless the authors feel that there is some merit in indicating briefly the historical structure of the advance to new knowledge. It is thus, by the historical aspect, that man and his achievements are perhaps best related. Consequently, each of the chapters in this textbook has a preamble consisting of a brief historical outline highlighting some of the names or events playing a principal role in the material discussed in the chapter.

Our present concept of the atomicity of matter was perhaps most significantly advanced by Dalton's work in chemistry and the discovery by the English botanist, Robert Brown, of the quivering of tiny spores in a drop of water. This work took place in the nineteenth century.

Near the close of the nineteenth century Wilhelm Conrad Röntgen, the discoverer of x-rays, already enters the picture; his discovery shortly led Henri Becquerel to the discovery of radioactivity. From the discovery of radioactivity followed much of our present-day understanding of the nature of the atom.

That most of the mass of the atom is concentrated at a very small central region which contains all the atom's positive electrical charge was first proposed by Ernest Rutherford in 1911 and experimentally confirmed by his co-workers in 1913 by what became one of the classical experiments in physics. This experiment required the use of radioactivity and thus, indeed, the discovery of radioactivity played a major role in man's attempt to comprehend the nature of matter.

Also in 1913, Niels Bohr, a student of Rutherford, developed the first tenable theory of a simple atom such as that of hydrogen. This theory was the first step toward a more complete wave-mechanical treatment of atomic phenomena such as we accept today.

Wave mechanics or quantum mechanics is, like all physical theories, an abstraction, a mathematical formulation, but unlike many other physical theories, it is one which does not lend itself to any tenable model or analogy in terms of phenomena observed in everyday life. However, this theory does lead to the observed experimental results in the realm of atomic physics in a very convincing manner. The two principal originators of this theory were Werner Heisenberg (1925) and Erwin Schrödinger (1926).

1.1 THE NATURE OF PHYSICS

When a nail is being hammered into a board, there is a transfer of energy from the moving hammer to the nail and ultimately also to the wood.

When two billiard balls collide, there is an exchange of energy and after the collision the two balls each move differently from the way they did before.

When you sit in the sunshine you become warmer.

When electrons, rushing through an x-ray tube, strike the target, the target heats up and also some x-rays are produced.

When a positive electron (positron) and a negative electron (usually just called electron) combine they annihilate one another. These small particles of matter disappear and energy, in the form of gamma rays (which are like x-rays but of higher energy), appears.

In all the previous examples, we note the interaction between matter and other particles. It is the nature of physics to deal with such interactions in an attempt to understand the behavior of matter and energy, employing as few basic assumptions as possible. It is the application of these basic assumptions and the consequently derived principles to electrical technology and to the biological sciences which makes medical radiography the powerful tool that it is today.

Physics, like all science, has a dual nature: It is at once a body of facts, of systematically organized knowledge, and at the same time it is a way of thought, a way of attacking problems. Its main objective is the formulation of general principles which lead to a better understanding of the world around us, and in fact the world within us.

In our concern with the physics relating to medical radiography we shall be mostly concerned with physics as a body of systematically organized knowledge. We shall be more deeply concerned with understanding the physical principles associated with medical radiography than with the actual quantitative analysis of problems in physics, or the rigorous derivation of general principles from basic assumptions. In short, we shall be concerned with applied physics, and that primarily from a descriptive rather than a quantitative viewpoint.

It is in the realm of physics to explain, on very basic assumptions, how the x-ray tube works. It is in the realm of technology to devise an efficient tube. And it is in the realm of the medical radiographer, or x-ray technician, to use this x-ray tube wisely and safely. It is the contention of the authors that such usage may be more effectively achieved if the x-ray technician has a basic knowledge of the physical principles underlying the production of x-rays and their interaction with matter.

This book presents the basic physics the technician needs to understand these principles. The treatment is by no means comprehensive. As has been indicated in the preface, this is a textbook, not a reference volume, and consequently the problem facing the authors has primarily been one of selecting and deploying a limited number of facts. We now tackle these facts. We address ourselves to the study of some elements of atomic and nuclear physics, certainly of electricity and magnetism, and—to a very limited extent—of heat and optical phenomena.

Students who have previously studied physics beyond the elementary school level may well be able to skim quickly through some of the material, since this book is not based on the assumption that senior secondary school and/or college physics be a prerequisite. However, the authors would caution all students against being satisfied with a peripheral understanding only. Students who have more than a minimal background for such a course as this book serves may well struggle with some of the deeper implications and thereby stimulate learning for themselves and their less-well-prepared classmates.

Stephen Leacock, Canadian humorist, of McGill University, reputedly once stated, "The real thing for the student is the life and environment that surrounds him. All that he really learns, in a sense, he learns by the active operation of his own intellect and not as the passive recipient of lectures. And for this active operation what he needs most is the continued and intimate contact with his fellows."

All students are reminded that a scientific book must not be read as a novel. You, the student, must pause, ask yourself questions, engage in debate, criticize, review, and, in our case, relate to medical radiography all that lies within these pages. What the authors mean by this admonition is perhaps best expressed in the New Testament, in James, Chapter 1, verse 22:

> *"But be ye doers of the word, and not hearers only, deceiving your own selves."*

The study of physics requires an inquiring and active mind, a characteristic which is also useful in the x-ray department!

1.2 THE NATURE OF MATTER

Brownian Movement

We have just stated that physics concerns itself with matter and energy. That matter is essentially granular in nature is not surprising to most people. However, that energy itself can be considered to consist of small discrete lumps is really not yet well established in our culture. We shall refer to this granular nature of energy shortly when we discuss the atom, and again in later chapters when we deal with such matters as the nature of x-rays. In the meantime, let us ask the question, "What evidence is there that matter is essentially of a granular structure; that the target of the x-ray tube, for example, consists of an aggregation of small individual particles, called atoms?"

As one piece of evidence we consider an observation such as you might make in your own classroom or laboratory (see Fig. 1.1). Here we have a small chamber into which we can draw some air, together with some smoke particles from a cigarette or a recently blown-out match. Then we shine

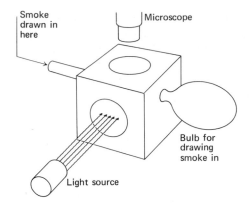

Smoke drawn in here

Microscope

Bulb for drawing smoke in

Light source

FIG. 1.1. Brownian movement. Smoke particles in air.

some light through this chamber and look into it through a microscope with the magnification somewhere in the region of 40–50 diameters. What do we see? We see very bright points darting hither and thither in a random fashion. These bright points are the smoke particles reflecting the light shining into the chamber. The interpretation that we make is that these minute smoke particles scatter about in a random fashion because they are continually being bombarded by other particles, which we assume to be discrete particles, the granular particles of air. These discrete small entities of air we shall refer to as *air molecules.*

In this experiment one actually uses indirect evidence of the presence of small particles of matter by having these bump into something which is small enough to be affected by the collision and yet large enough to be seen with an optical instrument. In this case we presume that small discrete entities of matter, that is, of air (known as molecules), are colliding with those particles which are visible, that is, the smoke. This particular type of random motion of small individual entities of matter, referred to as molecules, is known as the *Brownian movement,* after Robert Brown (1773–1858), an English botanist who first observed this sort of motion by peering through his microscope and noting the strange quiverings of tiny particles floating in a solution.

The interpretation we may give to these Brownian movements supports not only the idea of the granular nature of matter but also the so-called kinetic molecular theory of gases. These observations offer a basis for the idea that gases or liquids are composed of small particles and also for the idea that these small particles are undergoing some kind of random motion, a viewpoint which is one of the key assumptions of the kinetic molecular theory of gases.

Law of Definite Proportions

Is the Brownian movement the only evidence of the granular structure of matter? No. For instance, we might refer to the chemical *law of definite proportions.* Consider an example: It is always found, no matter who performs the experiment or where it is done, that 1 gram of hydrogen will combine with 8 grams of oxygen to produce 9 grams of pure water; that 21 grams of hydrogen will combine with 168 grams of oxygen to form 189 grams of water; that on the other hand, in attempts to combine 8 grams of hydrogen with 8 grams of oxygen, the law of definite proportions still holds true, in that 8 grams of hydrogen plus 8 grams of oxygen will yield 9 grams of water and leave over 7 grams of uncombined hydrogen. How does this support the idea of the granular nature of matter? Well, if each of the elementary substances (e.g., hydrogen, oxygen) were to consist of discrete particles, each of which particles of the same substance had the same mass, then assuming each particle of the more complex substance (e.g., water) to be the same, the mass ratios of the elementary components would always have to be the same. The ratio would not be altered if 1 discrete particle, 10 discrete particles, or 10 million discrete particles were to combine chemically with other discrete particles. (Incidentally, you may be more familiar with this principle expressed in terms of weight, as is generally done by chemists, since weight is proportional to mass.) This interpretation of the law of definite proportions is due to John Dalton (1766–1844) an elementary school teacher who made quite an impact on the world of science.

Before we leave this point we should look at modern research which indicates that the law of definite proportions, although correct in most ordinary chemical reactions, needs to be modified under certain circumstances. This modification arises out of the fact that we now know that not every discrete particle of a given substance has precisely the same mass as another one. (We shall discuss this point later in the chapter when we deal with isotopes.) Moreover, we now know that the mass of the reactants (e.g., hydrogen and oxygen) does not sum up exactly to the mass of the resulting compound (e.g., water). This fact is due to the energy which is either required by or evolves from a chemical reaction. Einstein's *theory of special relativity* led to the famous relation which shows the equivalence of energy and mass, $E = mc^2$, which relation we shall later employ in our discussion of x-rays and their interaction with matter. In this expression E is energy, m is mass, and c is a constant, the speed of light in vacuum. Now how does this relation affect the law of definite proportions? Well, if energy is evolved in the reaction, then this energy appears at the expense of an appropriate loss in mass, according to $E = mc^2$. In ordinary chemical reactions, however, this amount of mass is so small that the best chemical balance will not indicate any change between the masses of the reactants and the mass of the product. In nuclear reactions, however, such as are involved in the production of so-called "atomic" energy, the energy evolved is so great that appreciable mass changes are noted.

Field Ion Microscope

One more piece of evidence in favor of the granular structure of matter is in the form of a photograph (see Fig. 1.2). Here we have the first actual photograph of discrete particles of matter called *atoms*. (Such atoms in

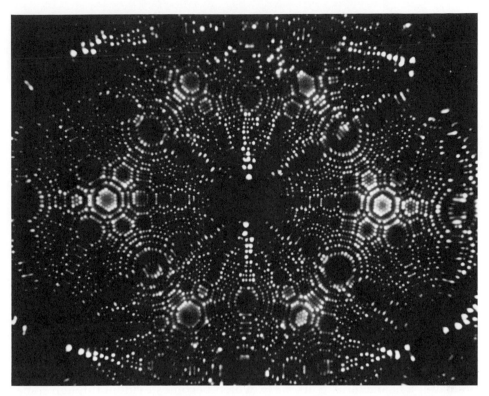

FIG. 1.2. Field ion microscope image of a tungsten needle tip, that is, a hemispherical tungsten crystal approximately 420 angstroms in radius. (Courtesy Dr. E. W. Müller, The Pennsylvania State University)

certain cases combine with other atoms to form larger discrete particles of matter, such as we have previously been talking about, namely molecules.)

This photograph dates back to 1957, when Dr. Erwin W. Müller of The Pennsylvania State University devised a sophisticated piece of apparatus known as a field ion microscope. What we see in this picture are small bright dots, each of the smallest of which is presumed to represent a single atom in the crystal of tungsten, while the larger dots represent clusters of atoms. That is, we are looking at the arrangement of atoms in a metal by means of Dr. Müller's device, which yields a magnification of two or more million diameters!

Perhaps we should look at one more piece of evidence (see Fig. 1.3). Here we can see the trails left by electrically charged particles (such as the nuclei of helium atoms) as they travel through a moist vapor. The nature of this trail is much like the vapor trail left in the sky by a jet aircraft. This type of evidence you can also see for yourself in the laboratory. All

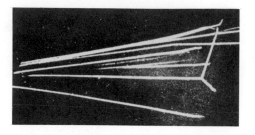

FIG. 1.3. Cloud-chamber photograph of the collision between an electrically charged particle and the nucleus of an atom. (From A. B. Arons, *Development of Concepts of Physics,* Addison-Wesley, 1965.)

you need is a simple cloud chamber and a source of small electrically charged particles, such as some radioactive material. Again this is a point to which we shall return later.

Matter and the Forces of Nature

Let us summarize: There are varieties of evidence which indicate that the structure of matter is granular, that is, that matter is composed of small discrete particles. Shortly we shall consider some of these small discrete particles individually, but before we do so we might raise one further question. We have talked about matter; but in effect, what *is* matter? This question can be answered from everyday experience in a more or less descriptive manner, involving both observation and intuition. We might add a little more rigor to our idea of matter by saying that we can ascribe to matter a characteristic, its *mass*, which becomes evident through something with which we are all familiar: its *weight*. Further, we might refer to this characteristic of matter which we have called mass as representative of the inertia that matter exhibits, its characteristic to oppose any change in the state of its motion. (Students with some physics background may note that we have referred here to both gravitational mass and inertial mass and implied their equivalence.) Consider a block of wood at rest on a table. To change the state of its motion means to speed the block up so that it is moving at say several feet per second along the table top. To achieve this change in motion we need to overcome the matter's inertia by exerting a push or pull, that is, a *force*.

Another characteristic associated with matter is the appearance of certain natural forces. These are *gravitational forces, electrical forces*, and *nuclear forces*. Electrical and nuclear forces will be referred to later. As for gravitational force, it hardly requires further elucidation, since we are all familiar with the fact that every object is attracted toward the center of the earth with a pull, which is gravitational force, and which we call weight.

Table 1.1 summarizes the forces of nature as presently conceived. You might now well ask, "Aside from contributing to general knowledge, does the information in this table have any relevance to radiography?" The answer is yes. These forces play a role in our understanding of the production of x-rays and their interaction with matter (Chapters 9 and 10).

Table 1.1

THE FORCES OF NATURE

Type	Relative strength	Action distance	Particles affected	Comments
Nuclear force	1	About 1×10^{-13} cm (nuclear radius)	Most of the "heavy" particles; e.g., neutron, proton, hyperon	Very strong force Short range Not yet well understood
Electric force (includes magnetic force)	1×10^{-2}	No theoretical limit	All charged particles	The binding force of molecules Strength follows an inverse-square law
"Weak" force	1×10^{-14}	About 1×10^{-8} cm (atomic radius)	"Light" particles; e.g., neutrino, electron, μ-mesons	Evident in processes such as β-decay Short range, but weak Not well understood
Gravitational force	1×10^{-39}	No theoretical limit	Anything having mass (including radiations such as visible light and x-rays)	The force involved when we speak of weight Strength follows an inverse-square law

Moreover the relative strengths of these forces play a very important part which is generally not considered. Compare the electrical force with the gravitational force and you will understand that your x-ray tube does not have to have a special orientation; that it works just as well pointing horizontally as downward. Such would not be the case if the gravitational force on the electron stream in the tube played a significant role.

We are now ready to look in more detail at some of the discrete particles of matter. Let us start with the molecule.

1.3 THE MOLECULE

In our previous reference to the small granular particles of matter we have, on occasion, used the word molecule and the word atom, relying on your previous contact with these words and indeed with these concepts. We now review these concepts briefly.

It is reported that Avogadro (Italian, 1776–1856) said, "We suppose that the particles of any simple gas are not formed of a solitary atom but are made up of a certain number of these atoms united by a traction to form a single molecule." Here the definitions of the two words atom and molecule are implied.

The Smallest Entity of A Chemical Compound

The atom is the smallest particle of an element to retain the chemical characteristics of the element; the molecule is the smallest particle of an element normally capable of independent existence. One must qualify this statement, however, since certain molecules are in effect atoms, in that they are *monatomic*, that is, *they consist of a single atom.* However, molecules of many elements are made up of more than one atom, and certainly molecules of chemical compounds consist of two or more atoms. Referring to our previous example of the compound, water, we now know that one elementary particle of oxygen—that is, one atom—combines with two elementary particles of hydrogen—that is, two atoms—to form a new entity, a molecule of H_2O, that is, water. We might say that *the molecule is the smallest entity of a chemical compound that can exist and still maintain all the characteristics of that compound.* The astonishing thing about molecules is that, if they are formed from different atoms, they (the molecules) have chemical and physical characteristics quite different from those of the constituent atoms. For example, is the molecule poisonous or not poisonous? Stable or highly explosive? Is an aggregation of these molecules, under normal conditions, a solid or a gas? These characteristics are not in general the same as those of the constituent atoms.

The States of Matter

Aggregations of molecules can be found in any one of three states: *gas, liquid,* or *solid.* Most solids are crystalline, as, for example, tungsten. Such solids have their molecules arranged in a fixed geometrical pattern. We shall find later (Chapter 9) that this characteristic of crystalline solids is essential to the process of measuring x-ray wavelengths. The molecules of a crystal oscillate about certain definite equilibrium positions, and the energy of oscillation of the molecules is related to the temperature of the solid. If heat energy is added and thus the temperature is increased, the amplitude of oscillation increases until, at a certain definite temperature, *the melting point,* molecular groups at the surface of the solid move completely away from their equilibrium positions and enter the liquid state. These molecular groups which have entered the liquid state do not necessarily position themselves much farther apart. Rather they merely display more random motion, sliding freely past one another, not being confined to the solid-state equilibrium positions.

Amorphous solids such as glass, or gelatin which is used in x-ray film, do not make a sharp transition from the solid to the liquid state as crystalline solids do, but do so over a range of temperatures, with the solid first softening and then turning into a thick viscous liquid.

An important question to raise when considering an aggregation of atoms or molecules forming a solid is: What is the origin of the forces holding these small particles together? A full answer to this question is well beyond the scope of this text. However, we can make a rather sweeping general statement, which is that *the binding forces are electrical in nature.*

This same answer will suffice to deal with the matter of molecular binding, that is, how atoms are held together to form molecules. Although our answer seems on the surface quite simple, the actual variations of the interaction of the electrical forces involved are considerably more complicated. The famous biochemist, Linus Pauling, was awarded a Nobel prize (1954) for the elucidation of the various aspects of the nature of the chemical bond, particularly with reference to the more complex molecules.

A liquid changes into the gas or vapor state by evaporation. The process of evaporation goes on at all temperatures, and continues until the liquid disappears, or until the space above the liquid has become saturated with the vapor. In this process those molecules in the liquid which have exceptionally high velocities approach the liquid surface at such a rate that they are able to break away from the liquid and form the vapor. Since, of all the molecules in the liquid, only those with higher than average velocity are able to "escape" into the vapor state, it follows that consequently the average velocity of the remaining molecules in the liquid is lowered. Since temperature is related to energy of molecular motion, evaporation is a cooling process, which fact is readily demonstrated if one places a drop of alcohol or ether on the skin.

A material which evaporates readily is said to be *volatile.* Ether is such a volatile liquid, and since it is also exceedingly explosive as a vapor, it poses operating-room problems, particularly for the attending x-ray technician, whose equipment therefore needs to be sparkproof to avoid possible explosions.

Molecular Size

Before we leave the molecule and consider its constituent, the atom, we might note that molecules, even though they may be composed of many atoms, are nevertheless exceedingly small entities; too small to be observed with an optical microscope, but in some cases large enough to be identified by the use of the electron microscope. Although small numbers in themselves, without comparison, are rather meaningless, we should note that experimental evidence is available to show that the diameter of many molecules is of the order of 1 *angstrom* (an angstrom is 10^{-8} centimeter or 10^{-10} meter). Incidentally, this length, 1 angstrom, is also approximately the length of the x-ray waves used in medical radiography.

1.4 THE ATOM

As mentioned before, the atom is the smallest entity of an element having the characteristic of that element. (It is perhaps excusable, at this point, that we become somewhat circular in our definitions, in that we use "element" to describe the "atom" and the "atom" to describe "element." Further usage of these terms will clarify their meaning by implication, although most readers no doubt already have these concepts in hand.) For example, tungsten contains only tungsten atoms, all of which atoms are chemically identical. We could smash the tungsten with a hammer; we could vaporize it, as we do when we overheat the target in the x-ray tube; we could heat it until it melts; we could grind it into a fine powder, but we would still have tungsten atoms, all with exactly the same chemical characteristics.

Atomic Size

Now what do we know about these atoms which constitute the elements? We cannot see them, except in the rather special case of the field ion microscope picture of Fig. 1.2. We must rely on indirect evidence of their existence such as has been implied in the previous discussion of the granularity of matter. Such indirect evidence, for example, might include the tracks left by ionized (electrically charged) helium atoms (or alpha particles) as they travel through a cloud chamber. (Figure 1.3 shows such tracks of electrically charged particles.)

The atom is exceedingly small. Its diameter is generally of the order of magnitude of a molecular diameter. In a multi-atomic molecule, of course, the diameter of the atom will be somewhat less than that of a molecule. In the event that you are more comfortable in the British system of measurement, let us consider again a diameter of around 10^{-8} cm, or 1 angstrom unit, and convert this into the British system of units. We note that 10^{-8} cm $\simeq 4 \times 10^{-9}$ inch. An atom of iron, for example, has a diameter of less than 1 hundred-millionth of an inch.

Although the head of a pin has a mass of only about 8 milligrams and its volume is maybe 1 cubic millimeter, this pinhead contains around 10^{20}, that is, 100,000,000,000,000,000,000 iron atoms!

Thinking at the Atomic Level

What do we know about the atom's composition and behavior?

First, a word of warning. In our discussions we shall take some liberties tending to oversimplification or to the use of analogies which are not completely satisfactory. We shall not always point out the "ifs" and "buts" for fear of making this textbook as large as an encyclopedia. Particularly when we are talking about the atomic region we tend to find comfort in macroscopic analogies, and sometimes these analogies are helpful and therefore of pedagogical merit. After all, our discussion of physical phenomena is bound to be dominated by our own direct experience. All of us find it relatively easy to comprehend those aspects of science which are more or less on the human scale in space and time. This fact is not too surprising, since our language originally developed for communication of the more obvious, macroscopic observations in human affairs. However, we have no adequate language for experiences far removed from the realm of everyday or "household" experiences. Although we have no trouble in expressing matter and/or energy relationships—that is, the laws of physics—of things that are "household" size and even thousands of times smaller or larger, we do find an insurmountable, or almost insurmountable, obstacle in comprehending with our language affairs in the realm of say 10^{-8} cm, which is the approximate diameter of an atom. Here we cannot get help from our senses, we cannot make a direct appeal. Thus we talk about these things in terms of analogies which may occasionally be misleading. Because of these deficiencies in our language and experience, we must tackle the realm of atomic and radiation physics with a concerted effort to keep an open mind. Professor D. H. Wilkinson, professor of experimental physics at Oxford University, suggests in "Towards New Concepts, Elementary Particles," a lecture published in *Turning Points in Physics* (Harper Torchbooks, 1961), that we need to be prepared for, at least, two changes in our attitude. First, the acceptance of new concepts which have no counterpart in the "household world," and second, an increased reliance on symbols and mathematics or (in our case at least) on the results derived thereby. We must be prepared to accept the fact that some of the things learned appear to run counter to common sense and that some of the concepts, since they have no real "household" counterparts, thus cannot be dealt with fully by any particular analogy. It may be necessary therefore to use several analogies which would on the "household" scale appear to be in conflict. One example of such a conflict is the wave-particle duality of nature. We shall before long come to grips with the fact that we need, on occasion, to describe x-rays as though they were constituted of particles which we call photons, and on the other hand we may need to describe certain phenomena in which we treat x-rays as though they behaved like waves. Furthermore we shall shortly see that sometimes a wave concept, which has no real meaning in our macroscopic world, has to be attached to an atom. We shall find that the most modern theory of the atom is a mathematical abstraction in which the waves themselves have no immediate physical meaning, but rather a mathematical one.

The Bohr Atom

The atom, and consequently matter, is essentially electrical in nature. For example, surprising as it may seem, the reason that you cannot push your hand through the desk in front of you is the presence of electrical forces.

For our purposes a planetary concept of the atom, somewhat as conceived by Niels Bohr in 1913, will suffice. (Bohr, a Danish physicist, was awarded the Nobel prize in physics in 1922.) We shall, however, have to make on occasion brief references to what has supplanted this simple "household" analogy.

Let us say that atoms are composed of tiny particles, which are referred to in the realm of physics as *elementary particles*. Although nowadays in physics laboratories more and more so-called elementary particles are appearing, the question is increasingly becoming: What is elementary? Well, for our purposes, we shall consider as elementary only those particles which are either stable—that is, are around by themselves for a long time—or else those that are at least not so transient in nature that they have lifetimes of only fractions of microseconds.

The particles composing the atom are of three kinds: (1) There is always at least one proton, carrying a unit positive charge of electricity.

(2) There may be some neutrons, which carry no electrical charge. (3) There are always as many electrons, carrying a unit negative charge of electricity each, as there are protons. Now it is impossible to say exactly what these little particles are. Sometimes they do indeed behave like tiny billiard balls, but on the other hand sometimes their behavior is best analyzed as though they behaved in a wavelike fashion. In the Bohr concept, however, we picture them as little balls.

The protons and neutrons are clustered very tightly together in the central part of the atom, called the *nucleus*. More than 99% of the mass of the atom is located here in the nucleus. The electrons circle in certain fixed orbits in the space about the nucleus. Since the electrons and the nucleus are both small compared with the size of the electron orbits, the atom, and hence matter, is mostly empty space. However, one might reasonably imagine that the electrons whiz around the nucleus at such great speeds that they in effect form a shell around the nucleus, somewhat as a fast-moving blade on a machine to all intents and purposes forms a solid disk.

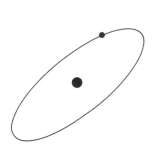

FIG. 1.4. Hydrogen, a simple atom.

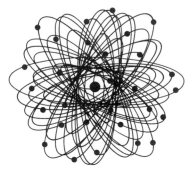

FIG. 1.5. A more complex atom.

Some atoms are quite simple. For example, an ordinary hydrogen atom has one proton in its nucleus and retains its electrical neutrality as an atom by having only one electron circling around the nucleus (see Fig. 1.4). On the other hand, copper, which is of some interest in the x-ray world as a good conductor of electrical current, has an atom which is much more complex. A copper atom has 29 protons and 34 neutrons in the nucleus, with 29 electrons circling around it (somewhat like Fig. 1.5).

We now look a little more thoroughly at the Bohr idea of the atom. Let us plunge right along and state two of Bohr's fundamental postulates and then see where these lead. First of all, Bohr said, "A bound atomic system can exist without radiating energy only in certain discrete stationary states." This means that in the hydrogen atom, for example, there are certain permissible orbits possible for the electron whirling around the nucleus. Not any orbit is possible, but just special orbits (labeled K, L, M, N, etc., where K refers to the innermost one). These orbits he calculated by virtue of the fact that for the electron to be able to whirl around the nucleus it needed a force to hold it in its path, somewhat as a string is required to pull on a rock whirling around in a circle, and further, that the force in this case, analogous to the string tension, would be the electrical attraction between the positively charged nucleus and the negative charge on the electron. Now the fact that only certain orbits are allowable leads us to the statement that the orbits are *quantized*, that is, that only definite orbits and not all the various in-between orbits are possible. Nowadays one refers to this in a slightly different way. One associates energy levels with the orbits. For example, since a positive charge will attract a negative charge, the orbit farther away from the nucleus is said to be of a higher energy, because work would have to be done on the electron to pull it away from the nucleus into a farther or outermost orbit. Presently therefore one says that the Bohr concept implies that the atomic, or electronic, energy levels are quantized, and one associates a definite number—that is, a *quantum number*—with a certain level.

Now the notion of the quantization of energy, that is, that energy comes in discrete chunks, first appeared in the realm of physics as the result of work done in 1900 by Max Planck (Nobel prize in physics, 1918). According to Planck's quantum theory, energy cannot flow in a continuous fashion from radiating bodies, but rather the energy, in the form of electromagnetic radiations, comes off in distinct and separate chunks, known as *quanta* or *photons*.

Emission Spectra

Now let us follow Bohr a little further. He goes on to postulate that when an atom undergoes a transition from an upper energy state to a lower energy state, electromagnetic radiation—that is, *a photon of energy*— is emitted, and that photon is therefore characteristic of the atom emitting it. This idea explains why, for example, when you excite mercury you get a light of a particular color, rather greenish; or if you somehow excite sodium you get a light which is predominantly yellow. (The latter may be achieved simply by placing some ordinary table salt into a flame.) The fact that these colors are different simply means that the energy levels in the sodium and in the mercury atom are different. Hence this Bohr postulate says that *the energy given off can only be, and is exactly, the difference between the energy levels*, or orbits if you like the older terminology, characteristic of the atom concerned. Figure 1.6 shows, on the one hand, an orbital representation, that is, some of the various orbits possible for a hydrogen atom, and second the associated energy-level diagram.

Atoms are sometimes excited (by heat or electrical energy, for example) to higher energies, only to return again to the ground state, that is, to the condition in which the electrons occupy the lowest possible energy levels available, with the radiation of energy as visible light. Some atoms may be excited to a greater or lesser degree and return to the ground state with the emission of invisible radiation. One example of this type of invisible radiation following great excitation are the so-called characteristic x-rays which will be discussed in Chapter 9. Another example is the ultraviolet radiation, given off by mercury atoms following their electrical

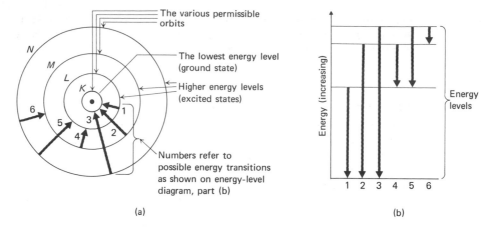

(a)

(b)

FIG. 1.6. (a) Bohr orbits. (b) Energy levels, showing some possible transitions of the electron of a hydrogen atom (not to scale).

excitation; this is the kind of radiation used in germicidal lamps for hospitals. However, if the energy jumps are too small to produce visible light, we may have infrared radiation or "heat waves"; these are the principal means for heat transfer from an open fireplace. This type of heat transfer was also the main mode for cooling of the original Coolidge x-ray tubes, and is still significant in more modern tubes used in medical diagnostic work.

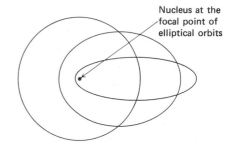

FIG. 1.7. The Sommerfeld atom. Elliptical orbits are permissible. (Note that the circle is a special case of the ellipse.)

Now Bohr's calculations agreed fairly well with the various spectra, that is, with the various colors that were observed when the light emitted by electrically excited hydrogen gas was separated into its constituent colors with a glass prism. However, as the field of spectroscopy (that is, the analyzing of the various colors or the analyzing of the so-called spectra) improved, some spectral lines (i.e., colors) were noted which were not completely in accord with the Bohr theory, and consequently at this point in the history of atomic physics a series of patching-up affairs took place. One such modification, proposed by Arnold Sommerfeld (1916), was that the electron orbits need not be circular, but could be elliptical (see Fig. 1.7). What this modification really meant was that additional permissible energy levels were introduced, in addition to those allowable ones suggested by the original Bohr theory. In this manner a second quantum number was first introduced in the specification of an electron's energy state.

Quantum Mechanics

However, when one begins to look at more complex atoms, the Bohr theory, even as modified by Sommerfeld, becomes progressively less capable of making the correct predictions of experimental observations. Although the Bohr theory is an essential and exceedingly helpful beginning and is, in effect, still a useful crutch quite adequate for our purposes, it had to be replaced by a theory which was more in accord with the experimental evidence relating to the more complex atoms.

Such a theory was the theory of *wave mechanics* or *quantum mechanics,* introduced in two conceptually and mathematically different ways by Werner Heisenberg and Erwin Schrödinger around the end of the first quarter of the twentieth century. Since wave mechanics is a mathematical abstraction, it is difficult at the level of this book to make much convincing sense out of it. In fact, it is often said in reference to atomic structure and behavior that there are two possible approaches: the *classical approach* (that is, the Bohr atom) which has the advantage of being readily visualized but is unfortunately not completely adequate; and the *quantum-mechanical approach* (that is, wave mechanics) which seems implausible but is entirely adequate.

Let us say simply that wave mechanics replaced the idea of the permitted circular orbits of Bohr and the permitted elliptical orbits of Sommerfeld with the idea of permitted waves. These waves, however, are not to be construed in the ordinary physical sense, such as water or sound waves, but rather in a mathematical sense. The permitted waves yield the knowledge of what is the most likely distribution of electrons around a given nucleus. It can be shown that these *permitted probability distributions* are related to definite permitted energy levels of electrons in a given atom. Hence, nowadays, rather than speaking of definite orbits, we speak of atoms in terms of definite energy levels. (These definite, permissible energy levels, as suggested before, are assigned numbers, called *quantum numbers,* of which present quantum theory assigns four to each electron in an atom; and further, no two electrons in any atom may have the same set of four quantum numbers. We shall refer to this matter later in our discussion of the periodic table.) In the case of a simple atom like hydrogen, wave mechanics yields exactly the same answers, or makes the same predictions, as the Bohr theory. This fact is really part and parcel of the development of a physical theory, namely that the newer or more modern concepts should be more encompassing than the older ones, but should include the older concepts as special limiting cases.

For our purposes it is fruitful to continue to sketch atoms in terms of the Bohr concept, and to use this representation later on, even when we are talking about the production of x-rays as electrons strike the target in an x-ray tube. But we must remind ourselves not to construe these diagrams as physical realities, that is, as "pictures of atoms," but rather as crutches to help us deal with the microcosmos of the atomic world. In terms of today's physics, we had better speak of the various energy levels of atoms and accept the fact that discrete energy levels exist, and that these discrete energy levels are different for different atoms, and therefore that the way that an atom (via its electrons) can pick up energy or give off energy can only be in terms of discrete chunks of energy. For example, if an atom, by some method of excitation, goes from energy level E_1 to the adjacent energy level E_2, it comes back down to the lower energy level giving off energy of an amount which is the difference between E_2 and E_1. This particular difference in energy—this lump, bunch, bundle, chunk, or quantum of energy—as was first proposed by Planck, can be related to the frequency (and hence the wavelength) of the radiated energy. In the visible region this fact means that the frequency can be related to the color of the light. The relationship is ΔE (the energy change between two levels) equals hf, where f is the frequency of the radiation and h is a fundamental constant, known as *Planck's constant*. We write this relationship as an equation,

$$\Delta E = hf,$$

or often simply as

$$E = hf, \tag{1.1}$$

where E now stands for the energy of the emitted photon. The higher the frequency the greater the energy. In the visible region this means, for example, that the frequency of violet light is greater than the frequency of red light, since violet light is of a higher energy.

Before we leave the idea of the quantization of emitted radiation, we should emphasize that this quantization is applicable to the energy input to an atom also. The atom can accept energy only in bundles of the same size as it may emit. The size of the energy bundles that an atom may accept, like the size that it may emit, depends on the differences between the various energy levels.

Now once more we should ask what all this has to do with medical radiography. Well, first of all, we are establishing a reasonably modern vocabulary in physics. Without this vocabulary and background we cannot sensibly discuss anything about x-rays in any serious fashion whatsoever. Second, we have already seen the direct application of these ideas, insofar as we have mentioned that in due course we shall use them to describe the production of characteristic x-rays. Also we shall find ourselves using these ideas when we talk about the photoelectric effect which enters the x-ray realm in the timing circuitry, that is, the photoelectric timer, and in the photoelectric absorption of x-rays in body tissue.

The Electron

Now is a good time to say something about the electron. The electron plays a major role in x-ray production and, of course, we have referred to it continuously in our discussion of the atom. The electron is one of the so-called *elementary particles* which is stable by itself, that is, it can exist by itself as well as exist as an integral part of an atom. Its mass is

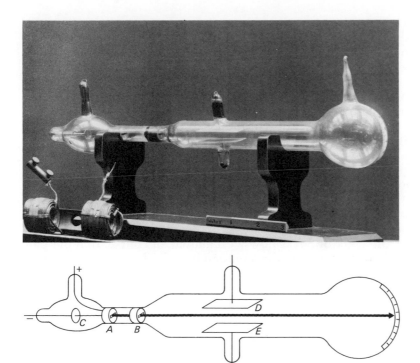

FIG. 1.8. Thomson's *e/m* experiment: the apparatus and its schematic illustration. The photograph shows the original equipment lent to The Science Museum, London, by J. J. Thomson, Esq., M.A., Trinity College, Cambridge.

9.108×10^{-31} kilogram, which is 1/1,837th the mass of a hydrogen atom, and its electrical charge has been identified as 16.02×10^{-20} coulomb of negative electricity. The electron as such was first identified by the Nobel-prize-winning English physicist, J. J. Thomson, in 1899. The famous experiment which J. J. Thomson performed, and which led him to the ratio of the electric charge to mass, that is, *e/m*, for the electron can be described with reference to Fig. 1.8. Although this experiment was first performed in 1897, it might well have been performed much earlier, except for one rather important requirement, and this requirement has a bearing on x-ray tubes. A look at the equipment shows that what is apparently involved is a glass tube; but what one really needs is a tube that has as little gas in it as possible, and therein lies the reason the experiment was not performed earlier. The experiment was dependent on technological improvements in vacuum techniques; the stream of electrons which is emitted by a hot filament, just like the one in the x-ray tube, at point *C* in the diagram, must not be appreciably disturbed by collisions with gas molecules in the tube.

Let us now have a look at the nature of this experiment, since it has a lot in common with what is going on in an x-ray tube. Cathode rays (that is, a stream of electrons) were emitted at point *C*, focused by means of the slits *A* and *B*, and then caused to pass between the plates *D* and *E*. It was noticed that when an electrical charge was placed on these plates the beam was deflected either upward or downward, depending on the nature of the charge on the plates. This fact suggested to Thomson that cathode rays must carry electrical charge. Further analysis (which you might make yourself after our discussion of the magnetic and electrical effects in later chapters) involving the application of magnetic fields permitted Thomson finally to calculate the ratio of the electrical charge of the cathode-ray particles to their mass. Now the value of this charge-to-mass ratio turned out to be much bigger than the corresponding values determined for *ions* (electrically charged atoms, or molecules) by means of electrolysis, in fact bigger by a factor of several thousands. The conclusion which Thomson reached was that cathode rays consist of particles with a mass much smaller than that of ions. He further deduced from his experiment that the particles composing the cathode rays have a negative charge. He called these particles corpuscles and their charge, which represented the basic unit of an electric charge, the electron. It is now well known, of course, that the particles themselves in later usage have come to be called electrons, and that the charge is simply referred to as the electronic charge, which, as we previously stated, is 16.02×10^{-20} coulomb.

The story of the electron is not yet complete. We have identified it as the negative charge carrier, but we have only its charge-to-mass ratio. The actual electrical charge on the electron, which we have already quoted, was not determined until sometime later, in another of the classical experiments of physics. That experiment was the *Millikan oil-drop experiment*. This work was done by the American physicist Robert A. Millikan (Nobel prize in physics, 1923), who began his studies of the electron charge in 1907 and several years later obtained a remarkably accurate result, well in accord with the presently accepted value we have previously quoted.

1.5 THE NUCLEUS

We now leave the whirling electrons and address ourselves to the central, dense part of the atom: the nucleus. Since it was well known in the early days that the atom itself was electrically neutral, one of the concepts of the atom was that it was somewhat like a plum pudding. The atom was assumed to be composed, in essence, of a homogeneous mass having a positive electrical charge, in which, like raisins in a pudding, were the electrons.

Rutherford Nuclear Atom

That the plum-pudding concept was not true was first proposed by Sir Ernest Rutherford (1911) and experimentally verified by H. Geiger and E. Marsden (1913), working in Rutherford's laboratory at the University of Manchester. Rutherford's proposal was the concept we used earlier in this chapter when we were discussing the Bohr atom. Actually we might have said in this earlier discussion that one of Bohr's postulates was the acceptance of the Rutherford concept of the nuclear atom, that is, that the mass of the atom is concentrated, along with its positive electrical charge, at a very small and very dense central part. Some comparison is in order.

If an atom had a diameter about equal to the length of an x-ray table, then the nucleus would have a diameter about twice that of a human hair. Thus the nucleus has a diameter about one ten-thousandth as large as the diameter of the atom, that is, the diameter of the nucleus is of the order of 10^{-12} cm. The simplest nucleus (hydrogen) is even smaller than that, the diameter of a single proton being about 10^{-13} cm.

How it is possible to measure this incredibly small diameter can be explained by various analogies, somewhat like the following. Consider an opaque box, the mass of the contents of which is known. We are asked to determine, without looking inside, the distribution of the mass inside the box. The box might, for example, be filled completely with a material of relatively low density such as putty, or it might contain only a couple of steel balls, held in place with a very fine thread so that shaking the box yields no information. What can we do? Shoot small bullets into the box. If the bullets all seem to emerge in the direction they were fired, then we might reasonably conclude that the box is filled with some relatively homogeneous material such as putty. If, on the other hand, a few bullets are significantly deviated from the direction of firing, it is fair to assume that this result must be due to collision with some small, hard, dense objects, widely separated.

Well now, for the box and contents substitute a thin gold foil, and for the bullets substitute alpha particles, the small particles shot out by a radioactive source (radon in this case), and you have the essence of the famous Rutherford scattering experiment (see Fig. 1.9).

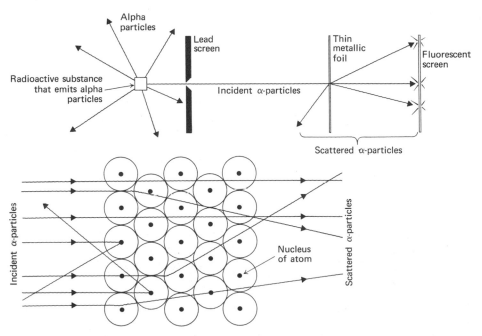

FIG. 1.9. The essence of the Rutherford scattering experiment, showing the experimental setup and the situation inside the thin metallic foil.

Geiger and Marsden observed some large scattering angles, and these were in accord with Rutherford's calculations. Consequently the concept of the nuclear atom was firmly established.

As mentioned in the previous section, it is now well known that the nucleus of an atom is composed of *protons*, which carry all the atom's positive electrical charge, as well as in some cases one or more neutrons. The proton itself was identified and named by Rutherford some time after his nuclear atom was confirmed.

Rutherford also predicted the existence of the *neutron*. (Other people who predicted the neutron were W. D. Harkins in the U.S.A., and O. Masson in Australia.) The year was 1920. Not until 1932 was the neutron identified by Chadwick (Nobel prize in physics, 1935) in England. The neutron's mass is about the same as that of the proton. However, unlike the proton, the neutron carries no electrical charge and it is not a very stable particle. A proton may exist indefinitely as a proton, but a free neutron has a *half-life* of only about 12 minutes. What this means is that if you had a handful of neutrons, then 12 minutes later you would have only half a handful; the rest of them would have decayed, each into a proton and an electron.

(Incidentally it is interesting to note that the neutron itself has entered the field of radiography. Pictures made using low-energy neutrons disclose some things which are not easily seen in x-ray radiographs. Although neutrons for radiography are limited to use with nonliving materials, new detection methods are making the use of neutrons an effective new inspection tool.)

The number of protons in the nucleus is referred to as the *atomic number, Z*. This number is characteristic of a particular element. Since the mass of a neutron is almost the same as that of a proton, the combined number of protons and neutrons—that is, the total number of *nucleons*— is referred to as the *atomic mass number, A*. For example, the ordinary oxygen nucleus could be represented by the symbol $_8O^{16}$. This symbolism indicates that the oxygen nucleus is composed of 8 protons ($Z = 8$) and 16 nucleons ($A = 16$), which implies that this nucleus includes 8 neutrons ($N = 8$). Consider hydrogen: $_1H^1$. The information shown is that this nucleus is no more than a single proton.

This symbolism makes it easy to describe complicated phenomena in simple shorthand, as in the following example:

$$_2He^4 + _7N^{14} \rightarrow _8O^{17} + _1H^1.$$

Here we have the alchemists' dreams come true: a "manmade" transmutation of the elements, as first achieved by Rutherford (1919). We see that a helium nucleus is made to interact with a nitrogen nucleus, thereby yielding a proton and an oxygen nucleus. Note that the atomic mass numbers (across the top) are balanced, that is, that they are the same before the interaction as after, and also that the atomic numbers (across the bottom) balance. In other words, the number of protons and of neutrons remains unchanged. Also note that the oxygen is not quite the same as the oxygen cited in the previous paragraph: There is a difference in the number of neutrons. The two types of oxygen are said to be *isotopes*. We shall discuss isotopes further later on in this chapter.

Theory of the Nucleus

Physicists are generally agreed that we now have a more or less complete and satisfying theory of the structure and behavior of the atom. But this is not yet the case with respect to the nucleus. Theoretical models of the nucleus have been proposed to account for the various nuclear phenomena, as, for example, the relative instability of certain large nuclei which split into parts when they are bombarded by neutrons, a process which is known as *nuclear fission* and is the basis of nuclear reactors, that is, "atomic" energy. However, none of the models proposed to date yields a complete and generally accepted theory.

The very force which holds nucleons (nuclear particles, protons, and neutrons) together is well enough identified, but yet poorly understood. Reference to Table 1.1 shows how tremendously large and yet short range this force is. A complete theory of this nuclear force must deal successfully with such phenomena as the fission referred to above, nuclear energy levels, so-called resonance absorption by the nucleus of neutrons striking it, and radioactivity, which we shall consider next.

1.6 RADIOACTIVITY

In 1901 Wilhelm Conrad Röntgen was awarded the world's first Nobel prize in physics for his discovery of x-rays. Two years later Antoine Henri Becquerel shared the Nobel physics award with the Curies, Marie and Pierre. Becquerel's share of the prize was for his discovery of the radioactivity of uranium and the Curies received their award for the discovery of other elements exhibiting radioactivity.

Discovery of Radioactivity

Becquerel's discovery of radioactivity (1896) was a rather immediate consequence of Röntgen's discovery of x-rays (1895). Röntgen's mysterious and marvelously penetrating rays were produced in the course of an electrical discharge through a gas-filled glass tube. As we understand it today, the x-rays were produced chiefly by electrons striking the walls of the tube. This electron bombardment also made the glass luminescent. Becquerel's first assumption was that x-rays were associated with this glowing or luminescence of the glass. He therefore embarked on a series of experiments to determine whether x-rays were emitted by materials that were caused to luminesce through the action of visible light.

Among the materials with which Becquerel experimented was pitchblende, a double sulfate of uranium and potassium which was known to be phosphorescent, that is, it was known to glow for some time after it was exposed to sunlight. What he did was to wrap a photographic plate in thick black paper so that no sunlight could get to the plate. Then he placed the wrapped photographic plate in the sunlight with the salt containing uranium on top of the black wrapper. And indeed the photographic plate appeared exposed under the salt crystals. The salt had taken a picture of itself! On the surface his premise had been upheld: Materials which glow after exposure to sunlight give off x-rays. Fortunately there was limited sunshine in Paris during March when he performed these experiments and hence he had occasion to prepare the experimental materials and then leave them in a dark drawer awaiting the sunshine's appearance. But no sun appeared for the following days, so he took the photographic plate out of the drawer and developed it, expecting to see only a negligible exposure. However, in his own words, "The silhouettes (of the uranium salt) appeared, to the contrary, with great intensity." He thus discovered that the effect on the photographic plate was apparently not dependent on the luminescent effects exhibited by the uranium salt. He confirmed this new idea by using other uranium compounds, some of which were not luminescent. He had discovered some new property of certain materials. He described this new property as the emission of *"radiations actives."* He had discovered radioactivity.

Early Radioactive Elements

Two years after Becquerel's discovery, Marie Sklodowska Curie involved herself and her husband, Pierre, in a search for other elements exhibiting these curious *"radiations actives."* In the course of these investigations they discovered the elements radium and polonium. (It was Madame Curie who coined the word "radioactivity" for the property exhibited by these materials.)

Further investigations by Marie Curie confirmed earlier conclusions by other scientists: that there were three different types of radiations emitted. In her doctoral thesis (1903) she summarized the different electrical properties of the radiations in the form of a diagram (see Fig. 1.10). The radioactive material is presumed to be in a deep well in a lead block. In the absence of external electric and magnetic forces the radiations would emerge as a single beam. Application of an electric or magnetic field,

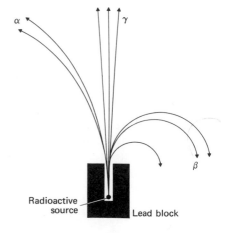

FIG. 1.10. The three types of radiation. Magnetic field is perpendicular to paper. This diagram must be approached with caution, for it is very schematic indeed. For example, the suggestion that all radioactive materials give rise to these three types of rays is false. Further, the radii of the beta-particle paths are much too large relative to the trajectories of the alpha particles.

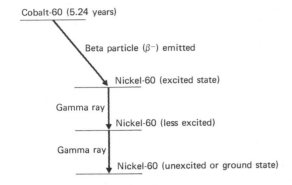

Cobalt-60 (5.24 years)

Beta particle (β^-) emitted

Nickel-60 (excited state)

Gamma ray

Nickel-60 (less excited)

Gamma ray

Nickel-60 (unexcited or ground state)

FIG. 1.11. Typical radioactive decay scheme. Cobalt-60 decays to stable nickel-60, giving off electrons and gamma-rays.

however, would cause the radiations to separate as shown. (The student might return to this diagram after we deal with electromagnetic phenomena in the following chapters.) The three types of radiations are referred to as alpha (α), beta (β), and gamma (γ) radiations, terms which were adopted by Sir Ernest Rutherford.

Most naturally occurring radioactive elements emit either alpha or beta rays, although in a very few cases both are emitted. Gamma rays accompany the other two radiations in some cases. An example of such a case may be seen in Fig. 1.11. Nuclei are sometimes left in an excited state after alpha (or beta) emission and the de-excitation may involve the emission of one or more gamma rays.

The Process of Radioactivity

Ernest Rutherford (1871–1937), who entered the field of physics just after the discovery of radioactivity, was the first to recognize radioactivity as the process of disintegration of the nuclei of unstable atoms. It was for this interpretation of the phenomenon of radioactivity and other discoveries concerning the chemistry of radioactive elements that he was awarded the Nobel prize in chemistry in 1908. Rutherford went on to identify the alpha radiation or alpha particle as the nucleus of a helium atom, composed of two protons and two neutrons. As we have already seen, Rutherford used these alpha particles to probe the atom, thus supporting the nuclear concept of the atom. His sources of alpha particles were the radioactive elements radon and polonium. The latter will serve as an example of the process of radioactive decay.

A polonium nucleus after it emits an alpha particle is no longer polonium. What has happened? The nucleus now has two fewer protons and two fewer neutrons. Since the number of protons in the nucleus determines the element, the resulting nucleus is that of lead.

On the other hand, one type of radioactive iodine decays by giving off a beta particle (an electron, that is) and the net effect is the same as if a neutron in the nucleus had been changed to a proton. Thus the new nucleus has one more proton than iodine; it is the nucleus of the element xenon. *Radioactivity is thus a process which results in the transmutation of one element into another.* This process is shown in the radioactive decay schemes of Figs. 1.11 and 1.12.

As mentioned before, some of the alpha and beta emissions are accompanied by gamma radiation. Gamma rays are electromagnetic radiations, such as visible light and x-rays, and since their emission results in no appreciable mass change in the nucleus and no change in the nuclear charge, or number of protons, they do not contribute to the transmutation process.

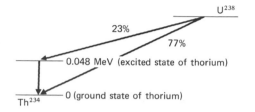

FIG. 1.12.   The emission of γ-rays in conjunction with the emission of α-particles.   (Energy of emitted γ-rays is 0.048 million electron volts.)

The question arises: Why should some elements be radioactive? It turns out that all elements with atomic number (Z) greater than 83 and/or atomic mass number (A) greater than 209, as well as some others, exhibit this property of decaying spontaneously into another element. A thorough treatment of why this is so is beyond the scope of this text. However, we may cite as a general condition of the instability of an atom (which may or may not lead to radioactivity, depending on further considerations) that the mass of the atom should be greater than the mass of any combination of components into which it may decay. If, on the other hand, the mass of an atom is smaller than, or equal to, the mass of the components into which one might conceivably consider it to decay, then the atom is stable and not subject to radioactive disintegration. The student is challenged to seek the plausibility of the above statements, by recourse to the Einstein concept of the equivalence of mass and energy ($E = mc^2$), referred to earlier in the chapter.

Penetrability of the Various Radiations

The student's answer to the question suggested above will, of course, depend on the realization that in radioactive decay, the alpha (or beta) particles are emitted with considerable energy. This *kinetic energy* (energy of motion) makes it possible for the particles to penetrate matter. Of the three types of radiation which occur, the α-particles have the least penetrating ability. They have a range of only a few inches in air and may be stopped by a piece of paper. Consequently, the danger associated with external α-particle sources is in some respects not serious, provided the sources are properly stored so that contact with personnel is avoided. On the other hand, some α-emitters, including radium, produce gaseous radioactive daughter products which may be readily spread about and absorbed by the body. In the latter case the α-particles may, indeed, cause serious injury. The moral of this story is: Treat *any* type of radioactive material with due respect.

Beta particles are more penetrating, being able to penetrate a few millimeters of body tissue. In fact, the more energetic β-particles may well penetrate as much as an eighth of an inch of aluminum. However, even this penetrating ability is still not very great, and hence the dangers from exposure to an external beta source are readily obviated by the use of light metal shielding.

Gamma rays are a different matter entirely. They are able to travel long distances through the air and penetrate deeply into the body. They may even substantially penetrate an inch of lead if they are of sufficient energy. In fact a study of the attenuation of γ-rays reveals that, although shielding with lead can reduce the γ-ray intensity to tolerable levels, there is always some penetration; a γ-ray beam can theoretically never be completely attenuated. In practice, however, if the absorber is sufficiently thick the beam may well be attenuated to the point at which no transmitted energy is readily detectable. Protection from these rays will be discussed later, when we deal specifically with radiations of this type produced when high-speed electrons strike a solid target; we are referring to x-rays, of course.

Half-Life

When α-particles and β-particles are emitted, the nuclei, as was pointed out earlier, are transformed into nuclei of different elements. This process goes on at a well-defined rate, characteristic of a given element. It is a statistical process. This means that although the rate of decay is well defined for an assembly of atoms, so that in a particular piece of material we can say quite definitely that within the next minute x number of atoms will decay, we have no way of knowing which ones of all the millions of atoms of this piece of material it will be.

The rate of this decay process may be expressed in terms of a decay constant, λ (the Greek letter lambda), which clearly "fingerprints" a given element, because it has a definite value for a particular element and is unaffected, to all intents and purposes, by any chemical or physical states imposed on the element. Another way of expressing this constant characteristic of a radioelement involves a concept introduced by Rutherford, *the half-life*, a term which we mentioned briefly in our earlier reference to the neutron. Let us now tie these ideas together.

Suppose that, at a given time, we have N atoms. The number of atoms that will decay in a short interval thereafter turns out, quite plausibly, to be proportional to N. The number of disintegrations, which is the change in N, we shall call ΔN, where the Δ simply means "change in" or "part of," and the relevant time interval is Δt. Since the number of atoms N is decreasing as time goes on, we could express the decay process as a proportionality,

$$\Delta N \propto N \, \Delta t. \qquad (1.2)$$

That is, the number of disintegrations is proportional to both the original number of atoms and the time interval under consideration. (Actually, one should use here a very, very, *very* small time interval, because N is continuously changing.)   Let us turn that proportionality (1.2) into an equation by supplying the appropriate proportionality constant. We then write

$$\Delta N = -\lambda N \,\Delta t, \tag{1.3}$$

where the proportionality constant λ is the previously encountered decay constant, which must be empirically determined for each radioelement, and the minus sign indicates that the number of atoms is decreasing. Using Eq. (1.3), we can show that the *radioactive decay law* has the form

$$N = N_0 e^{-\lambda t}, \tag{1.4}$$

where N is the number of atoms present at a time t, given that N_0 is the number present at a time $t = 0$, and e is the base of natural (or Napierian) logarithms. This type of equation is known as an *exponential equation*, and consequently one says that radioactivity follows an exponential decay law. We shall meet this type of equation again later when we consider the charging of a capacitor (Section 2.6) and the attenuation of x-rays (Section 10.1). [Those students who have the calculus at their disposal might try writing Eq. (1.3) as an ordinary differential equation and then integrating it to get Eq. (1.4); to derive the equation without the calculus is also possible, but to do so requires a little more labor.]

Next we relate the decay constant λ to the half-life. We recall that the number of radioactive atoms at $t = 0$ is N_0. Then, by definition, the half-life is the value of t when $N = (\frac{1}{2})N_0$. Using the symbol T to mean half-life, we can rewrite Eq. (1.4) as follows:

$$(\tfrac{1}{2})N_0 = N_0 e^{-\lambda T} \qquad \text{or} \qquad \frac{1}{2}\frac{N_0}{N_0} = e^{-\lambda T},$$

which gives

$$\tfrac{1}{2} = e^{-\lambda T}.$$

Now, taking logarithms (to base e, *not* base 10) of both sides, we have

$$\ln 0.5 = -\lambda T,$$

and when we look this up in the tables of natural logarithms, we get, for the value of $\ln 0.5$,

$$-0.693 = -\lambda T.$$

Finally we have

$$T = \frac{0.693}{\lambda}, \tag{1.5}$$

which is the relation between the half-life and the decay constant that we were trying to find.

We could now rewrite Eq. (1.4) as

$$N = N_0 e^{-(0.693/T)t},$$

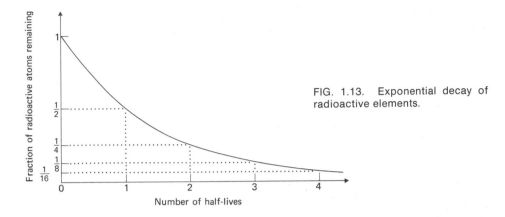

FIG. 1.13. Exponential decay of radioactive elements.

where the coefficient of t is, of course, a constant. We could also write

$$\frac{N}{N_0} = e^{-(0.693/T)t},$$

and plot this equation (see Fig. 1.13) to see what an exponential curve looks like.

Just to make sure we understand the concept of half-life, let us consider some radium used in the hospital. Suppose that one had 1 gram of radium (which is a relatively large quantity of this material, being perhaps all the radium on hand in a moderate-sized cancer clinic). It has a half-life of 1620 years. How much would be left in 3240 years? Simple. In 1620 years one would have one-half of 1 gram left, and in 3240 one-half of one-half, which is one-fourth of a gram. The therapy department does not have to worry too much about radium being used up! Table 1.2 gives the half-lives of some other radioelements of interest in medicine.

It is interesting to note that the half-lives of radioelements vary from around 10^{-9} second to 10^{10} years, truly an incomprehensible range! A look at these figures makes us realize why there are relatively few radioactive elements found in nature. Given that the earth has been in existence for some time (present estimates are about 5×10^9 years), we are not surprised to learn that it is primarily the radioelements with *long* half-lives that still appear in nature.

Table 1.2

Half-lives of some radioelements

Element	Half-life	Radiation emitted
Phosphorus-32	14.3 days	β^-
Cobalt-60	5.24 years	β^-, γ
Iodine-131	8.05 days	β^-, γ
Cesium-137	30 years	β^-, γ

The Curie

A student who put his mind to the preceding discussion would undoubt-edly come up with the conclusion that the shorter the half-life, the greater the activity (refer to Eq. 1.5), that is, the greater the number of radioactive disintegrations for a given number of atoms per unit time. The activity is assigned a unit called the *curie* (abbreviated Ci). One curie refers to an activity of 3.7×10^{10} disintegrations per second. This number derives historically from the fact that early experiments indicated this as the num-ber of disintegrations per second of 1 gram of radium. Table 1.3 shows the mass per curie of certain radioactive substances as compared with radium. For comparison, it is perhaps interesting to note that a cobalt therapy unit may have from 2000 to 5000 curies, while the activity of a radioactive sample you might use in elementary physics experiments is of the order of microcuries (abbreviated μCi), as is that of a luminous watch dial.

Table 1.3

Activity of certain radioisotopes	
Element	Milligrams per curie
Phosphorus-32	0.0035
Cobalt-60	0.88
Iodine-131	0.0081
Radium-226	1000

The form of Eq. (1.4) may be retained to represent the activity of a given radioactive sample. After all, the activity (that is, the number of disintegrations per unit time) depends on the number of atoms present. Hence, if we use the symbol A to represent activity, we have

$$A = A_0 e^{-\lambda t}. \tag{1.6}$$

Further, since the activity of a radioactive sample is measured by the in-tensity of the signal produced in some detection device, such as a Geiger counter, we could write

$$I = I_0 e^{-\lambda t},$$

where I is the intensity at some time t, while I_0 is the intensity at any chosen zero time. It thus seems entirely plausible that whenever the in-tensity of any radiation varies in a constant fractional manner, either with a change in time or a change in distance, such an exponential expression is valid. This point is worth revisiting when we read about x-ray absorption in Chapter 10.

Natural Radioactive Series

As we have previously pointed out, only relatively few radioelements occur in nature. There are 14 such elements with half-lives of the order of magnitude (or greater) of the age of the earth. Most of these elements decay to stable "daughters." However, three of them—thorium-232, uranium-235, and uranium-238—decay into daughters which are themselves radioactive. Final stability is achieved in these three cases only after a series of successive radioactive decays, which finally end in some stable form of lead. The radium which was discovered by Madame Curie, and which is used in medicine, appears as an intermediate product in the decay chain of the uranium series shown in Fig. 1.14. (You have undoubtedly noted that in these discussions we have made frequent use of a suffixed number after an element's name. This number, the atomic mass number, is affixed to distinguish different forms of the same element, a matter which has been peripherally touched on earlier and which we shall cover in more detail shortly in the section on isotopes.)

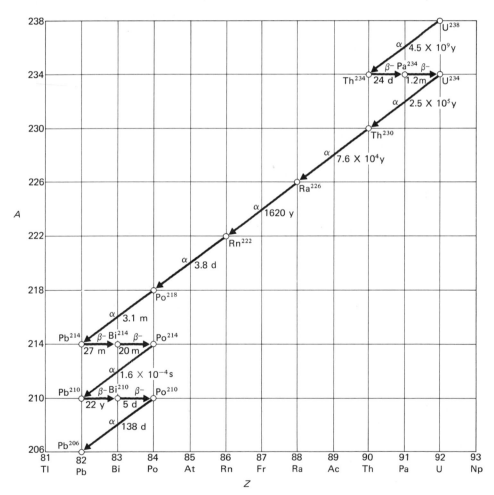

FIG. 1.14. The uranium series, showing the main decay modes leading to lead-206. The respective half-lives are shown in seconds (s), minutes (m), days (d), or years (y).

Radiography and Radioactive Sources

Radioactive sources may play roles in radiography in two distinct ways. First, one might ask, why not use the γ-rays from a radioactive source for radiography in place of the electrically generated x-rays? The answer is that in fact this is done, but primarily in industrial radiography, for such purposes as looking for flaws in metal castings. Gamma-ray radiography in medical diagnostic work suffers from two main drawbacks. One is that the energy of the available γ-rays is higher than that most suitable for medical diagnostic films. (Gamma-ray energies are in the million-electron-volt region, while medical diagnostic work involves x-rays in the kilo-electron-volt region.)

The second disadvantage of the radioactive source is the relatively low intensity of the beam. This fact leads to very long exposure times, which, although they pose no serious problem in industrial radiography, are obviously not suited to dealing with living beings. However, electronic image intensification may well remove this deficiency in due course.

Nevertheless, according to F. Jaundrell-Thompson and W. J. Ashworth in *X-Ray Physics and Equipment* (Blackwell Scientific Publications, 1965), some useful experiments have been made in dental radiography using small γ-ray sources.

The other way to bring radioactive sources to bear on radiography is to use some β-emitter. The β-particles may be directed toward a target and may thereby produce x-rays in exactly the same fashion as the electrons energized electrically in a conventional x-ray tube. This approach is also being industrially employed. The thickness and weight of inorganic coating layers on paper can be measured precisely by using an x-ray absorption technique, and for this type of analysis a radioactive x-ray source is sometimes used. For example, one may use hydrogen-3, which decays by β-emission. These β-particles (electrons) in turn strike a titanium target, thus producing x-rays in the 4 to 8 keV (kilo-electron-volt) region.

The preceding paragraphs suggest no great use of radioactive properties in medical radiography. However, in the following section on isotopes, we shall talk about the fact that the radioactive properties of many elements are finding many new medical applications.

1.7   ISOTOPES

We have already referred to two different nuclei of oxygen: O-16 (8 neutrons) and O-17 (9 neutrons). The first such same and yet different nuclei were identified in 1912 by J. J. Thomson. He found both neon-20 (10 neutrons) and neon-22 (12 neutrons). If we were to use the symbolism suggested earlier, we would write the nuclei of these isotopes as $_{10}\text{Ne}^{20}$ and $_{10}\text{Ne}^{22}$.

Isotopes: Stable and Radioactive

By inference we now have a definition of isotopes: Isotopes are nuclei (and hence atoms) of the same element; that is, they have the same atomic number Z but different atomic mass numbers A and hence different num-

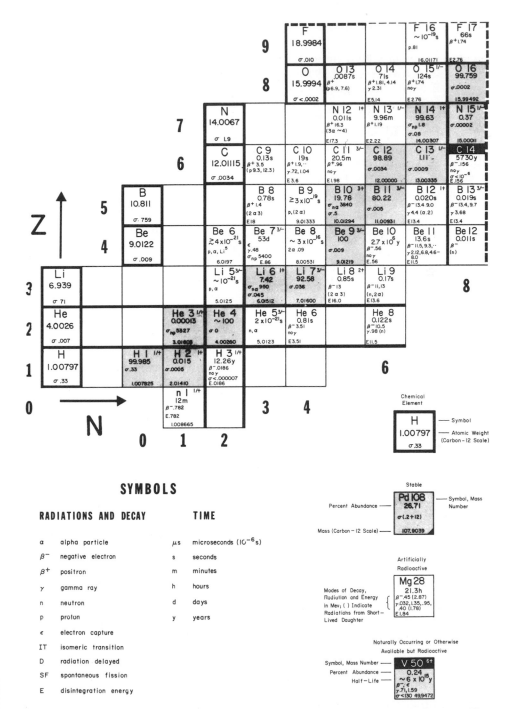

FIG. 1.15. Part of an isotope chart adapted from Chart of the Nuclides, 9th Edition. The horizontal number *N* refers to the number of neutrons, and the vertical number *Z* to the number of protons. (Courtesy Knolls Atomic Power Laboratory, Schenectady, New York. Operated by the General Electric Company for the United States Atomic Energy Commission.)

bers of neutrons. Hydrogen, for example, has three known isotopes: H-1, H-2, H-3. Of these, H-1 is the most commonly occurring hydrogen. Hydrogen-2 occurs only as 0.015% of the hydrogen in nature. This isotope, called *deuterium*, is the one used in the manufacture of so-called *heavy water*. H-3, or tritium, is artificially produced; that is, it does not occur in nature. It is radioactive, having a half-life of 12.26 years.

Figure 1.15 shows 6 of the 8 isotopes of carbon, of which the most abundant in nature is the stable isotope C-12. Note that C-14 is a naturally occurring radioactive isotope. It is the one involved in the radio-carbon dating of archeological specimens.

Now, although the isotopes of a given element have different numbers of nucleons, they have the same number of protons, and hence the complete atoms have the same number of electrons. Since the chemical characteristics of an atom are dependent on the number of orbital electrons, it follows that isotopes are chemically identical. Consequently isotopes cannot be chemically separated, and therefore all occupy the same place in the periodic table, which we shall discuss in the following section. The English physicist Soddy, noting this characteristic, coined the word *isotopes*, meaning "in the same place."

Up to the present time, almost 1500 isotopes have been identified. Although in the case of some elements, such as hydrogen, only a few isotopes have been discovered, in the case of others many isotopes are known. For example, we know of some 25 isotopes of tin (Sn), of which as many as 10 are stable ones. Cobalt, now familiar in medicine, lies somewhere between the extremities of tin and hydrogen, in that for Co we find 11 isotopes.

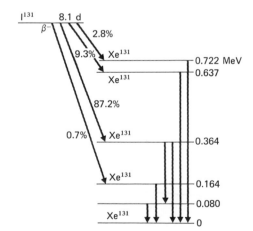

FIG. 1.16. Beta-minus decay of iodine-131.

Production

Those radioactive isotopes—or simply *radioisotopes*—which do not occur in nature are produced by engendering the appropriate nuclear reactions. This process involves bombarding certain nuclei with highly energetic charged particles, such as protons or α-particles, or with γ-rays or with neutrons. From the standpoint of large-scale production, the most suitable method is that employing neutrons; the reason is that there is a copious supply of neutrons associated with the many nuclear reactors in the world today. A typical reaction is the one involved in producing cobalt-60:

$$_{27}Co^{59} + {}_0n^1 \rightarrow {}_{27}Co^{60}.$$

Cobalt-60 is a β-emitter, as are most artificially produced radioisotopes. An example of a typical decay scheme is shown in Fig. 1.16, which deals with iodine-131. The β-decay processes of artificial isotopes may involve either *beta-minus* (electron) or *beta-plus* (positron) emission, although the decay of naturally radioactive nuclei seems restricted to beta-minus (β^-) decay.

Medical Use

As we implied earlier, radioisotopes are finding extensive use in both industry and medicine. Figure 1.17 shows examples of the range of their application.

We might recall that both the previously mentioned isotopes, Co-60 and I-131, are among the many radioisotopes used in medicine. The former isotope, in so-called "cobalt bombs," has replaced many high-voltage x-ray units in cancer clinics. It is estimated that Canadian-produced cobalt units alone are used for over 1.5 million treatments per year, in some 40 different countries.

The therapeutic use of radioisotopes is, of course, not their only medical application.

Medical use falls roughly into four main areas:

1) Research, including, for example, the metabolism of pharmaceuticals.

2) Therapy, such as radium implantations.

3) Sterilization of surgical instruments and dressings, especially of the disposable type, which can be made relatively cheaply, of non-heat-resistant materials. This sterilization method is based on the lethal effect of radiation on bacteria.

4) Diagnosis, in which the use of radioisotopes permits doctors to see body tissues as these tissues emit radiations from the isotopes with which they have been infiltrated.

Possibly the widest and most effective application of any radioisotope in hospitals at present is that of iodine-131. Sodium iodide (the iodine being I-131) is readily taken up by the thyroid. Thus I-131 is used diagnostically for measuring the degree of thyroid function, and indeed for measuring the basal metabolic rate of an individual, by means of measurements involving the γ-rays which are emitted (see Fig. 1.18). This radioisotope has a further therapeutic application in the treatment of hyperthyroidism.

Undoubtedly the scope of the medical use of radioisotopes is on the verge of large-scale expansion. This will probably mean that in due course the x-ray technician may well have to work closely with his colleague, the "isotope technician."

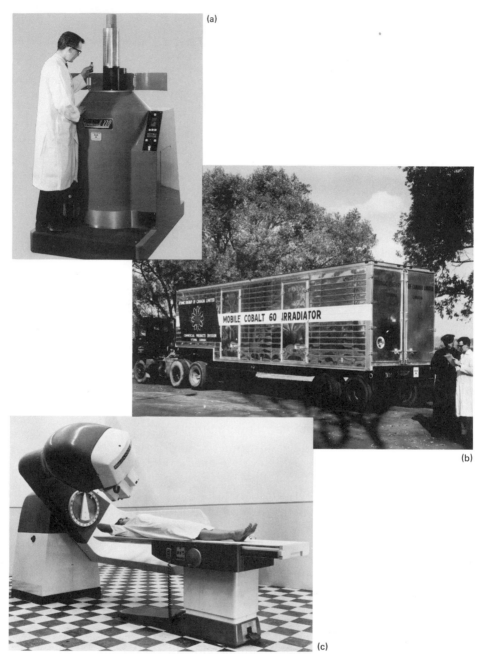

FIG. 1.17. Radioisotopes in industry, agriculture, and medicine. (a) The Gammacell is a portable irradiation unit designed for industrial and other research work. It is used to study the effects of γ-rays on various materials. (b) The Mobile Cobalt-60 Irradiator was designed to irradiate various foods with γ-rays to increase their shelf life or, in the case of potatoes and other vegetables, to inhibit sprouting. (c) Cobalt-60 used in cancer treatments (courtesy of Atomic Energy of Canada Limited).

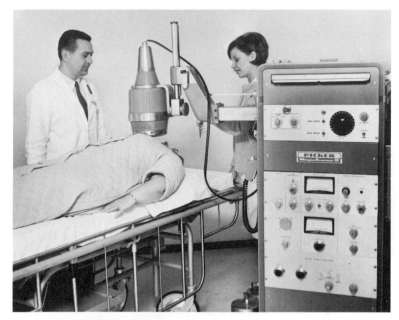

FIG. 1.18. A patient undergoing a thyroid scan. The patient has been given 50 microcuries of I-131 the previous day. (Courtesy Herbert A. Selenkow, M.D., Thyroid Laboratory, Peter Bent Brigham Hospital, Boston, Mass.)

1.8 THE PERIODIC TABLE

Now that we have spent some considerable time with matters essentially nuclear, let us complete our journey through the realm of atomic and nuclear physics by a further look at some atomic phenomena, those bounding on the realm of chemistry. We say chemistry because we shall concern ourselves with the number and arrangement of electrons in atoms, and it is these electron configurations which determine the ways in which an element will, or will not, combine with other elements; that is, these configurations determine the element's chemical properties.

Electron Configurations

Let us briefly recapitulate our earlier discussions by recalling that the electrons in the case of each element have particular energy levels, or orbitals, or shells and subshells, and that electrons will ordinarily try to be as close to the nucleus as possible, since this situation is the one in which the electron has the lowest energy.

One aside is perhaps useful here. The lower the electron's energy, the more energy would have to be given to it to remove it from its parent atom. Another way of expressing this idea is to say that the closer the electron is to the nucleus, the tighter it is bound there, that is, the greater its *binding energy*. Outer electrons are at higher energy levels and therefore exhibit less binding energy than inner electrons, and are consequently more easily removed from their parent atoms.

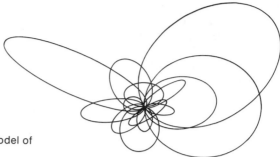

FIG. 1.19. Approximation of Bohr model of aluminum atom.

As one considers more and more complex atoms, more and more electrons are added in ever higher energy levels, much as water, when poured into a bucket, fills the bucket from the bottom up and not from the top down. Of course one might ask: Why do all the electrons not go into the lowest possible energy level or innermost shell? The answer to this question has also been previously indicated. It follows from the *Pauli exclusion principle,* which, roughly speaking, states that no two electrons in an atom may be in exactly the same energy state; or, more precisely, that no two electrons in an atom may have exactly the same four quantum numbers (this was mentioned in Section 1.4).

With this concept in mind, we can show by resorting to quantum mechanics (more specifically the four quantum numbers) that the inner or K-shell of an atom is filled with two electrons, while the next shell, the L-shell, is not filled until eight further electrons are added, and so on. In this manner we may explain the periodicity of that orderly arrangement of the atoms known as the *periodic table.*

Before we look at the periodic table, let us first note how this progressive addition of electrons in the various shells may be graphically represented. Figure 1.19 is a model of an aluminum atom (the element most frequently used for diagnostic x-ray filters). Note the large elliptical orbits of the three outer electrons of the M-shell, and the smaller orbits of the completely filled L-shell, and the still smaller orbits of the also completely

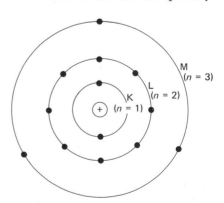

FIG. 1.20. Bohr schematic representation of the electrons in an atom of aluminum ($Z = 13$).

filled *K*-shell. Now we would note that it is still common practice, and useful, to schematically represent atoms in a simpler fashion than that of such a model, by drawing merely circular orbits which are indicative of the various (*K*, *L*, *M*, etc.) shells, but which do not indicate the energy level variations associated with elliptical orbits. Such a schematic representation of the aluminum atom is shown in Fig. 1.20.

The Periodic Table

The essence of the periodic table (Table 1.4) is: List the elements in order of increasing atomic number and hence increasing number of electrons. Then you can arrange row (or period) under row so that there appear vertical columns (or groups) yielding elements of similar chemical properties. This system works with all the 104 elements known to date. Let us see.

There are but two different atoms with electrons only in the *K*-shell. Hydrogen and helium are the sole elements in the first row, or period, of Table 1.4. In the second period of Table 1.4, there are eight elements, corresponding to the eight additional electrons permitted in the *L*-shell. When we look at the outer electronic structure of elements in the same column, or group, we see that the elements in the same column have the same electronic configuration. For example, lithium, sodium, and potassium are in the same group. They each have one outer electron, lithium in the *L*-shell, sodium in the *M*-shell and potassium in the *N*-shell. We assume that this similarity in outer electronic configuration accounts for the similarity in chemical properties.

Complete clarification of the periods in Table 1.4 becomes more complex in the case of the periods with more than eight elements, but is readily possible if we employ present knowledge of quantum mechanics: specifically the four quantum numbers used in conjunction with the Pauli exclusion principle.

Valence

Further, the combinatorial aspect of chemical properties now seems clarified. For example, atoms with completely filled outer shells and subshells and/or eight outer electrons are chemically relatively inert. One might say crudely that eight outer electrons (except in the case of the elements of the first period) cause a balance of electrical forces within the atom such that great stability is achieved. In fact, elements such as neon which fall into this category are known as *inert* or *noble* elements, because the completeness in their electronic configurations makes them extremely stable and not at all amenable to electron exchange with other elements. Not until 1962 was the first compound of one of these elements formed. The compound, xenon hexafluoroplatinate, was prepared by Neil Bartlett at the University of British Columbia.

Let us pursue this relationship between electron configuration and chemical behavior a little further. If the neon configuration is very stable, then perhaps sodium would readily give up its lone *M*-shell electron and thus achieve a more stable configuration, like that of neon. Readiness to give up an electron in an interaction with another atom suggests chemical

Table 1.4

PERIODIC TABLE OF THE ELEMENTS*

(Numbers in parentheses indicate the mass number of the longest-lived isotope of radioactive elements)

Outer electrons are in the	I	II	III	IV	V	VI	VII	VIII			0	Electrons per shell
First or K-shell	1 H 1.00797										2 He 4.0026	2
Second or L-shell	3 Li 6.939	4 Be 9.0122	5 B 10.811	6 C 12.01115	7 N 14.0067	8 O 15.9994	9 F 18.9984				10 Ne 20.183	2,8
Third or M-shell	11 Na 22.9898	12 Mg 24.312	13 Al 26.9815	14 Si 28.086	15 P 30.9738	16 S 32.064	17 Cl 35.453				18 Ar 39.948	2,8,8
Fourth or N-shell	19 K 39.102	20 Ca 40.08	21 Sc 44.956	22 Ti 47.90	23 V 50.942	24 Cr 51.996	25 Mn 54.9380	26 Fe 55.847	27 Co 58.9332	28 Ni 58.71		
	29 Cu 63.54	30 Zn 65.37	31 Ga 69.72	32 Ge 72.59	33 As 74.9216	34 Se 78.96	35 Br 79.909				36 Kr 83.80	2,8,18,8
Fifth or O-shell	37 Rb 85.47	38 Sr 87.62	39 Y 88.905	40 Zr 91.22	41 Nb 92.906	42 Mo 95.94	43 Tc (99)	44 Ru 101.07	45 Rh 102.905	46 Pd 106.4		
	47 Ag 107.870	48 Cd 112.40	49 In 114.82	50 Sn 118.69	51 Sb 121.75	52 Te 127.60	53 I 126.9044				54 Xe 131.30	2,8,18, 18,8
Sixth or P-shell	55 Cs 132.905	56 Ba 137.34	57–71 La series*	72 Hf 178.49	73 Ta 180.948	74 W 183.85	75 Re 186.2	76 Os 190.2	77 Ir 192.2	78 Pt 195.09		
	79 Au 196.967	80 Hg 200.59	81 Tl 204.37	82 Pb 207.19	83 Bi 208.980	84 Po (210)	85 At (210)				86 Rn (222)	2,8,18, 32,18,8
Seventh or Q-shell	87 Fr (223)	88 Ra (226)	89–103 Ac series**	104 Ku (260)								

*Lanthanide series:	57 La 138.91	58 Ce 140.12	59 Pr 140.907	60 Nd 144.24	61 Pm (145)	62 Sm 150.35	63 Eu 151.96	64 Gd 157.25	65 Tb 158.924	66 Dy 162.50	67 Ho 164.930	68 Er 167.26	69 Tm 168.934	70 Yb 173.04	71 Lu 174.97	2,8,18, 32,9,2
**Actinide series:	89 Ac (227)	90 Th 232.038	91 Pa (231)	92 U 238.03	93 Np (237)	94 Pu (244)	95 Am (243)	96 Cm (247)	97 Bk (247)	98 Cf (251)	99 Es (254)	100 Fm (257)	101 Md (256)	102 No (255)	103 Lw (257)	2,8,18, 32,32,9, 2

* Elements 102, 103, 104 have been added.

activity. And indeed sodium *is* chemically very active, and so is lithium, and so is potassium. Again, if a complete outer shell is most comfortable, then fluorine is perhaps very active in accepting another electron from elsewhere. It too is chemically very active.

We are now on the brink of *valence*. In fact, if we define chemical valence simply as the number of electrons an atom would readily yield or accept in a chemical combination, we have arrived. Numerically, valence turns out to be either the number of outer electrons (positive electronic valence) or the number lacking in the outer shell to make eight (negative electronic valence) which is the number of electrons in the outer shells of the stable "inert" elements. For example, Table 1.4 suggests that aluminum has a positive valence of 3. Why? Because Al has 13 electrons, of which two fill the K-shell and eight fill the L-shell, thus leaving three in the incomplete M-shell.

It must be added, however, that like many of the other concepts at the atomic level which we have discussed, the preceding statements may be criticized as oversimplifications. Indeed, we have not pursued what happens with respect to gain or loss of electrons when compounds are in solution, or are electrically charged, or even how it is that some elements form various compounds demanding different valences.

Transuranic Elements

In addition to giving interesting chemical information, the periodic table provides, of course, a listing of the known elements. As noted before, 104 elements have been identified to date. Of these, the one with the highest atomic number occurring in nature is uranium ($Z = 92$). Elements beyond 92 have no stable isotopes and all their radioisotopes would be expected to have half-lives which are short compared with the time of existence of the earth. These elements must consequently be produced in the laboratory.

The first of these *transuranic* (beyond uranium) elements to be produced and identified was neptunium ($Z = 93$). This feat took place at the University of California at Berkeley in 1940. It was the work of E. M. McMillan and P. H. Abelson, and involved the cyclotron of the Crocker Radiation Laboratory in the production of the required neutrons. Let us use our nuclear shorthand to describe the event:

$$_{92}U^{238} + {}_0n^1 \rightarrow {}_{92}U^{239} + \gamma.$$

The uranium-239 is radioactive and decays with a half-life of the order of minutes to neptunium-239.

$$_{92}U^{239} \rightarrow {}_{93}Np^{239} + {}_{-1}e^0,$$

where $_{-1}e^0$ refers to a β^--particle or electron. As suggested, neptunium has a short half-life, 2.35 days.

At the time this text is being written, the latest transuranic element to appear is element 104, kurchatovium, which was discovered in 1964 at the Dubna Laboratories of the USSR Academy of Sciences in Moscow.

1.9 SUGGESTIONS TO THE STUDENT

Early in this first chapter we, the authors, have indulged in some admonitions to you, the student. We apologize to the more experienced and mature student who may well have found these comments redundant and tiresome.

Nevertheless we press on to some final, and we hope useful, suggestions on the use of this text. Throughout the first chapter you will have noticed our habit of having subheadings within each subsection of the chapter. These subheadings are given in order to help the student review by facilitating the organization of the salient features. And a review is necessary, fairly soon after the material has been covered for the first time.

We would also suggest trying the questions at the end of each chapter. *By and large, the questions have been adapted from examinations of the Canadian Society of Radiological Technicians and the British Society of Radiographers.* The questions are by no means all-embracing. A good study procedure is for you to make up others; and to try them on your colleagues. Remember that you are faced with two tasks: One is to learn the relevant physics and the other is to pass a professional examination. It is possible to achieve the first goal without gaining the second, although the inverse is exceedingly unlikely. Therefore practice in answering questions clearly is of the utmost importance.

There are many diagrams, graphs, and pictures in this text. Squeeze all you can out of them. Do not be content with a peripheral comprehension of their significance. Sometimes we have omitted the "ifs" and "buts" and other extras; you should provide these for yourself with (or perhaps without) the guidance of your instructor. For example, refer to Fig. 1.15, which deals with isotopes: There is much information (to which we have made no direct reference in the text) to be gleaned from this small part of an isotope chart.

Finally, there is the suggested reading. Time is always of the essence when you are taking a course; therefore it is unrealistic for a student to attempt to seriously consider all or even a significant portion of the extra reading. Indulge in the reading to the extent that it will help you to master the present course and then use the suggested reading list after the course is over, to build a fuller background, to acquire a useful professional library, or to make preliminary preparation for a higher examination.

QUESTIONS

1. Describe briefly the structure of a simple atom according to the Bohr concept, and clearly define the terms "atomic number" and "mass number."

2. Describe how the Bohr concept of the atom accounts for the emission of monochromatic light.

3. What is a photon?

4. What is the relation between the energy of a photon and the frequency of the associated wave?

5. In what way does present-day quantum mechanics offer a description of atomic phenomena which is superior to the description offered by the original Bohr concept?

6. Which electrons have the greater binding energy, those of the outer shell or those of the inner shell? Explain.

7. Define: (a) molecule, (b) element, (c) electron, (d) neutron, (e) alpha particle.

8. Consider Becquerel's discovery of radioactivity. Was the exposure of his photographic plates due to the emission of α-particles by uranium? Explain.

9. What is the unit of activity of a radioactive material?

10. By reference to Eq. (1.3), define the radioactive decay constant, λ, in words.

11. "The radioactive decay process follows an exponential law." Explain this statement and write the appropriate equation.

12. What is meant by the term "radioactive series"? Name one of these series.

13. "Iodine-131 is a radioactive isotope having a half-life of about 8 days. It emits β-particles and γ-rays." Explain these statements, with particular emphasis on these terms: radioactive, isotope, 131, half-life, β-particles, and γ-rays.

14. A 5-gram source of cobalt-60 is installed in a beam therapy unit today. How much of this cobalt remains 5.3 years hence?

15. A certain sample of I-131 has an activity of 4 millicuries at 1 P.M. on January 1. What will be its activity at 1 P.M. on January 17 of the same year?

16. Write the nuclear reaction involved in making phosphorus-32 from phosphorus-31 by neutron bombardment.

17. Give a brief outline of the medical use of radioisotopes.

18. What might you expect to happen to film contrast if you made an exposure using a radioactive γ-ray source rather than a conventional x-ray generator?

19. What is meant by valence?

20. The periodic table is arranged in vertical groups and horizontal periods. What is the significance of this arrangement?

SUGGESTED READING

BOOTH, VERNE H., *The Structure of Atoms.* New York: Macmillan, 1964 (first edition). Very readable; essentially descriptive. Recommended for those who wish a relatively nonmathematical but considerably fuller discussion of the matters treated in our Chapter 1. Some relevance also to our Chapter 9.

QUIMBY, E. H., and S. FEITELBERG, *Radioactive Isotopes in Medicine and Biology: Basic Physics and Instrumentation,* Philadelphia: Lea and Febiger, 1963. For those readers with some physics background who wish a more thorough treatment of radioactivity. Some parts of this book also have relevance to our Chapters 9 and 10. Knowledge of elementary calculus is presumed.

JOHNS, H. E., *The Physics of Radiology.* Springfield, Ill.: Charles C. Thomas, 1964 (second edition, revised second printing). Chapter XV of this book offers an excellent summary of the clinical use of radioisotopes. Very profitable reading for those students who find themselves dissatisfied with the relatively short shrift this topic received in our Chapter 1. In fact, as an addition to a budding x-ray technician's professional library this book may be highly recommended, although one must bear in mind that it is directed primarily to the therapeutic rather than the diagnostic use of high-energy radiations. Johns has been a member of the International Commission on Radiological Units and Measurements (ICRU) for some years.

PAULING, LINUS, and ROGER HAYWARD, *The Architecture of Molecules*. San Francisco: W. H. Freeman, 1964. Beautifully illustrated introduction to the subject of how atoms are arranged and interconnected in molecules. The book's brief but lucid explanations, coupled with the concrete representations of molecular structures in the form of illustrations, clarify such diverse molecular properties as hardness, color, density, nutrient and toxic qualities. The explanations of Hayward's illustrations are by the Nobel Prize chemist, Pauling, who authored the definitive text on the nature of the chemical bond. Written particularly for the beginner in atomic and molecular science.

SEABORG, G. T., and E. G. VALENS, *Elements of the Universe*. New York: Dutton, 1958. Excellent authoritative treatment of the "building blocks of nature" in an elementary, nonmathematical manner. Particularly good on the historical development of the periodic table, and the discovery of transuranic elements. Seaborg shared the Nobel Prize in chemistry with E. M. McMillan in 1951 as the result of their work with the transuranic elements.

CHAPTER 2

Static Electricity

In 1961 the city fathers of Magdeburg, in Germany, renamed the local Technische Hochschule after Otto von Guericke; this was some 300 years after his many excellent contributions to science. Von Guericke deserves mention in x-ray physics on at least two counts. One is the fact that he started the world on an understanding of vacuum and the way to produce one; and a good vacuum is, as will be discussed in more detail in Chapter 7, a key requirement for the present day x-ray tube.

A spectacular experiment of Von Guericke's is probably the all-time classic of large public scientific demonstrations. It involved two halves of a heavy bronze sphere, approximately two feet in diameter. After air had been evacuated from the sphere, the two halves were so firmly held together by the external atmospheric pressure that two teams of eight horses each were required to pull them apart.

However, for the moment we are more concerned with a realization that von Guericke made many pioneer contributions to electrostatics, most of which lay dormant until rediscovered in America by Benjamin Franklin, who is usually associated with elementary matters of electricity. Among von Guericke's accomplishments was the invention of the first electric machine, a ball of sulphur mounted on a wooden axle so that it could be effectively rubbed.

As a starting point in "electrical history," the work by an English physician (not physicist) in the days of Queen Elizabeth is generally quoted. This extensive work was made public in 1600 in a treatise which its author, William Gilbert (1540–1603), entitled *De magnete*. In truth, this treatise was predominantly on magnetism, but the single chapter on the "amber effect," that is, static electricity, does lay some groundwork for the study of electrical phenomena. Probably his "versorium" was the first electrical instrument to be invented. (The versorium was simply a pointer, say of wood, well balanced horizontally so as to pivot easily; it was a form of electroscope.) Gilbert may also be credited with the word "electricity," in that he called "electrics" (from Greek for "amber") those substances which exhibited attraction forces when rubbed.

Electrical repulsion was not discovered until after Gilbert's death. The discoverer was Nicolo Cabeo (1585–1650), an Italian priest.

The French scientist Dufay (1698–1739) proposed a "two-fluid" theory to account for these and other electrical phenomena. Benjamin Franklin, on the other hand, countered with a "one-fluid" theory, and added an important postulate: that electric charge is conserved; that is, that it can neither be created nor destroyed.

Probably nothing put electricity more into the news in its infancy than the discovery in 1745, independently in Holland and in Germany, of the Leyden jar; that is, a capacitor, which permitted the accumulation of sufficient charge that spectacular shocks could be felt by the intrepid investigators.

The major *tour de force* in the quantification of electricity was the result of experiments in France by Charles Augustin Coulomb (1736–1806). Coulomb's law, as we shall soon see, helps to explain, both descriptively and quantitatively, many significant electrical phenomena.

2.1 ELECTRIC CHARGES

In the previous chapter we asserted point-blank that matter is essentially electrical in nature. You were expected to draw on your background knowledge to know what was meant by electricity. We now backtrack a little, before we make a further advance, in order to define terms and describe concepts, some of which have already been used earlier. If this approach seems strange to you, you might well meditate a moment on the problem of writing a dictionary. Look up any word. Then look up each word used to define the first one, then each of the ones used in these definitions, etc. Sooner or later, depending on the word you chose, you will come full cycle: The first word you looked up will appear in a definition of one of the words arising from your pursuit of the words used in the original and subsequent definitions. One has to start somewhere. It is no different in physics.

If we were to concern ourselves with physics in a more rigorous and fundamental manner, rather than in the applied sense of this text, we should spend considerable time on the discussion of "fundamental" quantities. To avoid the implied circularity of definitions, physicists generally have agreed to accept a number of terms, or physical dimensions, or entities, as undefined. The best one can do with these terms or entities is to describe how they can be measured, a procedure known as giving an *operational* definition. The fundamental, undefined entities often quoted are mass, length, time, electrical charge, and temperature degree. However, in electricity we shall actually define the electrical charge, using electrical current as the undefined quantity specified only in terms of an operational definition (which is more or less a cook-book rule telling how it is measured in terms of previously defined quantities). We shall return to this matter of the definition of electrical charge in the next chapter, when we deal with direct-current electricity.

Ionization

In the first chapter, we said that atoms and molecules are normally electrically neutral, and that, although the nucleus contains positive electricity, the associated electrons represent a balancing amount of negative electricity. What if this electrical balance is disturbed?

If by some means an electron is removed from an atom or a molecule, the electrical balance is disturbed; the atom (or molecule) has an excess of positive charge; the atom (or molecule) is now referred to as an *ion*, a *positive ion* in this case. If an extra electron should be added to an atom (or molecule), then the resulting particle, also electrically charged, is referred to as a *negative ion*. Examples of ions that we have previously encountered include the simplest of all positive ions, the proton, which is an ionized hydrogen-1 atom, and the α-particle, which is a doubly ionized helium-4 atom. *Doubly ionized* means either an excess or a deficiency of two electrons relative to the electrically neutral condition (see Fig. 2.1).

In general, ions do not exhibit all the properties characteristic of the element or compound from which they are formed. This fact, among others, makes ions of considerable interest in the fields of chemistry and solid-

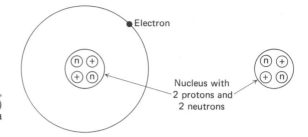

FIG. 2.1. Positive ions: helium-4, singly and doubly ionized. (a) Singly ionized atom. (b) Alpha particle: doubly ionized.

state physics. For example, x-ray diffraction studies (see Chapter 9), even in their early days, cleared up an amazing number of vague conceptions about mineral structures, on the basis of the concept of ions. One of the highlights of such x-ray analysis (which arose from the study of the structure of ordinary table salt, NaCl) was that one must in general abandon the idea of the molecule in the realm of inorganic chemistry, and replace it with the concept of a "mix" of ions. Linus Pauling, who was mentioned in Chapter 1 in the discussion of the nature of the chemical bond, gave theoretical support to this idea. He determined that in stable structures like minerals the ions take up positions such that the energy associated with the electric field (see Section 2.2) between them is a minimum.

The processes of forming these electrically charged particles, the ions, are varied. As implied above, in solids electric forces are involved more or less directly, as is the case with ionic solutions. An example which requires us to rush on ahead of ourselves a little (Chapter 3) may nevertheless be instructive. When a simple electric circuit such as is shown in Fig. 2.2 is set up, the light will not go on because the water normally has only neutral molecules. However, when some table salt is poured into the jar, the NaCl, under the influence of the associated electrical forces, dissociates itself into positive sodium ions (Na^+) and negative chloride ions (Cl^-), and these electrically charged particles now serve to transport electrical charge; they constitute under these circumstances an electric current; the light goes on.

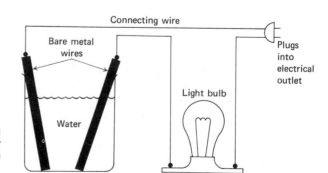

FIG. 2.2. Experiment showing electrical charge transfer (electric current) through ionized solution.

A more important way of creating ions, as far as radiography is concerned, involves knocking electrons from atoms or molecules by means of radiation energy. This matter will crop up in several places later in this book, particularly in the chapter dealing with the interaction of x-rays with matter. It is probably fair to say that all the radiologically useful properties of x-rays are associated with their ionizing effects.

Fundamental Charge

We shall now focus a little more closely on the idea of electrical charge. We recall that in our previous discussion of atomic levels, two kinds of electrical particles were extensively involved: *the proton*, which we said is positively charged; and *the electron*, negatively charged. In other words, on the basis of our present knowledge, the "two-fluid" concept of Dufay is upheld; and yet could we not also describe a positive ion, for example, simply by saying that it lacks some negative electricity? In short, we could also build up much, but not all, of present-day electrical theory on the basis of Benjamin Franklin's "one-fluid" concept, by ascribing a second name to the condition of the lack of a single "fluid." It is for this reason that some of Franklin's work is as useful today in the light of new knowledge as it was in the middle of the eighteenth century.

Again referring to earlier discussions, we should now reiterate that the experiments by the American physicist, Robert Andrews Millikan, in the early 1900's, established that the electrical property, or charge, of a *single electron* seems to be the smallest quantity of this electrical property, or charge, which exists in nature. (In other words, electrical charge, like light or radiation energy, comes only in discrete chunks. That is, electric charge is also *quantized*.) We said before that therefore this amount of electricity is considered to be the fundamental electric charge, and that in terms of the more practical and universally accepted unit of electric charge, the coulomb, the charge on an electron is 16.02×10^{-20} coulomb of *negative electricity*. Further, the proton, although it has a much larger mass than the electron, has exactly the same amount of positive charge as the electron has negative charge; that is, the charge of a proton is 16.02×10^{-20} coulomb of *positive electricity*. And the coulomb, as mentioned earlier, will be defined quantitatively later, in our discussion of current electricity.

Triboelectricity

So far, we have dealt essentially in the microscopic realm, in the atomic and the subatomic world. It is useful, however, to consider electrical phenomena also from the directly observable, the "household" or macroscopic viewpoint. We shall now define the two types of electricity in macroscopic terms. The definitions are quite arbitrary and, once agreed upon, lead to the fact that an electron is said to be negatively charged. Different definitions might well have been employed, as might different words; there is nothing intrinsically significant in choosing the words "negative" and "positive," although there is perhaps some mathematical simplicity in this choice, as opposed to, for example, "green" and "red" electricity.

Negative electricity is the kind of electricity that predominates in a body composed of resin after it has undergone electrification by rubbing with wool. (From our current understanding this means, of course, that the wool, having given up some electrons to the resinous body, is now positively charged.)

Positive electricity is the kind of electricity that predominates in a body composed of glass after it has been rubbed with silk. (Again this means that the silk is thereupon negatively charged.)

Note that in both these definitions an electrification process quite common to all of us is involved. The process demands two different materials, called nonconductors or insulators, in which electrons do not easily move from one atom to the next. This fact allows the accumulation of charge, if some can somehow be transferred fron one body to another; that is, the charge does not "flow" away readily; it accumulates and remains at rest. It is "static." Hence the term *static electricity.*

Further, the charge transfer from one body, say wool, to an ebonite rod or a hard rubber comb, although it requires only the contact of the two surfaces, is enhanced by rubbing the two materials together. Hence the term *triboelectricity* (Greek: *tribein,* to rub), or frictional electricity. Although the details of the electric charge transfer involved are not completely understood at present, one can say that the phenomenon rests on the fact that different types of atoms have different affinities for their electrons and that the rubbing is probably only significant in that it increases the surface contact area. Be that as it may, the phenomenon exists, as we often witness when we take off sweaters; furthermore, this method of accumulating electrical charges poses several problems for the radiographer. For example, later in this chapter (Section 2.5) we shall have more to say about related operating-room hazards.

In the meantime, we might point out that, since it is quite possible for us to pick up considerable electric charge when walking (particularly with rubber-soled shoes) along many types of floors, it is often useful (particularly in dry climates) to touch a radiator before touching a patient. This procedure allows the accumulated electric charge to leak off, thereby sparing the unsuspecting patient from the unpleasantness of a noticeable electric shock.

The Electroscope

It is now reasonable to ask how one may detect the presence of triboelectricity, or any static electric charge, without waiting until the accumulations are large enough for the unpleasantness of a personally felt electric shock to furnish the evidence. The answer lies in the use of an *electroscope.* We have already made brief reference to Gilbert's versorium earlier in this chapter. We leave the student to meditate on how an instrument such as Gilbert's would work, and address ourselves to some of the simplest types of electroscopes in use today.

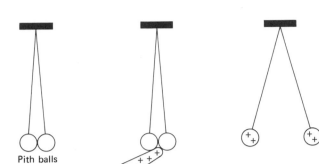

FIG. 2.3. Charging a pith-ball electroscope by contact. Some electrons from the pith balls migrate to the positively charged rod, leaving both pith balls with a positive charge.

Pith balls

Charging rod

Suppose that we were to have two very light spheres suspended from two threads. Further, we stipulate that the threads be of a nonconducting material (that is, one in which electrical charges do not readily move), so that if we place an electric charge on a ball, this charge will not leak off through the threads. Now, if a glass rod is rubbed with silk and we then touch both the small suspended spheres with this glass rod that is (by definition) positively charged, the spheres will fly away from the rod and will also repel one another (see Fig. 2.3). The inference we make is that the spheres each acquired some of the electric charge of the glass rod and that like electric charges repel one another. Certainly the presence of an electrical charge is noted, in that the two spheres, before they were electrified, were quite content to hang together in contact, but after they had been electrified, they kept well apart. This instrument, therefore, indicates the fact that there is an electrical charge on the glass rod. It is a very simple electroscope, known as a *pith-ball electroscope*, because the small spheres are frequently made from the pithy central part of the stem of some plants, such as elderberry, for example. The student could well construct such an electroscope himself, and with it perhaps achieve some personal conviction of the matters discussed in these pages, including the fact that if a positively charged pith ball is approached by a negatively charged body (e.g., an ebonite rod rubbed with wool) the pith ball will be attracted toward this oppositely charged body (see Fig. 2.4).

Such a pith-ball electroscope (and, of course, many other types of electroscopes) could also serve as an instrument for the detection of x-rays.

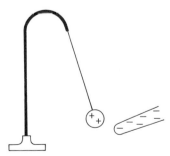

FIG. 2.4. Pith-ball electroscope used to show that unlike charges attract.

We have said that x-rays have the property of causing ionization. If the air around the electroscope becomes ionized, there is a mechanism for the transfer of charge. For example, negative air ions would be attracted to a positively charged pith ball, thus neutralizing the charge. In other words, the charge "leaks off" the pith balls and they come back together. This experiment may be performed in the x-ray department simply by placing a charged electroscope on an x-ray table and making an exposure.

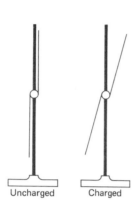

FIG. 2.5. The Braun electroscope.

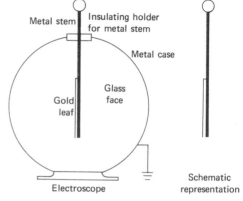

FIG. 2.6. Gold-leaf electroscope.

Other electroscopes are shown in Figs. 2.5 and 2.6. Of these, the second one, generally referred to as a gold-leaf electroscope (although the movable leaf is sometimes of another metal, such as aluminum), is the more sensitive. Let us embark on a thought experiment with a gold-leaf electroscope. If we bring a positively charged rod near to the knob of the metal stem, we observe the gold leaf swinging away from the stem. What is happening? The positive charge on the rod attracts electrons toward it and, since electrons in a metal (that is, a conductor) are relatively free to move, some electrons migrate to the knob, leaving a temporary deficiency of electrons, or a positive charge, on the lower part of the stem and the gold leaf. The stem and the gold leaf, since they are of the same charge, exert a force of repulsion on each other. Now, without having touched the knob with the charging rod, we remove the charging rod. What should happen? Since we neither removed electrons nor added them to the electroscope, the net charge on the electroscope should have remained zero, as it was at the beginning. Hence the leaf will fall back against the stem, as electrons return to that part of the electroscope from which they came.

What if we had touched the knob of the stem with the charging rod? Then some electrons from the electroscope stem would have migrated to the positively charged rod, leaving a deficiency of electrons on the electroscope, and thus causing the electroscope to be positively charged. When we then removed the charging rod, the leaf would stay repelled from the stem. We would have placed a charge on the electroscope by contact.

Charging by Induction

It is also possible to use a charged object to charge any number of nearby objects by the process of induction rather than by contact. This process is most readily effected if the objects to be charged consist of conducting materials (in which electrons are relatively mobile), such as metals.

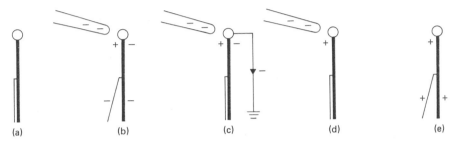

FIG. 2.7. Charging an electroscope by induction.

Figure 2.7 shows the charging of a gold-leaf electroscope by this process of induction. At (a) the electroscope is in its original electrically neutral condition. At (b) the negatively charged rod has brought about a redistribution of charge as shown (the plus and minus signs indicate the nature of the charge only in the region concerned; these signs are not to be construed as a quantitative indication of the charge distribution). Touching the knob allows electrons to escape from the electroscope into the ground, under the influence of the repulsive forces due to the negative charging rod. [This process is referred to as *grounding*, and is generally indicated by the symbol employed in (c).] Now the electroscope actually has lost some electrons, leaving a net positive charge on the instrument. Removal of the charging rod (e) allows the redistribution of the electrons in the stem and leaves and, since there is a deficiency of them, the net positive charge appears evident in that the leaf is now repelled from the stem. Note that the final charge on the electroscope is positive, while the charge on the charging rod was negative. This is just the opposite of the situation we encountered previously in charging by contact. There we saw that the charge on the object charged was of the same kind as the charge on the charging rod.

It is useful to pursue the matter of induced charges further, for a thorough understanding of this phenomenon will stand the student in good stead in most aspects of electrical study. We pose the question this time as to whether it is possible to electrically charge two metallic spheres by induction. Yes. The answer is implicit in Fig. 2.8.

We are now in a position to understand an observation made in charging a pith ball by contact (which observation we chose to ignore earlier).

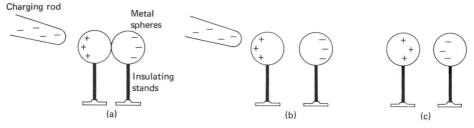

FIG. 2.8. Separating electrical charges by induction.

When one first brings the charging rod very close to the uncharged pith ball, one notices a mild attraction before the contact is made and the pronounced repulsion becomes evident. As the charging rod is brought very close to the pith ball, a charge distribution is induced in the pith ball, causing the side nearer a positive charging rod to be slightly negative, and the far side consequently slightly positive. Since the negative side is closer to the positive charging rod, the attraction is slightly greater than the repulsion, due to positive charges on the far side (see Fig. 2.9). Now, as a matter of fact, the preceding argument presumes the pith ball to be coated with a material which permits the mobility of electrons, say a metallic paint.

But will we not also see this effect even if the pith ball is not coated and electrons cannot readily move about, on, or through it? The answer is yes. And the explanation is the same as that which clarifies why one may rub a comb through one's hair a few times and then pick up small (about $\frac{1}{8}$ of an inch square) pieces of electrically uncharged paper with the comb. We shall dramatize the effect by a little oversimplification. We say that the electrons cannot move about in the pith ball, but we admit that they have some mobility in their own particular atom. This means that in the presence of a negative charging rod, for example, in each atom the electrons tend to be as far away from the charging rod as possible. So-called electric dipoles are formed, that is, are induced. (Further, some atoms are naturally electric dipoles and thus behave similarly to those whose polarity is induced; see Fig. 2.10.) We thus see that on the average

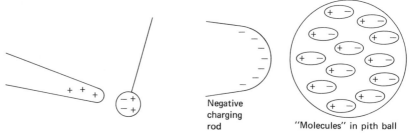

FIG. 2.9. Charge distribution
induced on a pith ball.

FIG. 2.10. Molecular dipoles.

the negative charges in the pith ball are farther from the charging rod; thus the attraction due to the closer positive charges causes the pith ball to be attracted to the charging rod or the paper to the comb. On contact, of course (since some charge is transferred by contact), the pith ball becomes negatively charged and flies away. Similarly, the paper pieces will fly off the comb after a brief interval.

2.2 THE COULOMB FORCE

Although the Greeks knew as long ago as 600 B.C. that amber, when rubbed, temporarily acquired some attracting force, a quantitative understanding of this force awaited the experiments of Coulomb in 1785.

Coulomb's Law

Coulomb employed a torsion balance (see Fig. 2.11). The two pith balls, A and B, were initially in contact; then both were given an electrical charge of the same sign, whereupon the movable ball B was repelled by the fixed ball A.

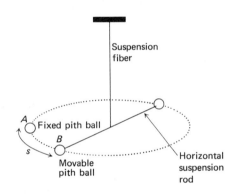

FIG. 2.11. Coulomb torsion balance.

The ball B came to rest when the twisting effect of the electrical force of repulsion between B and A was equal to the opposing twisting force exerted by the suspension fiber as it was disturbed from its normal equilibrium condition by the rotation of the horizontal suspension rod.

Now Coulomb had earlier carried out studies which showed that the angle through which such a suspension fiber is twisted (providing a certain limit is not exceeded) is directly proportional to the twisting force applied to the ball B on the end of the horizontal suspension rod. Consequently, he was able to relate the electrical repulsion force (which balanced the restoring force or twisting force exerted by the suspension fiber when the ball B was at rest) to the angle of twist, an angle which could be readily measured. He found that if he wanted the balls A and B closer together, he needed to twist the suspension fiber more. (With reference to Fig. 2.11, the twist applied at the top of the suspension fiber would have to be clockwise, as seen from the top, to bring B closer to A.) By means of this experiment, Coulomb was able to conclude that, with a given electrical charge on A and B, the electrical force of repulsion varied inversely as the square of the distance s between the centers of the balls. In other words, if s were cut in half the force would become, not twice as large, but four times as large.

This same torsion balance also lent itself to another investigation, one in which the relationship between the electrical force and the electric charge was revealed. As a consequence of this investigation, Coulomb concluded that the force varied directly as the product of the charges on A and B. That is, if the charge on B, for example, were to be made twice as large as it was formerly (that is, if it were to be increased by a factor of 2), then the force would become twice as large (that is, it would also be increased by a factor of 2).

The results of this work may be expressed succinctly in an equation which is known as *Coulomb's law:*

$$F = K \frac{q_1 q_2}{s^2}, \tag{2.1}$$

where q_1 and q_2 refer to the electric charges, s is the distance between them (see Fig. 2.12), and K is a proportionality constant dependent on the material between the charges.

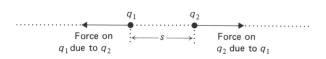

Fig. 2.12. Coulomb forces on charges of the same sign.

We now emphasize that F in Eq. (2.1) is the force exerted by one charge, say q_1, on the other, q_2. The force exerted in turn by q_2 on q_1 is of the same magnitude as that of q_1 on q_2, but in the opposite direction (see Fig. 2.12). This pair of forces obey Newton's famous third law: Whenever one body exerts a force on another, the second always exerts on the first a force which is equal in magnitude, is opposite in direction, and has the same line of action.

If the q's are given in coulombs and the distance s in meters, we are working in the so-called mks system (meter, kilogram, second; refer to Table 2.1) of units, in which the unit of force F is the *newton*. In this case, for air $K \approx 9 \times 10^9$ N-m²/coul².

Two other points might yet be made. First: We shall use Eq. (2.1) for calculating only the magnitude of the force; we shall therefore not use the minus sign which is commonly employed to designate a negative charge. The direction of the force we shall consequently obtain simply by recalling that like charges repel and unlike charges attract. Second: Note that this law is one of electrostatics because it gives only the force between charges *at rest* with respect to each other. We shall find later, in Chapter 4, that another force, a magnetic one, makes its appearance as well, when the charges are in relative motion.

Coulomb's law will aid us (descriptively at least, insofar as it will show the plausibility of many subsequent phenomena) in understanding most of the basic electricity to follow. We may even invoke this law now to support the plausibility of the Bohr atom of Chapter 1. The Coulomb attractive force acts as the "string" to keep the electron in orbit about the positively charged nucleus. Moreover, this law also suggests that the outer electrons are less tightly bound to the nucleus than the inner ones, a fact borne out by experiment. When woven into the elements of quantum mechanics, this law of electrostatics leads to presently accepted descriptions not only of the forces that bind the electrons to an atomic nucleus, but also of the forces that bind atoms to form molecules and, indeed, bind molecules and atoms to each other to form liquids and solids.

Some readers may now wonder how, on the other hand, a nucleus composed of more than one proton can exist. What about the repulsive force between two protons? For example, the Coulomb repulsive force exerted by one proton on another in an iron nucleus is about 14 newtons, that is, about 3 pounds in the British system of measurement; and yet these protons hold together in the iron nucleus. The answer may be deduced by reference to Table 1.1. The nuclear force which holds the protons (and neutrons) together is established to be about two orders of magnitude, that is, 10×10, or 10^2, larger than the electric force, but acts only at exceedingly small distances.

As an example of the application of Coulomb's law in the atomic realm, let us calculate the electrical force of attraction by the proton on the electron in a hydrogen atom. The distance between the two particles is about 5.3×10^{-11} meter, and the charge on each is, of course, in magnitude the electronic charge, that is about 16×10^{-20} coulomb. Thus, if we use

$$F = K \frac{q_1 q_2}{s^2}, \qquad (2.1)$$

we have

$$F = \frac{(9.0 \times 10^9 \text{ N-m}^2/\text{coul}^2)(16 \times 10^{-20} \text{ coul})(16 \times 10^{-20} \text{ coul})}{(5.3 \times 10^{-11} \text{ m})^2}$$

$$= 8.2 \times 10^{-8} \text{ N}$$

Electric Field

In our previous discussions of the pith balls A and B of Fig. 2.11, for example, we noted that a force is exerted by A on B even though the two may be widely separated in space. This mysterious "action at a distance" was quite repugnant to early investigators, and thus the ancient Greek philosophers conceived of a material cloud or "effluvium" (later to reappear in a somewhat different guise as the "ether" conceived to fill all space) that somehow extended out from an electrified object and in some way made contact with the attracted object. Present day physical theory has no need for such effluvia, nor for ether. The classical theory of electromagnetism on which our present electrical technology is based is essentially a *field* theory.

FIG. 2.13. Electric field: electric charge experiences a force. (a) No electric field. (b) Electric field present.

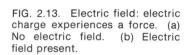

(a)

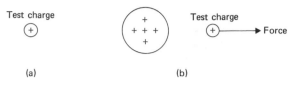

(b)

The field concept was first applied to the realms of electricity and magnetism by Michael Faraday (1791–1867), whose work provided the basis of the electrical advances which ultimately made medical radiography possible. This notion of a field, and those of effluvia and ether, are conceptually among the cornerstones of physical theory. It is naive to accept or reject these ideas glibly. However, we are not engaged in studying the philosophical aspects of physics, but rather are interested in practical results. Therefore, now that we have indicated that there is more here than meets the eye, we shall simply make some unadorned definitions and proceed. Readers who find themselves interested in the basics of this transmission of force without contact are referred to the book by Holton and Roller listed in the Suggested Reading section at the end of this chapter.

Suppose that we have a small positive electrical charge, a test charge, and we bring it to rest in some region far removed from other electrical charges. It experiences no electrical force. Let us remove it. Then we bring some positively charged body into the region (see Fig. 2.13) and now explore this region again with our test charge. This time the test charge experiences a force. The positively charged body has somehow endowed the space around it with this property: that an electrical charge experiences a force. A region in which a static electrical charge experiences an electrical force is called an *electric field*. We commonly represent this region by means of lines, so-called *lines of force*, the direction of which indicates the direction of the force on a positive charge introduced into the field. The density of these lines of force (that is, how close they are together or, more precisely, the number of lines per unit area) is representative of the strength or intensity of the electric field (see Fig. 2.14). Consequently, diverging lines indicate that the field is growing weaker.

We must emphasize at this point that these lines of force have no real physical meaning. Certainly we couldn't cut them with scissors! These

FIG. 2.14. Lines of force representing the electric field of a positively charged sphere.

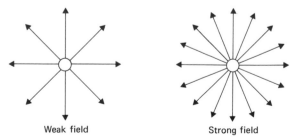

Weak field   Strong field

lines are abstractions designed to help to give meaning to the concept of electric field by means of a visual crutch. This visual aspect can, however, be related to the electric field in that pieces of thread, sawdust, grass seeds, etc., when they are placed in an electric field, in a manner relatively free to move, will assume definite positions through which one could draw lines which we call the lines of force.

We define the magnitude of the electric field strength, E, as follows:

$$E = F/q, \tag{2.2}$$

where F is the force on the test charge, q. This equation states that the electric field strength E is equal to the force per unit charge experienced by a charge (which itself is not significantly changing the electric field) placed in the field. The unit of E would thus be newton/coulomb in the mks system.

As to the direction assigned to the electric field; is there any significance in the fact that we say that it is the direction of the force on a positive test charge? No. This matter is quite arbitrary, but this direction is the universally accepted convention in classical electromagnetic theory.

The direction and configuration of an electric field are, of course, dependent on the charged body, or bodies, setting up the field. Figure 2.15 shows various examples of electric fields. Of those shown, case (c) best approximates (but very crudely) the electric field in an x-ray tube.

The student might now pause and ask in what direction electrons will move through the field, between the charged bodies, in this latter case.

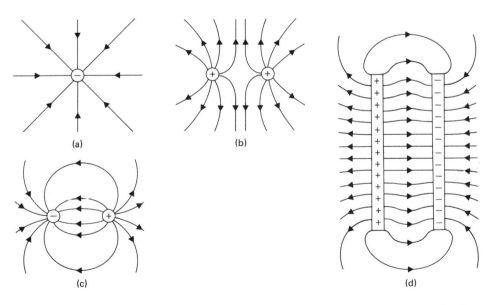

(a)

(b)

(c)

(d)

FIG. 2.15. Various electric fields represented by lines of force. Compare case (a) with Fig. 2.14. Compare case (d), which represents the case of two charged insulator plates, with Fig. 2.27, the case of two charged conductor plates.

Since to produce x-rays we require the electrons to strike the target with considerable energy (that is, high speed), the electric field in the tube is made quite strong. A typical value for the speed of the electrons is 100,000 miles/second, for which the electric field E must be of the order of 10^6 newtons/coulomb. (Students who wish to check out this calculation for themselves must realize that at the high speeds involved account must be taken of the associated mass increase of the electron, in accordance with Einstein's Theory of Special Relativity.)

Electric Shielding

Faraday, experimenting with an ice pail, confirmed an observation reported earlier by Benjamin Franklin: that the electric charge placed on an electrically insulated metal object (that is, an object supported by a material in which electrons are tightly bound to their respective atoms) resides entirely on the metal object's outer surface. Reference to Fig. 2.16 shows that this observation supports Coulomb's law: Like charges repel each other, and thus the charge spreads out as much as it can. This means that the charge must reside on the outer surface. Careful experiments with closed metallic vessels have indeed quantitatively verified Coulomb's law in this manner.

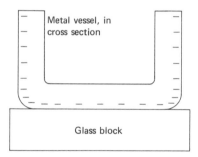

FIG. 2.16. Metal vessel charged negatively. Charge resides on outside surface.

A useful adjunct of this phenomenon is that, with the charge residing entirely on the outside of a hollow metal body, the electric field is zero inside the body. Thus one may protect oneself from lightning by simply staying inside a hollow metal body, such as a car. In fact, the metal does not have to be continuous. A wire cage will do. Inside the cage one will be blissfully free from outside electrical disturbances (except for the noise, of course).

Thus one frequently employs electric shielding to protect delicate electronic equipment, such as radio tubes, by enclosing it (or them) in a metal shield.

Van de Graaff Generator

One other aspect of this fact that charges will reside on the outside of a metallic vessel is that it is consequently possible to place an almost unlimited amount of charge on a hollow metal sphere by bringing the additional charge to the sphere from the inside. This charge immediately

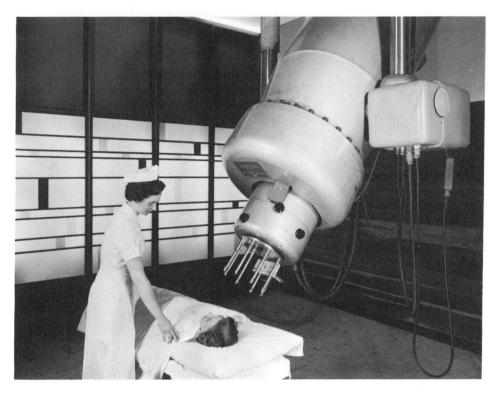

FIG. 2.17. Two-MeV medical Van de Graaff installation at the University of Pennsylvania Hospital. (Courtesy High Voltage Engineering Corporation, Burlington, Mass.)

spreads to the outside, permitting more charge to be brought inside. By this procedure one builds up exceedingly large charges on the hollow sphere. This behavior is the basis of an electrostatic high-voltage generator, the Van de Graaff machine (Fig. 2.17), which is finding extensive use in the production of high energy x-rays for therapy. (For a discussion of this device, see Johns, H. E., *The Physics of Radiology.*)

2.3 DIGRESSION ON WORK, ENERGY, POWER

It is sometimes said that x-ray technicians could well profit from a course in unarmed combat! Be that as it may, it is certainly obvious that it is easier to correctly position a light patient than a heavy one. More force is required for the heavier one. The fact that it is easier (takes less force) to get a wheeled stretcher with a cat on it from rest to normal speed than to achieve the same for a stretcher with an elephant on it is, at the very least, intuitively obvious. One may also draw on one's experience to realize that it takes more force to get a certain mobile x-ray unit from rest to a fast rolling speed in a given time than to just get it barely rolling in the same time interval. These conclusions are summarized in Sir Isaac

Table 2.1

Some Systems of Units

System	Force	Mass	Length (Distance)	Work or Energy	Power
British (engineering)	pound (lb)	slug	foot	foot-pound (ft-lb)	ft-lb/sec
cgs	dyne	gram	centimeter	erg	erg/sec
mks	**newton** (N)	**kilogram** (kg)	**meter** (m)	**joule**	**watt**

Newton's (1642–1727) famous second law of motion

$$F = ma,$$

where F is the net force, m is mass (of elephant, or of cat, for example) and a is the acceleration, that is, the rate of change of the speed of the mass m. The units associated with this equation are of some consequence. Although we shall restrict our subsequent discussions to only one system of units, two others are also shown in Table 2.1. Our main concern is with the system printed in bold-faced type, the so-called mks system, because it readily leads to the common, "practical" units of electricity such as the volt, which the reader will be using in x-ray work.

One can see from the application of Newton's second law, $F = ma$, that the mks unit of force, the newton, is simply another name for a kilogram-meter/sec². That acceleration a may be expressed in meter/sec² follows, of course, from the fact that

$$\text{speed} = \frac{\text{(change in) displacement, or distance}}{\text{time}},$$

which can therefore be measured in m/sec, and that

$$\text{acceleration} = \frac{\text{(change in) speed}}{\text{time}},$$

which thus has the units

$$\frac{\text{m/sec}}{\text{sec}},$$

which is the same as m/sec².

Work and Energy

The physical definition of the work done by a force is the product of the force and the displacement, or distance, through which the force is exercised, where the displacement is in the same direction as the force. If you are standing still, waiting for the hospital elevator, while holding a

big bag of barium sulfate, you may get tired, but the force you exert on
the bag is not doing any work! However, if you get tired of waiting for
the elevator and carry the barium sulfate upstairs yourself, the force you
exert on the bag does some work, in the sense that we have defined it.

Let us consider a simple numerical example. Suppose that it takes
a force of 100 N (about 23 lb) to push a stack of film cassettes along a bench.
How much work is done by this force in pushing the cassettes 2 m (about
6.6 ft)? (See Fig. 2.18.)

$$\text{Work} = \text{Force} \times \text{Distance},$$

which may be expressed in the shorter form

$$W = FD \tag{2.3}$$
$$= (100 \text{ N})(2 \text{ m}) = 200 \text{ N-m}.$$

The product unit, newton-meter, comes up so often in physical calculations that it is assigned a name, the *joule*, after James Prescott Joule, a
famous pupil of the John Dalton we mentioned in Chapter 1. (Refer to
Table 2.1.) The answer to our question is thus that 200 joules of work
have been done by the applied force.

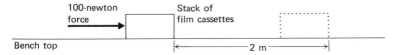

FIG. 2.18. Work done by an applied 100-N force in pushing an object along a level surface.

In doing this work, someone had to expend energy. Where did this
energy go? Since we may assume that the bench was level, the stack of
cassettes is no higher than it was before; it has not gained energy by virtue
of being farther removed from the center of the earth. In this case, the
energy expended when the work was done by the applied force was used
in overcoming friction between the cassettes and the bench, thereby
heating both the cassettes and the bench. You can convince yourself of
the plausibility of this fact easily enough by rubbing your finger rapidly
over a bench top. The key point to note is that energy was expended, that
is, work was done by some force, and that the energy consequently appeared in another form. In other words, energy transfers are accomplished
by the performance of work. And moreover we have implied the idea of
the conservation of energy, so that we could say that 200 joules of work
were done by an applied force, and 200 joules of heat energy were produced in the cassettes and bench.

Suppose now that you were to use a force of 20 N to lift a box of processing chemicals, weighing 20 N, from a shelf 1.0 m above the floor to
one 2.5 m off the floor. Then you would do, at least, 30 joules of work.
(At least that; because we are neglecting the small effort required to
overcome air friction and also the various accelerations involved.) This

result is arrived at by employing Eq. (2.3):

$$W = FD,$$

where F = force = 20 N and D = displacement = (2.5 − 1.0) m = 1.5 m. Hence

$$W = (20 \text{ N})(1.5 \text{ m}) = 30 \text{ joules.}$$

This time the energy expended—that is, the work done—is evidenced in an increase in the gravitational potential energy of the box. The box now has more energy than it had before the lift because it could fall to the lower shelf and in the process do some work; for example, turn a wheel of some kind. If the box falls down without doing work in turning a wheel, where does its potential energy go? It gains speed and thereby increases its energy of motion, its kinetic energy. Just before impact with the lower shelf, the kinetic energy of the falling box is 30 joules. We leave you with the question of what happens to this energy at the moment the box strikes the lower shelf.

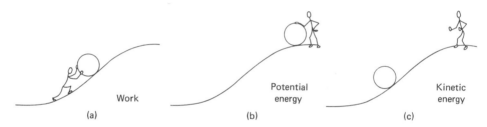

FIG. 2.19. Work is done on the large snowball by the x-ray technician pushing it up the hill; its potential energy is increased; finally the original work done appears as kinetic energy at the bottom of the hill.

What we have said about work and energy, potential and kinetic, may be summarized without further words by reference to Fig. 2.19, for which the electrical analog follows.

In the case of the x-ray tube, the electrical company does work on electrons(a), giving them potential energy (b) and hence kinetic energy (c), some of which produces x-rays as the electrons strike the target, but most of which is converted to heat energy, thus increasing the temperature of the target. (More about this important heating problem will appear in Chapter 7.)

Power

One other quantity of interest relates to how fast work is being done, or the rate at which energy is expended. This quantity is called power. We may define it as follows:

$$P = \frac{W}{t}, \tag{2.4}$$

where P = power, W = work or energy, and t = time. The power of doing one joule of work in one second is called a watt (see Table 2.1); that is,

$$1 \text{ watt} = \frac{1 \text{ joule}}{1 \text{ sec}} \cdot$$

The watt is the common unit of electrical power. For example, a bright lamp obviously uses more energy per unit time than a dull one. The bright one has a higher power; it may be a 150-watt bulb, while the relatively dull one may be only a 25-watt bulb. (Incidentally, the watt itself is a much smaller unit of power than the commonly employed horsepower: 1 hp = 746 watts.)

Now if you are paying your home electrical bill, should you pay for power or for energy? A moment's reflection should convince you that the important thing is how much work the electrical company did for you, that is, you should pay for the total energy consumed. Take a look at the light bill and you will see that you are being charged not for kilowatts (power), but for kilowatt-hours (energy = power × time).

Consider now an x-ray film of a hand. This might involve 60 kV, 100 mA, at $\frac{1}{15}$ sec. The power required here, as will be shown later in the next chapter, is 6000 watts or 6 kilowatts, and since the time of the exposure is $\frac{1}{15}$ sec, the energy used is obtained by applying Eq. (2.4):

$$W = Pt = (6000)(\tfrac{1}{15} \text{ sec}) = 400 \text{ joules.}$$

(*Note:* The power calculation of this example is actually correct only for a constant-potential x-ray unit. This fact will become clear after we discuss direct and alternating currents, in Chapters 3 and 6.)

2.4 ELECTRIC POTENTIAL

The concept of electric potential is probably the most commonly employed concept in electrical technology. We must understand this idea because it contains the key to much of what is to be discussed in the following chapters. The x-ray student must acquire a very firm understanding of such terms as potential difference, volt, energy, and electron volt.

Difference of Potential

We shall address ourselves first to the difference of electric potential, commonly called voltage, measured with an instrument called a *voltmeter* and expressed numerically in terms of a unit known as the *volt* (after Alessandro Volta, Italian physicist, 1745–1827).

Voltages encountered in the hospital may range from the microvolt (1 microvolt = 10^{-6} volt) potential difference, found between two electrodes placed on the scalp in the case of electroencephalography, to the kilovoltages (1 kilovolt = 10^3 volts) of the x-ray department.

We shall use the concept of electric field to establish the notion of potential difference. Any electric charge placed in a region in which there is an electric field experiences a force. If the charge moves under the influence of this force, the electric field is said to do work on it. This

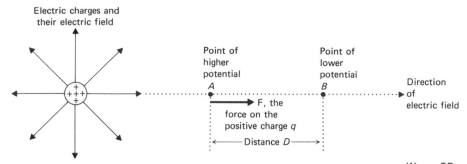

FIG. 2.20. Potential difference (V) between A and B: $V_{BA} = V_A - V_B = \dfrac{W_{BA}}{q} = \dfrac{FD}{q}$.

situation is analogous to the snowball of Fig. 2.19 rolling down the hill under the influence of a gravitational field. The electric charge on the one hand, and the snowball on the other, have themselves less potential to do work after this trip than before. Their potential energy is decreased. There is a potential difference between their initial locations and their final locations. Moreover, since at their initial positions they were able to do more work, their potential energy at the original position (before the electric or gravitational field has done work on them) is said to be higher.

Now, unlike the case of a mass in a gravitational field, the electrical case offers two possibilities. That is, we know of no snowballs which roll uphill, but we do know that if positive charges run down an "electrical" hill, then negative charges placed in the same field would go in the opposite direction. Therefore, to give meaning to "higher" and "lower" potential, we must make a decision. A convention must be established. Again, we choose to consider what the situation is with respect to a positive test charge. If a positive charge would move from point A to point B (see Fig. 2.20) under the influence of an electric field, then we say that point A is of a higher potential than point B.

So far we have discussed work and the resulting differences in energy. It is common practice in electrical work, however, to refer not to the total energy changes involved but to energy changes per unit electric charge. Thus by difference of potential (loosely called voltage), we mean the work done on electrical charges per unit charge. The total work done by the electric field on an electrically charged particle would hence be the product of the potential difference and the total charge on the particle (see Fig. 2.20). In terms of symbols, we write

W (work or energy) = V (potential difference) × q (electric charge).

This statement is, in effect, the definition of potential difference; that is,

$$V \text{ (potential difference)} = \frac{W \text{ (energy or work)}}{q \text{ (charge)}}. \tag{2.5}$$

Furthermore, Eq. (2.5) leads to the definition of the unit of potential difference. The potential difference between two points in an electric

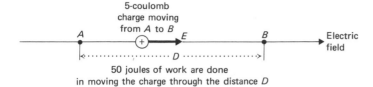

FIG. 2.21. Work done by electric field, E, in moving charge from A to B. V_A (the potential of point A) is higher than V_B (the potential of point B) and $V (= V_A - V_B) = 10$ volts.

field is said to be one volt if one joule of work is done on each coulomb of charge in moving it from one point to the other. That is,

$$1 \text{ volt} = \frac{1 \text{ joule}}{1 \text{ coulomb}}.$$

It is sometimes convenient to refer various potential differences to a common reference point, arbitrarily assigned zero potential. This practice will be of particular interest in our discussions of current electricity (Chapter 3) in which we shall arbitrarily assign zero potential to any circuit part connected to the ground; that is, a part which is grounded (or earthed). Assigning an arbitrary zero value for electric potential leads to the use of the term "potential" rather than "potential difference." For example, if the potential difference between two points A and B is 15 volts, where A is the point of higher potential, and if we assign zero potential to point B, we say that the potential, or rigorously, the absolute potential, of point A is +15 volts. If A were at a lower potential than B, which is at zero potential, then the potential of A would be −15 volts.

Let us summarize the above ideas by means of an example (see Fig. 2.21). Let us say that a body having a positive charge of 5 coulombs is moved under the influence of an electric field from point A to point B. The work done by the electric field is 50 joules.

Questions:

a)   What is the potential difference between points A and B?

b)   Which point is of the higher potential?

c)   What happens to the energy expended by the electric field?

d)   What is the potential (absolute potential) of point B if point A is grounded?

We describe the absolute potentials of points A and B by $V = V_A - V_B$, where V is the potential difference between points A and B and V_A, V_B are the absolute potentials of points A and B, respectively. One way of defining the absolute potential of a point is simply to say that it is the potential difference between that point and infinity.

Answers:

a) $V = \dfrac{W}{q} = \dfrac{50 \text{ joules}}{5 \text{ coulombs}} = 10$ volts.

b)   Since the positive charge can move from A to B under the influence of the electric field E, by definition A is at a higher potential than B.

c)   If the charged body is not subject to any forces other than electrical ones, the energy becomes evident in increased kinetic energy of the body; that is, by an increase in the body's velocity. In our case the charged body acquires 50 joules of kinetic energy through the work done by the electrical forces.

d)   Since by convention we arbitrarily assign zero potential to a grounded point, the potential of point A is zero. Thus

$$V_A - V_B = 10 \text{ volts,}$$
$$O - V_B = 10 \text{ volts,}$$
$$V_B = -10 \text{ volts.}$$

That is, the potential at point B is -10 volts.

As a second example, we apply the above ideas to an x-ray tube, in which there is a potential difference (voltage) maintained between the anode (target) and the cathode (filament). One may get an idea of the energy imparted to an electron accelerated through the vacuum from the anode to the cathode by simply stating the voltage. If the voltage is 40 kV (kilovolts), for example, the electrons strike the target with less energy than if the voltage is 100 kV. Moreover, since electrons are negatively charged, they move oppositely to positive charges in an electric field and hence by our definition of "high" and "low" potentials, they roll up the potential hill. In other words, the place they come from—that is, the filament—must be at a lower potential than the place they go, the target.

Electron Volt

This latter example also serves to introduce another useful quantity, the electron volt (eV). If we are interested in the total energy of an electron striking the target we need to know not only the potential difference between the filament and the target but also the charge of the electron. Using Eq. (2.5) and a potential difference of 40 kV, we have

$W = Vq = (40{,}000 \text{ volts})(16.02 \times 10^{-20} \text{ coulomb}) = 64.08 \times 10^{-16} \text{ joule.}$

This latter number, representing the total energy imparted to one electron when it is accelerated through a potential difference of 40 kV, is a rather small number. Hence it has become common practice to use another energy unit, a much smaller one. We are then able to work with larger numbers. Such an approach is sometimes convenient. In any case, it is accepted practice at present. This smaller energy unit is the electron volt.

An electron volt (eV) is the work done by the electric field on a single electron which is transferred through a potential difference of one volt. Hence, using Eq. (2.5), we get

$$W = Vq$$

Table 2.2

Some Energies in Electron Volts

Phenomenon	Energy, eV
Lattice vibration in a crystal at room temperature	$\sim 10^{-2}$
Average kinetic energy of air molecule at room temperature	4×10^{-2} (=0.04)
Photon of red light	~ 2
x-ray photon (maximum for 70 kV)	7×10^4
Gamma ray photon (from Co-60)	1.33×10^6
Energy required to remove a nucleon from the nucleus	$\sim 10^7$

and

$$1 \text{ eV} = (1 \text{ volt})(16.02 \times 10^{-20} \text{ coulomb})$$
$$= (1 \times 16.02 \times 10^{-20}) \text{ volt-coulomb.}$$

But from the definition of the volt, that is (1 volt)(1 coulomb) or (1 volt-coulomb) = 1 joule, we get

$$1 \text{ eV} = 16.02 \times 10^{-20} \text{ joule.}$$

As has been stated, the electron volt is a unit of energy; a very small unit. It takes $[1/(16.02 \times 10^{-20})]$ eV, that is, 6.24×10^{18} eV, to yield one joule of energy. (For those readers who feel more comfortable in the British system of units: 1 eV = 11.8×10^{-20} foot-pounds, or 1 foot-pound $\approx 10^{13}$ MeV (million electron volts).)

The electron volt is so commonly employed in electronics, atomic and nuclear physics, as well as in the realm of x-rays, that it is a good idea to have some familiarity with this unit. Table 2.2 gives some examples of energies in terms of electron volts.

Charge Concentration and Leakage

We have previously made plausible the fact that the electric charge on a conductor resides on its *outside* surface. In the case of a spherical conductor, this charge distributes itself uniformly over the surface of the conductor. Hence, for a given charge, the charge density is uniform, and is less on a large sphere than on one of a smaller radius because, in the former case, the charges are more spread out. Consequently the electric field in the region of the larger sphere is weaker than the electric field near the smaller one, even though it carries the same charge.

Now although air does not readily permit a transfer of electric charge (that is, air—dry air particularly—is quite a good insulator), there is nevertheless a continuous leakage of charge from any charged body because there are always some ions being produced in the air by such agents as cosmic rays. This means that a negatively charged object will attract positive ions from the surrounding air, thus neutralizing itself. The charge "leaks" off. As is to be expected, the leakage is greater in the region of the greater electric field. This means that in the case of the two similarly charged spheres, the one that has the smaller radius (that is, the one that has the greater electric field associated with it) loses its charge more readily than the larger one.

If it so happens that the charge density is sufficiently great, the associated electric field can produce an exceedingly rapid leakage, called a *spark*.

Let us consider two equally but oppositely charged spheres. There exists an electric field between them, such as is depicted in Fig. 2.15(c). Since work can be done on an electric charge between the spheres by the electric field, one says that there is a *potential difference* between the spheres. What is now of interest is how *large* a potential difference between the spheres is required so that the insulating property of the air breaks down, permitting a very rapid leakage of charge, or spark, from one sphere to the other. It turns out that in dry air at normal pressure, the potential difference required for a separation of one centimeter between such spheres is about 30,000 volts. (The exact voltage depends on such parameters as the humidity and pressure of the air and the radius of the spheres.) With the same spheres a larger potential difference is, of course, required to produce a longer spark.

Figure 2.22(a) shows how the above notions were applied in the early days of medical radiography to measure the kV. W. D. Coolidge (see Chapter 7), in his experiments involving the development of the hot cathode x-ray tube, used a device based on this same principle, and expressed the tube kV simply in terms of the length of a spark gap.

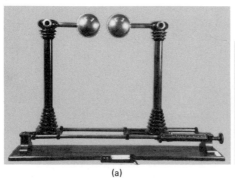
(a)

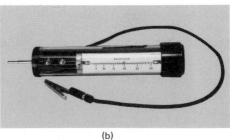
(b)

FIG. 2.22. Sphere-gap instruments for indicating high voltages by means of spark lengths. (a) Sphere gap of the type used in x-ray equipment in the past (up to 250 kV), shown in comparison with a small modern sphere gap. (b) Small modern sphere gap, used up to 30 kV; note the small spheres at the left end.

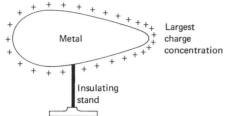

FIG. 2.23. Charge distribution on an irregularly shaped conductor.

Although our previous discussion of charge distribution and leakage may at each stage be made plausible by reference to Coulomb's law, we can rigorously prove an even more important aspect relating to the charge distribution on irregularly shaped bodies by applying this law (albeit with some relatively complicated analysis): On any given irregularly shaped conductor, the largest charge concentration, or charge density, is at the point of least radius (see Fig. 2.23). Outside the conductor near such a point, one encounters the largest electric fields. This fact means that if one wants charge to leak off readily, one should construct the conductor with a sharp point (hence sharp points on lightning rods). If, on the other hand, leakage is to be inhibited, there should be no points or sharp corners on the conductor. In the case of high-voltage equipment, such as x-ray machines, sharp points could result in a so-called corona discharge, evidenced by a continuous bluish glow around the point of discharge.

2.5 ELECTROSTATIC PROBLEMS IN RADIOGRAPHY

Some knowledge of electrostatics is a necessary tool for the study of current electricity that is to follow. In addition, a knowledge of electrostatics has an intrinsic practical value, because certain problems in medical radiography are electrostatic in nature.

Static Markings on Films

One problem relates to the static markings on x-ray films (see Fig. 2.24). There are in essence three kinds of static markings found on films: *crown static, tree static,* and *smudge static.* The first two types of markings are presumed to be caused directly by electric discharges (not involving production of visible light) occurring along the surface of the film emulsion. These discharges, like those involved in causing smudge static, are essentially triboelectric phenomena. They may come about as a result of rapid motions such as occur when one removes interleaving papers or perhaps as a result of contact with the fingers of the x-ray technician. In terms of the physics we previously discussed, these film problems arise from the accumulation of enough charge for the associated electric fields to be strong enough to effect an electric discharge.

When there are smudge and spot markings on film, they are assumed to be caused by film exposure due to visible light produced by electric discharges. What is presumed is that a relatively low potential discharge

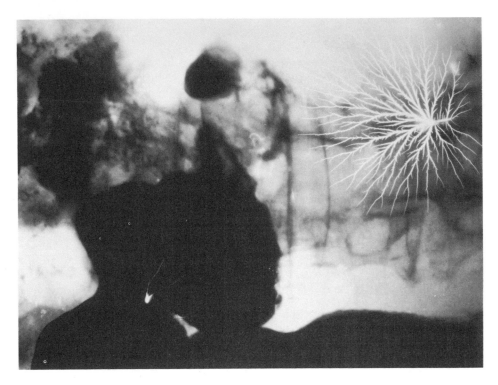

FIG. 2.24. Static markings on a radiograph.

occurs over a large area, and that this discharge tends to follow a path of dust, lint, or roughened intensifying screen surface.

A knowledge of the fundamentals of static electricity should permit the x-ray technician to formulate practical rules which would substantially reduce such static film markings. It is obvious that somehow charge accumulation should be avoided. In general, all such rules would therefore lead to a reduction in the rubbing together of different materials, and/or allow for rapid leakage of any accumulated charges. Electrically grounding any equipment (by connecting it to a water pipe, for example) with which the film cassette comes into contact would be such a rule.

Operating-Room Hazards

An entirely different aspect of electrostatic problems is associated with explosive hazards in the operating theatre. Many of the volatile agents used in anesthesia form highly explosive mixtures with air.

Now it is true that mobile x-ray units for use in operating rooms may be quite safe, in that dangers from the electricity involved in their operation have been eliminated by having the units hermetically sealed and flash-proofed for use in explosive atmospheres. However, the dangers arising from the accumulation of static charge still exist. It is quite possible for something to acquire relatively small charges and yet achieve relatively high potential differences. (This fact will perhaps become more obvious to you after you read the following section on capacitors.) And static electricity of high voltage on an insulated conductor such as a metal stretcher with rubber casters, or a mobile x-ray unit on rubber wheels, can discharge through the air if another object (such as an x-ray technician) of different potential comes near. The spark involved in such a discharge may contain more than enough energy to ignite an explosive anesthetic mixture, even though the spark may be much too small to be seen.

Tests have shown that potential differences between the floor and an operating table of as much as 10,000 volts can be generated by the mere act of stripping a wool blanket from a rubber mattress. All these effects, of course, are worse in places of low relative humidity. The moister the air, the more readily the accumulated charge leaks off before a high potential difference sufficient to cause a spark may be built up. To aid this charge leakage, it is not uncommon practice to drape a wet towel around the base of an operating table, thus ensuring better electrical contact with the floor.

This is not to say that moisture itself makes the air electrically more conductive. Actually, pure water is more or less an insulator, although not a good one, because it is usually very slightly ionized. However, if the air is relatively moist, condensation on surfaces such as clothing, floors, and equipment of all kinds takes place. ("Relatively moist" means that the relative humidity is fairly high; "relative humidity" means the ratio of the actual amount of moisture in the air to the maximum amount the air can hold at the given temperature.) The thin film of moisture on these articles, like the water on the wet towel referred to above, usually dissolves a certain amount of material, thereby rendering itself conductive, as in the example referred to in Fig. 2.2.

Naturally the x-ray technician in the operating room is wise to avoid wearing clothing of the type which is highly subject to building up static charges (e.g., wool, silk, certain synthetic fibers). Cotton has been found to be a relatively safe material.

Finally, it should be noted that recognition of these static electricity problems in the hospital has resulted in many improvements in both equipment and procedures. For example, the use of a special conductive rubber for wheels on rolling stock is now relatively common, and the periodic checking of the conducting properties of such stock and the extent of accumulation of static charge is part of the regular procedures of the electrical maintenance departments in many hospitals.

2.6 CAPACITORS

Let us close our discussion of electrostatics with the consideration of the device which permits the accumulation and storage of electrical charge; the *capacitor*. Recall that in the preamble to this chapter we pointed out that the development of the first capacitor, the Leyden jar, considerably heightened interest in matters electrical in those early days. Today it is safe to say that capacitors form a mainstay in our electronic way of life. Without capacitors our sophisticated communication systems would be impossible, since capacitors are used in the generation and detection of radio waves. Capacitors—as we shall discover in later chapters when we consider their behavior in electric circuits—also find much use in providing time delays. It is in this latter role that capacitors appear in various timing circuits of diagnostic x-ray machines. What are capacitors? Why study them in this chapter?

The answer lies in the fact that although we shall later look at the capacitor as a circuit element in current electricity, its operation is nevertheless essentially electrostatic. We explain its behavior in terms of charges at rest.

Capacitor Operation and Types

We have said that a capacitor stores electric charge. But so can any insulated conductor, such as a metal plate supported on a glass stand. What makes a capacitor different? It can be shown that if we approach the first plate with a second metal plate of an equal but opposite charge, then the amount of charge on each plate can be substantially increased. And only a small increase of potential difference between the plates will be noted as the plates come closer together. A description that is perhaps not quite rigorous but is at least plausible is that the positive charges on the one plate on account of coulomb attraction help to hold the charges on the other so that one can keep on loading up more and more charge and the work required to bring more negative charges to the negative plate is reduced because of the attractive influence of the nearby possitively charged plate. This description implies the construction of a capacitor. A parallel-plate capacitor is simply two conducting plates separated by an insulator, that is, a dielectric (see Fig. 2.25).

The Leyden jar fulfilled this capacitor requirement in that it consisted of a glass jar with some metal foil on the inside and some on the outside

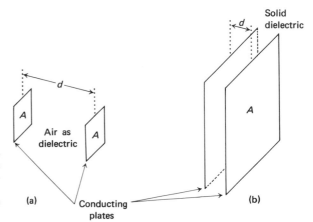

FIG. 2.25. Parallel plate capacitors.   (a) Small capacitance: small plate area (A), large separation (d), low dielectric constant.   (b) Large capacitance: large plate area (A), small separation (d), high dielectric constant.

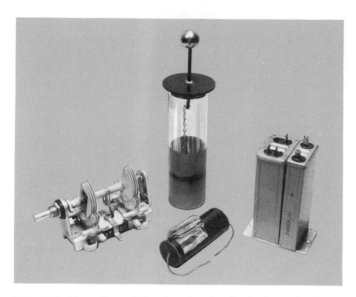

FIG. 2.26. Capacitors. The glass Leyden jar is shown in the center. To the left is a radio tuning capacitor, to the right an oil-filled capacitor, and in front center (partially cut open) a metal-foil capacitor.

surface. Hence the dielectric of the "capacitor sandwich" in this case was the glass of the jar.

Other forms of capacitors, although they seem quite different on the outside, must all have this same characteristic; that is, they must be composed of two conducting materials separated by a dielectric. One common form is composed of metal foil and wax-paper strips rolled up. Such an arrangement effectively gives a larger capacitor area but uses very little space. This and other types of capacitors are shown in Fig. 2.26. One particularly interesting type shown there is the variable capacitor used in radio tuning. When you select different stations, you are actually altering the capacitance of the capacitor by changing its effective area as the one set of vanes is moved in and out of the other. What is the dielectric in this case?

Let us now look at the electric field of the parallel-plate capacitor (Fig. 2.27). Note that, unlike the case of Fig. 2.15(d), there are, to all intents and purposes, no lines of force outside the capacitor plates. That is, just outside the plates of a charged capacitor the electric field is prac-

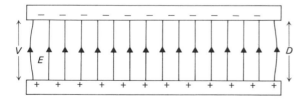

FIG. 2.27. Idealization of the lines of force representing the electric field (E) associated with a parallel-plate capacitor. The potential difference between the plates, which are separated by a distance D, is V, where $V = ED$.

tically zero. This situation derives from the fact that, since the capacitor plates are conductors, the negative charges placed on one plate will move to be as close as possible to the positive charges placed on the other, and that the electric field inside the conducting plates themselves is zero. The result is that outside the capacitor the contribution to the electric field of the positive charges more or less cancels the contribution due to the negative charges, and vice versa.

Note that, except for the fringing at the ends, the electric field between the parallel plates is uniform. This characteristic of parallel-plate capacitors is a very useful attribute in electrical technology.

Capacitance

We have earlier used the word capacitance on the grounds that its meaning is implied in the context. We define capacitance, C, as follows:

$$C = \frac{q}{V}, \qquad (2.6)$$

where q is the charge on either of the plates and V is the potential difference between the plates. The unit for capacitance is thus coulomb/volt, a quantity known as the farad; that is

$$1 \text{ farad} = \frac{1 \text{ coulomb}}{1 \text{ volt}}.$$

In actual practice this turns out to be a rather large value of capacitance, and the microfarad (μf) is more frequently encountered.

What affects the capacitance? The parameters involved are all quite plausible. Let us consider a parallel-plate capacitor. First of all, it seems quite reasonable that increasing the area of the plates would increase the capacitance. After all, there is then more place to store the charges. Secondly, the capacitance is increased by bringing the plates closer together. Thus we might expect

$$C \propto \frac{A}{d},$$

where A is the area of the plates and d is the distance between the plates. With the appropriate proportionality constant, the above proportionality turns into the equation

$$C = \epsilon \frac{A}{d},$$

where ϵ is a constant, characteristic of the dielectric material (and proportional to its dielectric constant). Thus it is possible to vary capacitances by changing the geometry (that is A and/or d) of the capacitor or by inserting a different dielectric (see Fig. 2.25).

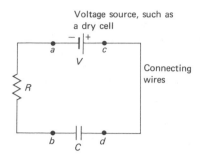

Voltage source, such as a dry cell

V

R

a c

b C d

Connecting wires

FIG. 2.28. Capacitor (C) connected to a constant voltage source (V), showing the usual circuit symbols for the capacitor, the voltage source, and the resistance to charge flow (R).

Charging and Discharging the Capacitor

From the standpoint of coulomb forces (like charges repel), it is expected that the higher the charge already on a capacitor, the more work would have to be done to add more of the same charges. In other words, when the capacitor is "empty" it is easy to add charge; and this process of adding charge becomes successively harder as the capacitor becomes more and more charged.

If we charge a capacitor by applying some kind of a constant voltage source, such as an ordinary dry cell, for example (see Fig. 2.28), the charging rate (current, see Chapter 3) will be rapid at first, and will finally come to a halt as the voltage across the capacitor becomes the same as that of the dry cell. At this time, since there is no longer any potential difference between points a and b and points c and d, no work can be done in moving further charges. It can be shown that the charging current falls to zero in an exponential fashion; that is, the "decay" of the current follows a law of the type encountered in Section 1.6 (on radioactivity).

Similarly the charge on, and the voltage across, the capacitor grow to a maximum in an exponential fashion; that is, rapidly at first, and slowly as the final value is approached. How fast the voltage across the capacitor grows depends not only on the capacitance C but also on the resistance R (Section 3.2) of the circuit. The product RC is thus quite sensibly called the *time constant* of the circuit; this product is of major importance in electronic timers (Section 8.5).

The discharge of a capacitor also follows an exponential law. If R is sufficiently small, the discharge occurs exceedingly rapidly at first, giving a large pulse or surge of charge. This principle is used in some capacitor-discharge circuits employed for the production of x-rays. The advantage of a capacitor over all other electrical-energy-storage devices is that it can deliver its stored energy in a short and easily controllable time interval. In other words, this device can provide a controlled nonpulsating unidirectional voltage (kV) and charge surge (current, or mA) to the x-ray tube. (For a discussion of this apparatus see the book by Jaundrell-Thompson and Ashworth, mentioned in the Suggested Reading at the end of this chapter.)

QUESTIONS

1. What is meant by the term "ionization"?

2. Define negative electricity (in macroscopic terms).

3. a) Explain why a charged electroscope loses its charge when a lighted candle is brought near it.
    b) Does this phenomenon have any relationship to discharging the electroscope by exposing it to x-rays? Explain.

4. Describe fully what is inferred by each of the observations made in charging an electroscope by induction according to steps (a) to (e) in Fig. 2.29.

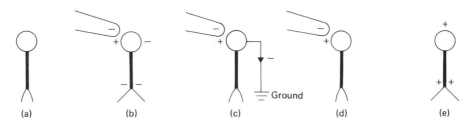

(a)   (b)   (c)   (d)   (e)

Fig. 2.29. Charging an electroscope by induction.

5. A point charge of $+5 \times 10^{-4}$ coulomb is 0.50 meter from another point charge of -3.0×10^{-4} coulomb.
    a) Sketch the lines of force representing the electric field due to these charges.
    b) Using the value of K given in this chapter, calculate the force of the first charge on the second and indicate the direction of this force.

6. What would happen to the force in Question 5, above, if
    a) the second charge were also positive;
    b) the distance between the charges were made twice as large?

7. Explain fully what is understood by "lines of force."

8. Define "electric field strength" and describe fully what is understood by this concept.

9. If 10^5 joules of energy are employed in 10^3 seconds, what is the average power consumption in watts?

10. a) If 10^5 joules of energy are employed by an external force in moving a positive charge of 50 coulombs from point A to point B in an electric field, what is the potential difference between points A and B?
     b) Which point is at the higher potential?

11. Suppose that one were to connect, on the surface of a conductor, a series of points which had this in common: The points were all at the same electric potential. A line through these points is called an *equipotential line*. What is the direction of the electric field, if one exists, near such an equipotential line?

12. a) If an electron is accelerated through a vacuum (Coolidge) x-ray tube from the filament to the target, the potential difference between filament and target being 70 kV, what is the energy (in electron volts) of the electron as it strikes the target?

    b) What would you expect the maximum possible energy of the produced x-ray to be (in electron volts)?

13. About how large an air gap in the old type spark-gap high-voltage measuring device would indicate 60 kV in dry air?

14. Explain why using a vacuum cleaner instead of a dry cloth to clean an intensifying screen might result in better films.

15. A common piece of advice regarding the handling of x-ray film which has interleaving papers is to let the interleaving paper fall away from the film rather than sliding it off. What is the main reason behind this advice? Explain.

16. Would it be better to wear leather-soled or rubber-soled shoes while performing x-ray duties in an operating theatre? Comment.

17. Describe the structure and electrical property of a capacitor.

18. Define capacitance and give the unit in which capacitance is usually stated.

19. A charged capacitor (0.15 microfarad) is connected across an x-ray tube for a certain time during which the potential difference across the tube falls from 95 kV to 50 kV. What charge in coulombs has passed through the tube? Draw a circuit diagram including the capacitor and the x-ray tube.

20. a) What is meant by the "time constant" of a circuit including a capacitor?

    b) In what part of x-ray circuitry is this time constant of particular interest?

SUGGESTED READING

EFRON, ALEXANDER, *Magnetic and Electrical Fundamentals*. New York: John F. Rider Publisher, Inc., 1959. As the publisher states, this small book is written "to provide a rigorously accurate but nonetheless readable and interesting coverage . . . from a level suitable to the general reader, to the point reached by the junior college student." One might quarrel with the last part of this statement if the junior college student is different from the general reader in that he/she has previously studied some physics. Perhaps it is just this objection that recommends this small book (124 pages) to readers who have not had any physics before entering their x-ray training and wish to review the basic elements of electricity and magnetism by consulting another book, while they study our Chapters 2 to 5.

GUEST, P. G., V. W. SIKORA, and BERNARD LEWIS, *Static Electricity in Hospital Operating Suites*. Washington: U.S. Government Printing Office, 1962 (reprint). A report by the investigators of hospital electrostatic problems such as might lead to explosions in the presence of certain anesthetizing agents. Excellent example of the practical application of the concepts discussed in the present chapter. Recommended reading for all x-ray technicians.

HALLIDAY, DAVID, and ROBERT RESNICK, *Physics for Students of Science and Engineering*. New York: John Wiley, 1962 (second edition). Part II of this book is for advanced students with a good background in secondary school physics, who have a knowledge of calculus, and who wish to quantitatively analyze many of the phenomena only qualitatively discussed in the present text. For example, in Chapter 28 of Halliday and Resnick, Gauss' law is used to prove what we have simply stated: that the electric field strength, E, inside a hollow metal sphere is zero.

HOLTON, GERALD, and D. H. D. ROLLER, *Foundations of Modern Physical Science*. Reading, Massachusetts: Addison-Wesley, 1958. Excellent treatment of physics at an elementary level, employing an historical approach. Part VII is highly recommended as an adjunct to our Chapters 2–5 for readers interested in the historical and philosophical aspects of electricity.

JAUNDRELL-THOMPSON, F., and W. J. ASHWORTH, *X-ray Physics and Equipment*. Oxford: Blackwell Scientific Publications, 1965. This book is mentioned as a reference regarding capacitor-discharge x-ray units. It contains a wealth of information on the details of x-ray equipment and the associated physics. For this reason, this book is one of two books in the realm of physics to be highly recommended to the x-ray technician establishing his/her own professional library. (The other book is Johns, H. E., *The Physics of Radiology*, described at the end of Chapter 1.)

RODERICK, J. F., and BRUCE SUTHERLAND, *A Study of the Static Electricity Problem in the X-ray Darkroom*. St. Paul, Minnesota: The X-ray Technician, **23**, March, 1952. A 7-page paper enlarging on the problem sketched in our Section 2.5. Includes a bibliography of interest to those who wish to pursue this matter further. (*The X-ray Technician* was the forerunner of the journal presently published in Baltimore under the title of *Radiologic Technology*.)

CHAPTER 3

Direct Current Electricity

So far we have examined the essentially electric nature of matter and specifically certain phenomena associated with electrical charges, primarily when these charges were assumed to be "at rest." We now turn to a study of electrical charges in some sort of continuous motion or flow. The simplest of such considerations involves a steady drift of charge, always in the same direction, so-called direct current (DC) or, more precisely, steady direct current.

Our concern in this chapter consequently finds its historical root in some experiments performed in England around 1730 by Stephen Gray. His discovery, which opened the door to the world of electricity that we are now dependent on, was that electricity, and consequently electrical energy, could be transferred or conducted from one body to another over fairly long distances. Thus out of experimentation was born the distinction between conductors and non-conductors.

A real impetus to the era of current electricity may be ascribed to the subsequent invention of the voltaic pile. Alessandro Volta's (Italy, 1745–1827) discovery permitted the production of fairly steady continuous currents.

The important mathematical relationship which underlies electrical technology as far as conductors are concerned came a century after Gray's discovery of conduction when a German physicist, professor, and high school teacher, Georg Simon Ohm (1789–1854), formulated the law now known by his name. Ohm's work on this topic of the flow of electric charge in a conductor was apparently derived by using an analogy with heat flow, a topic which had been worked out a few years earlier by the French mathematician, Fourier.

People had to wait another century in order to achieve an understanding of the basic (microscopic) processes underlying the distinction among conductors, insulators, and semiconductors. The present so-called band theory of solids is based on the quantum mechanics mentioned in Chapter 1. Relevant theories, with a quantum-mechanical basis, were advanced independently by the physicists W. Heitler and F. London (1927), and F. Bloch (1928).

3.1 CURRENT ELECTRICITY

The term *current electricity* refers to a continuous transfer or drift of electric charge through a conductor. By direct current, as has been stated before, we mean that the average motion of the electric charges is always in the same direction.

Mechanism of Charge Transfer

What is the mechanism involved in an electric current? What, if anything, undergoes motion?

Contrary to the notion arising from Benjamin Franklin's assumptions, it is not the positive electrical charges which move in a solid conductor (such as a metal), but rather the negative charges, that is, the electrons. An ingenious experiment known as the Hall effect (E. H. Hall, 1879) conclusively demonstrates that in metallic conductors only the electrons are free to move. Positive charge in a piece of copper, for example, is as immobile as it is in glass or any other insulating material.

Now it should not be construed that in a metal wire all the electrons pass along in a nice orderly fashion from one end to the other, depending on the direction of the electric field established in the wire. Rather, in the absence of an electric field, some electrons, the so-called free electrons, undergo a random motion through the metal, much like the Brownian movement mentioned in Chapter 1. For this reason one sometimes speaks of an "electron gas" in a metal. However, as soon as an electric field is applied, say from one end of the wire to the other, although the electrons do not entirely give up their random motion, there is nevertheless a drift, or average motion, through the wire in a direction specified by the applied electric field.

The speed of this drift is surprisingly low. For example, even in a wire carrying a quite reasonable current the drift speed may be so low that it takes some 30 sec for the conduction electrons to drift a distance of 1 cm. It is important at this point to emphasize that the drift speed of the electrons is not the speed with which electric field disturbances pass along the wire. This latter speed is close to the speed of light in a vacuum. And it is for this reason that one obtains almost instantaneous response when one switches on and off electric appliances.

Although in metallic conductors the mechanism of charge transfer involves only electrons, it is quite true that in certain cases positive charges may also move. Such is the case in electric currents through electrolytes (such as the salt-water solution of Section 2.1) and through ionized gases such as we shall discuss in reference to x-ray tubes in Chapter 7. A difference between conducting solutions and gases is that in conducting solutions there are no free electrons present, as there are in gases. In solutions negative charge carriers, like positive charge carriers, are all in the form of ions.

Further, when we consider materials called *semiconductors*, which are in the limbo between conductors and nonconductors, we find that the explanation of charge transfer in these cases involves both electron motion and the motion of quasi-positive charges, that is, holes (places in the material where electrons are lacking).

Conventional Current Direction

Since a positive charge moving in one direction is mathematically equivalent to a negative charge (of the same magnitude) moving in the opposite direction, one may continue with the Franklin convention of assuming all charge carriers to be positive, the Hall effect notwithstanding. Consequently, we shall always draw current arrows in the direction a positive charge would move were it the charge carrier (see Fig. 3.1 and Fig. 3.2). This direction is commonly called the *conventional current direction*, and is used almost exclusively in the world of physics and electrical engineering, although for a time there was a move afoot to introduce electron flow as a standard convention.

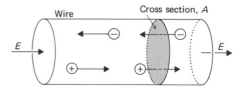

FIG. 3.1. Negative charges drifting to the left are equivalent to positive charges drifting to the right, in the direction of the electric field E. Conventional current direction is that of the drift of positive charges, that is, in the direction of E.

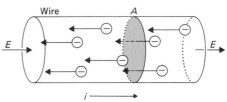

FIG. 3.2. Electric current. The charge carried by the electrons drifting through the cross section, A, of the wire per unit time is called the *current*. Note that i, indicating the current, is in the conventional direction, as though positive charges were moving.

Current and Charge

We now state in mathematical terms what is meant by electric current:

$$I = \frac{q}{t},$$

(3.1)

where I is the current, q the electric charge, and t the time involved in the drifting of the charge, q, through any given cross section of the conductor (see Fig. 3.2).

Equation (3.1) may also serve as a definition of the unit of charge, the coulomb, for we shall later (Chapter 4) independently define the unit of current, the ampere:

$$1 \text{ ampere} = \frac{1 \text{ coulomb}}{1 \text{ second}} .$$

In other words, when we say "a current of one ampere," we mean that a charge amounting to one coulomb drifts past some point in an electric circuit (that is, through a given cross section of a conductor) in one second.

In medical radiography we are mainly concerned with tube currents which are much smaller than 1 ampere, and hence the milliampere (mA) is generally employed:

$$1 \text{ mA} = 10^{-3} \text{ amp.}$$

Although Eq. (3.1) is adequate as a definition of electrical current for steady direct currents, this definition would not make sense for varying direct currents (e.g., pulsating DC) or alternating currents (AC). Why not? Because the current in these cases may have many different values at different instants, and consequently we must make a distinction between average and instantaneous values of the current. This situation is entirely analogous to the case of an x-ray technician driving a car from home to the hospital. If he/she takes the total distance from home to the hospital and divides it by the total time this trip takes, he or she obtains the average speed for the trip. But somewhere during the trip there may well be stops (zero speed) and some places along the route the speed may be up to 60 miles per hour, and along most of the route it would probably be around 30 mi/hr. Therefore, if one wants to find the instantaneous speed at a given point in the route, one cannot write

$$v \text{ (speed)} = \frac{s \text{ (total distance)}}{t \text{ (total time)}} .$$

On the contrary, one would have to look at a very, very small time interval and a correspondingly small distance. One would let the time interval approach zero. And so it is with current. The more general definition, which will hold in all cases (steady DC, varying DC, and AC), is

$$i = \lim_{\Delta t \to 0} \frac{\Delta q}{\Delta t} , \qquad (3.2)$$

where Δq refers to the amount of charge drifting past a given point in a circuit in the time element Δt, and the lower-case i is used, as is standard convention, to indicate the instantaneous value of the current. (Students who have some acquaintance with the calculus will note that i is defined by $i = dq/dt$, that is, i is the first derivative of charge with respect to time.)

We shall have occasion to refer back to this small digression on the definition of current when we deal with pulsating and alternating currents in Chapter 6. In the meantime, Eq. (3.1) is quite sufficient, since in steady DC the instantaneous current values are, from the definition of "steady," the same as the average values.

Let us try an example. Suppose that, in a case such as that shown in Fig. 3.2, a charge of 20 coulombs drifts through the cross section, A, in 2 sec. What is the current?

$$I = \frac{q}{t} = \frac{20 \text{ coul}}{2 \text{ sec}} = 10 \text{ amp.}$$

How many electrons would pass through this cross section in 1 sec to produce this current of 10 amp?

$$10 \text{ amp} = \frac{10 \text{ coul}}{\text{sec}}.$$

But the charge on one electron is about 1.6×10^{-19} coul; hence

$$10 \text{ amp} = \frac{10 \text{ coul/sec}}{1.6 \times 10^{-19} \text{ coul/electron}} = 6.3 \times 10^{19} \frac{\text{electrons}}{\text{sec}}.$$

Conductors, Semiconductors, and Insulators

Our previous discussion of the mechanism of charge transfer has dealt with the concept of electrical conduction. The best and most important electrical conductors are metals. It is a characteristic of metals that they contain free electrons: free to move through the crystal, not bound to a particular nucleus.

In the case of *insulators* (or *dielectrics*), on the other hand, there are no such free electrons. This is not to say that all the electrons in an insulator are entirely bound to their own atoms, but rather that the motion they may perform is one of simply exchanging places. This motion, of course, is of no merit in the conduction of a current.

The above is not to be construed as implying that there is some magic cutoff point which separates conductors from insulators. On the contrary, materials fall in line in a sort of conduction spectrum, from very good conductors to very good insulators; but there is no such thing as a perfect conductor (one which offers no opposition to current), nor is there a perfect insulator. If the voltage across any dielectric material is made large enough, the dielectric will break down and, even though it is basically an insulator, this material will now conduct. It is this fact which has posed many serious insulating problems in the development of high-voltage equipment associated with x-rays.

The difference in electrical-conducting properties of materials—that is, the extent of the spectrum mentioned above—is tremendous. Table 3.1 shows that the difference in electrical conductive (or resistive) properties between a good conductor, such as copper, and a good insulator, such as rubber (particularly hard rubber), is as much as 23 orders of magnitude. Or, in other words, a given piece of hard rubber poses a resistance to

Table 3.1

Approximate resistivities of certain
materials at room temperature (20°C)

Material	Resistivity, ohm-meter
Silver	1.6×10^{-8}
Copper	1.7×10^{-8}
Aluminum	2.7×10^{-8}
Tungsten	5.6×10^{-8}
Lead	2.1×10^{-7}
Constantan (Ni and Cu alloy)	4.5×10^{-7}
Carbon	3.5×10^{-5}
Salt water (sea water)	$2. \times 10^{-1}$
Germanium	$5. \times 10^{-1}$
Copper oxide (CuO)	$1. \times 10^{3}$
Distilled water	$5. \times 10^{3}$
Glass (varies widely with type of glass)	$1. \times 10^{12}$
Transformer oil	$2. \times 10^{14}$
Rubber (varies widely with type of rubber)	$1. \times 10^{15}$

electric current 10^{23} times that of a piece of copper of similar size and shape.

Our present-day electrical technology is becoming increasingly dependent on a group of materials in the middle of the conduction (or resistance) spectrum. These materials are the semiconductors, which are used in the manufacture of transistors, which in turn have to a large extent replaced vacuum radio tubes. Semiconductors are also finding more use in the construction of rectifying equipment in x-ray units. We shall discuss this aspect of semiconductor use in Chapter 6.

Some semiconductors are elements, such as germanium and selenium; others are the oxides and sulfides of certain metals, for instance, Cu_2O and PbS.

We can explain the fact that certain materials behave like conductors, others like semiconductors, and still others like insulators in quantum-mechanical terms by means of the so-called *band theory of conduction*.

In materials with a regular lattice configuration (that is, materials in which atoms are arranged in a regular and repetitive manner), there exists a grouping of permissible energy levels into so-called bands. The fact that, for an aggregation of atoms, there are energy bands instead of single energy levels, such as those which exist in a single atom, is the result of the interaction of the electric fields of the various atoms. This interaction causes modifications of the original single-atom electric potential situation. One way of looking at this idea is to realize that in a single atom the elec-

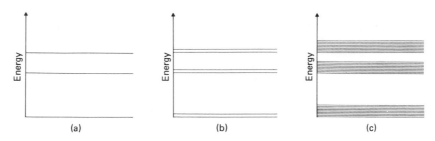

FIG. 3.3. Permissible electron energy levels: (a) a single atom; (b) two atoms together; (c) an aggregation of many atoms.

trons are restricted to a certain region due to the positive nucleus. Now when two atoms come together, some electrons might exist in the proximity of either nucleus. There is a reduction in the restriction of possible energy levels: The number of permissible energy levels is increased.

As an example, consider a system of two similar atoms. By itself (or far distant from the other atom), each atom's energy level diagram is like that of Fig. 3.3(a) or Fig. 1.6. When two atoms are brought together, the original single levels are split into two, as in Fig. 3.3(b). As more atoms are added to the system there are further splittings. That is, in a large aggregation of atoms, instead of the single energy levels of the isolated atom, we find many closely spaced levels, called *bands*, as shown in Fig. 3.3(c).

The case of metals is illustrated by the energy-band scheme of Fig. 3.4(a). According to the Pauli exclusion principle, no two electrons in a system in which the electrons are close enough to significantly interact with one another may have the same energy. Therefore the following situation holds in metals: There are in this case more electrons than can be accommodated in the lower band (or bands), and thus a partially filled band exists. Such a partially filled band is called a *conduction band* because, with the many closely spaced energy levels available to electrons, applying an electric field easily brings about the electron mobility required for conduction. This is so because the electrons are able to accept the relatively small amount of energy supplied by the electric field, since many just slightly higher permissible energy levels are yet unfilled. And conduction requires that electrons receive kinetic energy from the electric field in order that they drift through the conductor in a common direction.

The case of an insulator is shown in Fig. 3.4(b). There is normally no partially filled conduction band. In the filled band none of the electrons can gain energy from an electric field (no vacant energy levels), and hence there is no conduction. If the material absorbs sufficient energy (depending on the size of the band gap), an electron might be excited to the conduction band. But unless this relatively large excitation energy is supplied, there are no electrons free to roam about the crystal; the material is an insulator.

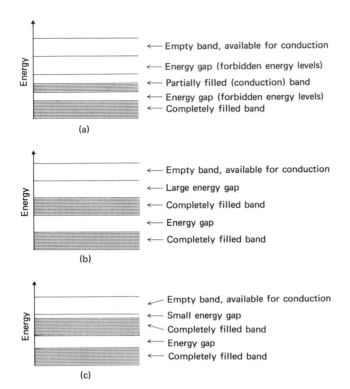

FIG. 3.4. Energy bands and gaps in (a) conductors, (b) insulators, and (c) semiconductors.

Figure 3.4(c) shows the case of a semiconductor. The narrow gap width above the filled band shows that, with a little urging (that is, absorption of energy), electrons could be shifted into a conduction band. Applying a normal electric field may suffice for this purpose.

At the risk of repeating what we said in Chapter 1, let us emphasize that in the preceding discussion the idea of energy levels provides us with a useful method of classification. The scheme does not imply that the electrons themselves literally move from one level to another; they do not, for example, jump up from the lower to the higher line in Fig. 3.3(a)! Rather they move within the lattice composed of many atoms. In a way, the concept of energy levels is a concept of categories. Let us risk an analogy: If two men go down the street, one running and one walking, we have two categories of men (the men are at different energy levels). If the walking man then runs, he moves from one category to the other. He is raised to a higher energy level, as may readily be described in terms of energy-level diagrams, such as in Fig. 3.3. But, in reality, he is running down the street.

Readers who wish to look deeper into this matter will find that they can gain some further understanding, even without recourse to the complex mathematical structure of quantum mechanics, by referring to the book by Alan Holden, listed at the end of this chapter.

3.2   **THE COMPLETE CIRCUIT**

The x-ray technician has frequent cause to speak of the x-ray circuit, the timing circuit, etc. Implicit in the term *circuit* is the notion that there is a complete, closed path for the electric charges in order that they may drift through the circuit continuously, like a runner around a looped race-track.

Circuit Symbolism

In order to facilitate an understanding of electrical circuits, people use certain conventional symbols. Let us now look at those symbols that are pertinent at the moment (see Fig. 3.5), and then add to them as we advance further in the direction of x-ray circuitry.

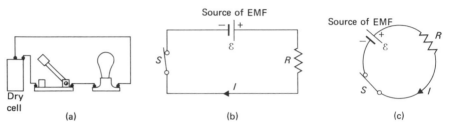

FIG. 3.5. Complete circuit, showing a resistor which has resistance R, a source of electrical energy, that is the source of EMF, which has an EMF $\mathscr{E}$, and a switch S. The direction of the current, I, is indicated by the arrow on the connecting wire. Diagram (b) is electrically equivalent to diagram (c); both are representative of the pictorial arrangement (a).

Note that the conventional way is to draw circuits in more or less rectangular configurations, as in Fig. 3.5(b), but there is no electrical significance to this. The circuit of Fig. 3.5(c) also has a switch, a resistor, and a source of EMF connected in series; it is entirely equivalent to the circuit of Fig. 3.5(b).

When we say *resistor*, we actually mean a specific circuit component designed to offer a certain resistance or opposition to charge flow, that is, current. However, the symbol employed for resistors, as shown in Fig. 3.5, is also used in a more general sense to denote any circuit resistance. For example, the same symbol might be used to indicate the presence of a light bulb, which offers a resistance to current. Sometimes we may also see such a symbol next to a source of EMF to indicate the internal resistance of the source. Such a symbol may even be employed to represent the resistance of connecting wires if this resistance is not negligible. In short, the symbol for a resistor is employed any time one wants to denote resistance to current. However, unless otherwise stated, the connecting wires represented by the single connecting lines in a circuit diagram are assumed to offer no resistance to the flow of electric charge.

Source of EMF

Let us now look a little more closely at the electrical component called the source of EMF in Fig. 3.5.

First we might look back at Fig. 2.8(c). If the two spheres in this figure were joined by a piece of copper wire, electrons would migrate from the right sphere to the left one. We would say that there is an electric current (conventional direction) from left to right. The reason this current is possible is that work was first done in charging the spheres. As soon as the charge from one sphere has neutralized the charge on the other sphere, the current stops. To keep the current going, we would have to remove electrons from the left sphere as fast as they arrive and replace electrons on the right sphere as fast as they drift off. We could do this job using a glass rod and an ebonite rod, rubbing them with the appropriate cloths, and then separating the rod and the cloth. This would require work. We would act like a source of EMF, a source of energy which is required to keep a steady flow of charge going, that is, to produce a continuous current.

A source of EMF is any device which changes other forms of energy (such as the physical energy involved in the cloth and ebonite rod case, above) into electrical energy.

In your flashlight the source of EMF is a dry cell in which chemical energy is converted into electrical energy. The source of EMF that provides the electrical energy for your x-ray unit may quite possibly be created by water falling and thus turning some electrical generators.

Although the source of EMF is a source of energy, by the actual EMF (indicated by $\mathscr{E}$), we mean the energy (or work) per unit charge done by the source. Consequently, EMF is measured in volts and, like potential difference, is sometimes called voltage. After all, the source of EMF provides the necessary potential difference (see Fig. 2.19) to permit the charges to flow, the current to exist. The EMF of your flashlight dry cell is probably 1.5 volts, this voltage being characteristic of the two commonly employed electrodes, zinc and carbon.

An Analogy

The following analogy may help to clarify some of the key electrical concepts associated with an electric circuit such as that of Fig. 3.5. The analogy, like any analogy, is bound to be somewhat imperfect. For example, students with a good physics background may note that the analogy cannot deal with capacitors. However, shortcomings notwithstanding, some insight into electrical affairs may be gained by a perusal of the mud-and-marble analogy. (The student is urged to take particular care to obtain some understanding of, and feeling for, the following electrical terms: potential difference, EMF, current, and resistance.)

You can best study the analogy by following (across pages 92 and 93) each of the headings, such as, for example, the *schematic representation* for the mud-and-marble situation followed by the *schematic representation* of the case of the electrical current. Students with considerable physics background might consider the challenge of finding any possible shortcomings in the analogy.

Schematic representation:

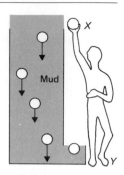

FIG. 3.6. Marble-lifter system: mud, marbles, and marble lifter.

The situation	1. The marble lifter lifts the marbles up, and drops them into the tube, containing thin mud, at point X (see Fig. 3.6). 2. The marbles ooze down through the mud from point X to point Y, giving up their energy to the mud (by heating it). 3. The marbles are lifted up again.
Particle involved	Marble
Quantitative unit of particles	Mass: A number of marbles have a total mass equal to some mass unit; for example, one kilogram.
Current	Current refers to the number of mass units passing through the cycle per unit time.
Unit of current	kilogram/second
Energy source	The marble lifter is the energy source. He does a certain amount of work per unit mass in lifting the marbles from Y to X (see Fig. 3.6).
Unit of energy	We concern ourselves not with the total work done by the marble lifter, but rather with the work per unit mass. The unit would thus be joule/kilogram.
Potential difference	The work per unit mass the marbles can do at X minus that they can do at Y may be called the difference in gravitational potential between points X and Y.
Resistance and its variation	If the mud is thin, the resistance is small, the marbles ooze down rapidly, and consequently the rate of motion of the marbles through the cycle is fast. Many marbles—that is, many mass units—pass through the mud per unit time.

Conversely, few mass units per unit time will go through the cycle if the mud is thick, that is, if the resistance is large.

[To keep this analogy more or less correct, we must assume that the number of marbles in the circuit is fixed *and* that the marble lifter lifts each marble immediately upon its arrival at the bottom.]

Schematic representation:

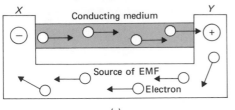
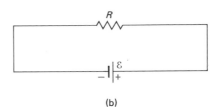

(a)   (b)

FIG. 3.7. Conducting medium, electrons, and source of EMF. (a) Electrical model corresponding to marble-lifter system. (b) Electrical circuit symbolism for (a), showing R, the
resistance of the conducting medium, and $\mathscr{E}$, the EMF.

The situation	1. The source of EMF forces electrons from positive termi-nal in source to negative terminal at X (see Fig. 3.7). 2. The electrons drift through the wire from the negative terminal X to the positive terminal Y, gaining energy from the electric field set up by the source and losing it to the con-ducting medium, that is, the wire (by heating it). 3. The electrons are again moved from the positive terminal to the negative terminal inside the source of EMF.
Particle involved	Electron
Quantitative unit of particles	Charge: A number of electrons have a total charge equal to some charge unit; for example, one coulomb.
Current	Current is defined as the number of charge units passing through the circuit per unit time. If I is the symbol for cur-rent, q for charge, and t for time, then $I = q/t$.
Unit of current	(coulomb/sec) = ampere
Energy source	The energy source is a source of EMF, such as a dry cell or a generator, for example. The source of EMF does work per unit charge in transporting the electrons from the positive terminal Y to the negative terminal X inside the source of EMF (see Fig. 3.7).
Unit of energy	The work per unit charge done by the source is called the EMF, which is symbolized by $\mathscr{E}$ or E, or sometimes V. The unit is (joule/coulomb) = volt.
Potential difference	The work per unit charge the electrons can do when at X minus that they can do when at Y defines the electrical po-tential difference between points X and Y. The symbol for potential difference is V; and since it represents work per unit charge, V is expressed in volts.
Resistance and its variation	If the electrical resistance is low, that is, if the loss of energy to the conducting medium is low, the electrons will pass through it readily. Consequently with a given energy source many charge units pass through the circuit per unit time; that is, the current is large. Conversely, the electrical cur-rent will be small if the electrical resistance is large.

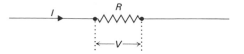

FIG. 3.8. Resistance, *R*, is defined in terms of the potential difference, *V*, across it and the current, *I*, through it.

Resistance

The last electrical term appearing in the preceding analogy bears some dwelling upon. We have already discussed conductors and insulators, and in that discussion we inferred that conductors have a low electrical resistance and insulators a very high one.

We define resistance as follows:

$$R = \frac{V}{I},$$
(3.3)

where *R* is the resistance of some circuit element to the flow of charge, *V* is the potential difference across the circuit element, and *I* is the current through it (see Fig. 3.8). This definition seems to make sense, for with a fixed potential difference, *V*, across a given circuit element, it seems reasonable to expect that if *R* were small (little opposition to current), the current, *I*, ought to be large.

Equation (3.3) may also serve to define the unit of resistance, the ohm, in this way:

$$1 \text{ ohm} = \frac{1 \text{ volt}}{1 \text{ ampere}}.$$

Thus, if a potential difference of 1 volt across the resistor in Fig. 3.8 results in a current of 1 ampere, the resistor is said to have a resistance of 1 ohm. (The Greek letter omega, Ω, is generally used as the symbol for ohm.)

Upon what does the resistance of a material, say a piece of wire, depend? First: It is quite obvious from our earlier discussion that the resistance depends on the nature of the material; that is, whether it is copper or iron, for example.

For the moment let us neglect that knowledge and simply concern ourselves with some given piece of wire. It has a certain resistance. It seems quite reasonable to assume that, if another piece of the same wire is joined to the end of the first piece to make a single longer piece, the total resistance of the two joined pieces will be greater than that of the original piece, since the second piece also is bound to have a resistance. It is plausible that

$$R \propto L,$$

where *L* is the length of the wire.

Now the current certainly depends on the availability of conduction electrons. A bigger volume of wire would furnish more conduction electrons. With a given length, *L*, of conductor, the way to increase the volume would be to increase the cross-sectional area of the wire. Thus increasing

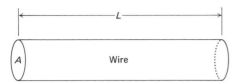

FIG. 3.9. The resistance of a wire is given by $R = \rho L/A$.

the cross-sectional area, A (see Fig. 3.9), would increase the availability of conduction electrons and thus decrease the resistance; that is,

$$R \propto \frac{1}{A}, \qquad \text{for a given } L.$$

Combining this result with our previous one, we get

$$R \propto \frac{L}{A}.$$

If we now supply the appropriate proportionality constant, we can turn the above expression into the equality

$$R = \rho \frac{L}{A}, \qquad (3.4)$$

where the proportionality constant, ρ, is (as you might guess) characteristic of the material of which the wire is made. This constant, ρ (Greek letter rho), is known as the *resistivity*. Perusal of Eq. (3.4) shows that if L is in meters, A is in m², and R is in ohms, then the unit for ρ must be the ohm-meter. Table 3.1 gives various values of ρ.

Now the resistivity has been referred to above as a constant. It is a constant, at a given temperature. That is, *the resistivity of a material varies with temperature.*

In the case of conductors, one may easily visualize how it might be that the resistivity of a material might change with temperature. Consider the conduction electrons colliding continuously with the randomly vibrating ionic cores of the conductor. The more frequent such collisions are, the more difficult the progress of the conduction electrons. Increasing the temperature of a material increases the lattice vibrations (see Section 1.3) and causes increasing distortion of the regularity of the lattice, so that electrons are progressively more involved in ionic collisions. Thus we note an increase in resistance with an increase in temperature. (The basic assumption here, of course, is that with perfect regularity in the lattice there would be no resistance. This concept is tenable according to present theory.) Although the following analogy must not be taken too literally, it is perhaps instructive: One may compare the ease of passing through a large group of soldiers lined up for parade with the frustrating difficulty of making one's way through a crowded department store, where the position and movement of people has no regularity. (We can obtain a more satisfactory explanation of this effect by resorting to a careful quantum-mechanical interpretation.)

The story with semiconductors and insulators is different. Here we must resort to our quantum-mechanical energy levels (see Fig. 3.4). An increase in temperature in these cases results in a decrease in electrical resistance. How can this be?

Let us look at semiconductors [Fig. 3.4(c)]. What conduction electrons there are certainly would suffer effects similar to those described for conductors. But there normally aren't many conduction electrons. Applying heat provides energy for some of the electrons in the filled band to "jump" the energy gap into the higher-energy vacant (conduction) band. Thus increasing the temperature of a semiconductor increases the number of conduction electrons, and thus the resistance of the material decreases.

To summarize, conductors have positive temperature coefficients; that is, their resistivities increase with temperature. Semiconductors and insulators have negative temperature coefficients: Their resistivities decrease with temperature increases. Such effects may be quite pronounced in semiconductors.

3.3   OHM'S LAW

Ohm's discovery that at any instant the ratio of the potential difference, V, between the ends of a metallic conductor and a current, I, through this conductor is a constant finds wide application in electrical matters.

Ohmic Circuit Elements

Let us express Ohm's law in terms of symbols:

$$\frac{V}{I} = \text{constant.}$$

But we have previously defined resistance, R, as the ratio V/I (Eq. 3.3). Thus we might say that if the resistance of a conductor is constant, Ohm's law applies; that is,

$$\frac{V}{I} = R, \qquad \text{where } R \text{ is a constant,}$$

is an expression of the law. More commonly, Ohm's law is stated in this form:

$$V = IR. \tag{3.5}$$

(Sometimes one finds Ohm's law also written as $E = IR$. It should be noted that the E in this case stands for voltage and not for electric field.) The units would be as previously employed in our discussion of resistance; that is, if I is in amperes and R is in ohms, then V is in volts.

If we were to make voltage and current measurements involving a metallic resistor, a tungsten light-bulb filament, for example, what would

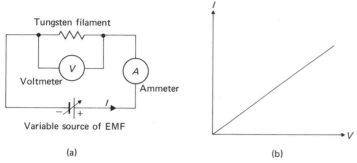

(a)   (b)

FIG. 3.10. Verification of Ohm's law. (a) Circuit for measuring voltage-current relationship. (b) Graphical representation of the results of voltage-current measurements made in a circuit such as (a).

the results yield? Consider a circuit such as that shown in Fig. 3.10(a). Assuming that we start our measurements when the filament is hot (so that no pronounced temperature-dependent changes in resistance are effected), we note that as the voltage across the filament is increased, the current through this filament increases correspondingly. For example, when the voltage is doubled the current will be doubled. (You can per- form such an experiment yourself with dry cells, a resistor, a voltmeter, and an ammeter.) Plotting the readings of the voltmeter on the abscissa and the corresponding ammeter readings on the ordinate results in a straight line, as in Fig. 3.10(b). The fact that this line is straight shows at a glance that the ratio V/I is constant; that is, R is constant. The tungsten filament is therefore said to be an *ohmic circuit element;* it obeys Ohm's law. Since this information is implied by the straight line on the graph, ohmic circuit elements are also called linear circuit elements. Many com- ponents of the x-ray circuit (e.g., conducting wires, resistors in the mA control) are ohmic or linear circuit elements.

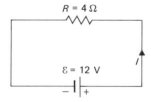

FIG. 3.11. Ohm's law: the current, I, is 3 amp.

Ohm's Law: An Example

Suppose that a 12-volt battery, having a negligible internal resistance (internal resistance is the resistance to current within the source of EMF itself), is connected to a 4-ohm resistor by wires of negligible resistance (see Fig. 3.11).

a)   What is the EMF?

$$\mathscr{E} = 12 \text{ volts.}$$

b)   What is the voltage, or voltage drop, or *IR* drop (*IR* because $V = IR$) across the resistor?

Since the battery is stated to have zero internal resistance, all the energy per unit charge (EMF) it provides is used up in the resistor; hence the voltage drop across the resistor equals the EMF; that is, $\mathscr{E} = V = 12$ volts.

c)   What is the current in the circuit?
Ohm's law: $V = IR$; hence

$$I = \frac{V}{R} = \frac{12 \text{ volts}}{4 \text{ ohms}} = 3 \text{ amp.}$$

d)   What would the, current be if a 6-volt battery were used in place of the 12-volt one?

$$I = \frac{V}{R} = \frac{6 \text{ volts}}{4 \text{ ohms}} = 1.5 \text{ amp.}$$

Nonlinear Circuit Elements

Many conductors do not follow Ohm's law. This means that their resistances are not constant, but vary with the applied voltage. A voltage-current graph of such devices does not yield a straight line as does that of Fig. 3.10(b). Rather, the graph is a curve of some kind, depending on the particular circuit element concerned. For this reason, such conductors are called nonlinear circuit elements.

Figure 3.12 shows examples of the voltage-current curves of two nonlinear or nonohmic devices. Figure 3.12(a) refers to a vacuum tube such as a radio tube and (b) is the case of a rectifier, a device which readily passes current in one direction but has a high resistance to current in the opposite direction. (Changing the polarity of the applied voltage of metallic, or ohmic, conductors simply changes the current's direction but not its magnitude.)

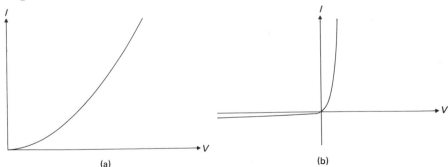

(a)   (b)

FIG. 3.12. Nonlinear circuit elements. (a) Vacuum tube. (b) Selenium rectifier.

In x-ray circuitry the valve tubes, the mA meter rectifying diodes, and the x-ray tube itself are examples of nonlinear circuit elements.

3.4 VARIOUS CIRCUITS

We shall now look at two circuit arrangements that are basically different and state some characteristics of the combinations of EMF's and resistances involved. We shall make no attempt to prove the stated results. To provide the appropriate proofs, we must refer to two laws of electricity (Kirchhoff's laws) which will not be treated in this text, although we shall actually use some of the ideas expressed in these laws as being intuitively obvious.

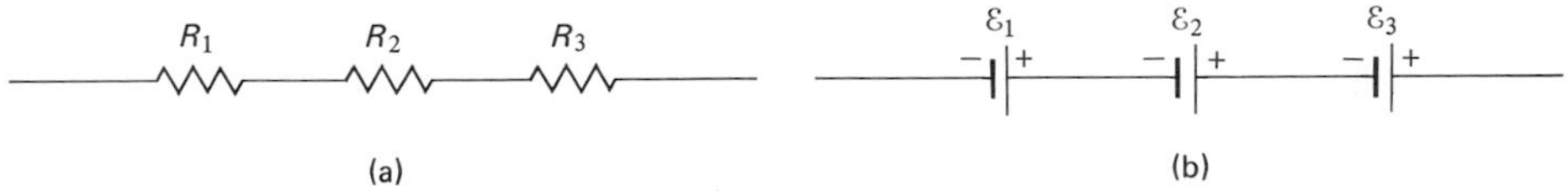

FIG. 3.13. Series connections. (a) Resistors in series: R (total) $= R_1 + R_2 + R_3$. (b) Sources of EMF in series: $\mathscr{E}$ (total) $= \mathscr{E}_1 + \mathscr{E}_2 + \mathscr{E}_3$.

Series Circuits

Circuit elements are said to be connected in series when they are connected end to end, as shown in Fig. 3.13.

The total resistance of a number of resistors connected in series equals the sum of the individual resistances:

$$R = R_1 + R_2 + R_3 + \cdots \tag{3.6}$$

The total EMF of several sources of EMF connected in series is the sum of the individual EMF's:

$$\mathscr{E} = \mathscr{E}_1 + \mathscr{E}_2 + \mathscr{E}_3 + \cdots \tag{3.7}$$

It should be noted that when EMF's are connected in series, this normally means that the positive terminal of one source is connected to the negative terminal of the next one. If two equal sources were connected in series with their like terminals joined, then, of course, the one would oppose the other and the net effect would be that $\mathscr{E} = 0$.

In the x-ray circuit the x-ray tube is connected in series with the mA meter and the source of EMF, in this case the secondary of the high-voltage transformer. Ammeters must always be connected in a circuit in series, and the mA meter is, of course, an ammeter.

Parallel Circuits

Parallel connections are "side-by-side" connections, as shown in Fig. 3.14.

A moment's reflection on our earlier discussion on resistance should make it plausible that if two resistors are in parallel, then their total resistance should be less than that of either one of them. The situation is en-

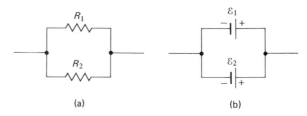

FIG. 3.14. Parallel connections. (a) Resistors in parallel:

$$\frac{1}{R \text{ (total)}} = \frac{1}{R_1} + \frac{1}{R_2}.$$

(b) Sources of EMF in parallel ($\mathscr{E}_1 = \mathscr{E}_2$): $\mathscr{E}$ (total) = $\mathscr{E}_1 = \mathscr{E}_2$.

tirely analogous to what happens to the resistance of a wire as one increases the wire's cross-sectional area. It can be shown that parallel resistances add in the following way:

$$\frac{1}{R} = \frac{1}{R_1} + \frac{1}{R_2} + \frac{1}{R_3} + \cdots \tag{3.8}$$

A simple numerical example will suffice to show that the above addition theorem gives a total or equivalent resistance which is indeed less than the resistance of the smallest of the individual resistances. Let us consider just two resistances, of 5 and 10 ohms, respectively, connected in parallel.

$$\frac{1}{R} = \frac{1}{R_1} + \frac{1}{R_2} = \frac{1}{5\,\Omega} + \frac{1}{10\,\Omega} = \frac{3}{10\,\Omega}.$$

Therefore

$$R = \frac{10\,\Omega}{3} = 3.3\,\Omega,$$

which is less than 5 Ω!

Parallel-connected EMF's (positive terminal to positive terminal, and negative to negative) are a different matter: Sources of EMF in parallel should always be of the same voltage. Their total voltage is then simply the voltage of any one of them.

Parallel circuitry appears in many places in an x-ray machine. For example, the prereading kV meter is in parallel with the source of EMF (primary of the high-voltage transformer). Voltmeters are always connected in parallel across the circuit element whose voltage is to be measured, and the kV meter is, of course, a voltmeter.

Grounding (or Earthing)

In electrical terminology, a *ground* is a conductor connected to the earth, the absolute potential of which is arbitrarily taken as zero. A common electrical symbol for a ground (or earth) is shown in Fig. 3.15.

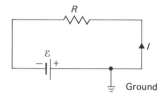

FIG. 3.15. Grounding one side of a circuit.

An important aspect of grounding relates to safety. In an x-ray machine, all the electrical components with which the radiographer may come into contact should be properly grounded. Why? Because if the x-ray technician accidentally touches uninsulated parts, or if the insulation should break down on insulated parts, the technician does not want to inadvertently become part of the electrical circuit and thus suffer a possibly dangerous electrical shock. If the equipment is properly grounded, then, since the technician is also grounded, there exists no potential difference between him and the equipment, and hence he suffers no passage of current. For this reason, for example, the mA meter, which is on the control panel, is connected with one terminal at ground potential (see Chapter 8).

A question that is sometimes raised is why no current flows into the ground in a connection such as that shown in Fig. 3.15. Recall that for a continuous charge flow (current), one needs a complete, continuous path. This is not provided if only one side of a circuit is grounded, as in Fig. 3.15.

3.5 LINE VOLTAGE DROP

We are now in a position to make an analysis which has a direct bearing on x-ray equipment. We employ Ohm's law.

Consider what happens to the voltage, say 240 volts, supplied to the x-ray equipment when an exposure is made. (We refer to Fig. 3.16, and recall that, even though copper is a good conductor, if the connecting wires ab and $a'b'$ are sufficiently long they will exhibit a measurable resistance.)

1. Voltage supply from the mains = 240 volts = $V_{ab} + V_{bb'} + V_{b'a'}$.

2. Normally, even when the mains switch of the x-ray machine is closed, there is practically no current in the circuit $abb'a'$; hence the voltmeter across bb' is as if connected across aa', that is, $V_{aa'} = V_{bb'} = 240$ volts (since $V_{ab} = V_{b'a'} = 0$).

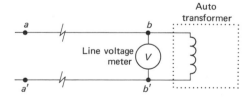

FIG. 3.16. Line voltage drop: input voltage to autotransformer, $V_{bb'}$, is less than voltage, $V_{aa'}$, supplied by the electric power company at the local distribution center.

3.   When an exposure is made, that is, when the x-ray switch is closed, the x-ray equipment draws energy from the autotransformer; a certain amount of electrical energy is being used and this results in an appreciable current through $abb'a'$. Thus V_{ab} and $V_{b'a'}$ are no longer zero. There is now a noticeable voltage drop across both ab and $b'a'$. In short, $V_{ab} = IR_{ab} \neq 0$ and $V_{b'a'} = IR_{b'a'} \neq 0$.

Therefore from (1) we see that $V_{bb'}$ (voltage across the x-ray equipment) must now be less than it was before the x-ray switch was closed. The difference between the "before" and "after" values is the line drop. Hence the actual operating voltage turns out to be less than the voltage originally set according to voltmeter V.

Let us summarize. The line voltage drop (or line drop) is the voltage drop along the connecting line to the x-ray equipment, due to the fact that the resistance of the line is not entirely negligible. This means that the equipment connected at the end of the line is operated at a voltage which is less than the supplied voltage by an amount equal to the line drop. In the case of a line (or mains) voltage of about 240 volts, the line drop may be of the order of 5 volts when a 200 mA exposure is made. This would mean that all the various x-ray machine parts get a lower voltage than they would if the input voltage remained at 240 volts. A 100-kV exposure would actually be a 98-kV exposure. The line drop increases, of course, as a greater mA is used, since then more energy is drawn by the high-voltage part of the x-ray circuit and consequently more current is required in the line to supply the extra energy. (We shall discuss the relation between energy and current in Section 3.7.)

Should further equipment be connected in parallel, the current drawn will increase, of course, because the total equipment resistance decreases in accordance with Eq. (3.8). And thus the line drop will increase. This fact suggests that it is probably wise to have not more than one piece of x-ray equipment on the same line. For example, suppose that two mobile units are plugged into the same line and operated at the same time. The voltage in the first will drop when the second is turned on, and vice versa.

Even starting the rotor of a rotating anode x-ray tube requires a large enough current to result in a small but quite measurable (for example, 1 volt) line voltage drop. Of course, once the rotor reaches its operating speed, the line voltage returns to normal (for example, 240 volts). This effect is entirely analogous to the occasional dimming of house lights when an electric appliance such as a washing machine starts up, that being the time when an electric motor draws the largest current.

From our previous discussions it is apparent that one can reduce line drop by making the line as short as possible and/or using as thick a wire as is economically and technically feasible.

Modern x-ray equipment, particularly the larger units, now has circuitry which automatically supplies the appropriate compensation in the kV meter so that the voltage indicated on the kV meter before the exposure is actually the voltage applied to the x-ray tube during the exposure.

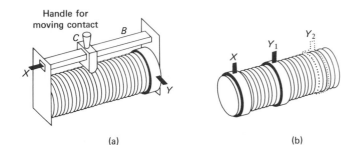
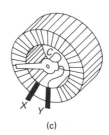

Handle for
moving contact

(a)   (b)   (c)

FIG. 3.17. Various types of rheostats. (a) If this rheostat is connected to the circuit by terminals X and Y, then sliding contact C to the right decreases the resistance, since B is a bar of copper of negligible resistance. (b) Moving connecting terminal Y_1 into position Y_2 increases the resistance. (c) If this rheostat is connected to the circuit by terminals X and Y, then rotating the contact C clockwise increases the resistance. Cases (a) and (c) are continuously variable resistors, while case (b) is an adjustable fixed resistor such as might be used to control the current in an x-ray valve tube filament circuit (shown in more detail in Fig. 3.18).

3.6 RHEOSTATS

A rheostat is a device whose electrical resistance may be adjusted. Hence such a device may be used to control the current in a circuit, in accordance with Ohm's law, simply by either increasing or decreasing the resistance of the rheostat. A common way this current control is achieved is by having a resistor made of many windings of a type of wire which, although it is essentially a conductor, has a reasonably high resistivity (e.g., constantan; see Table 3.1). This wire is wound around an insulating material, such as porcelain, and different lengths of this resistance wire can be tapped off by means of a sliding connection, as shown in Fig. 3.17(a).

Rheostats may also be made of carbon (the resistance of which varies with pressure), and electrolytic solutions. The electrical circuit symbol for continuously varying rheostats is as shown by R_3 in Fig. 3.21.

It is also possible to have various fixed taps (although these taps may, in some cases, be moved with the aid of a screwdriver to obtain various resistances), the connection to each of which then results in a different resistance [see Fig. 3.17(b)]. This type of rheostat is often used in x-ray units to establish the proper heating current for the valve tube filaments (see Chapter 7). Adjustments to these rheostats are not in the hands of the radiographer, but are carried out periodically by the x-ray equipment serviceman.

Another alternative is shown in Fig. 3.17(c). Here again, as in the case of Fig. 3.17(a), a continuous variation of resistance is possible. The main difference between (c) and (a) is that in (c) the resistance coil is wound around a circular core, and thus one may make the resistance adjustment by rotating a knob. Such rheostats also find use in x-ray equipment; in electronic timing circuits, for example.

Another way of changing circuit currents is by simply incorporating a switch in the circuit which makes connections to different resistors. In a way, such an arrangement can also be considered as a rheostat but, of course, this system allows for only discrete, stepwise changes (see Fig. 3.18a). This type of current control is employed in most large x-ray units. In order to change the mA, you actually change the heating current of the x-ray tube filament by selecting different resistors in the filament heating circuit.

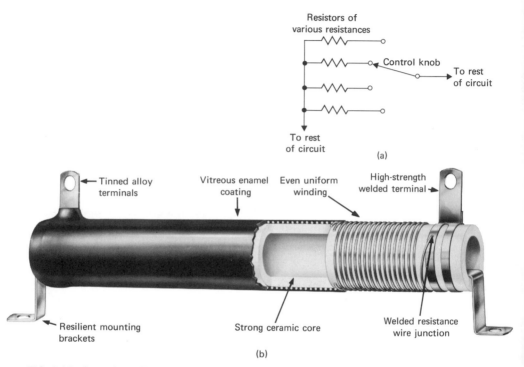

FIG. 3.18. Stepwise adjustment of circuit resistance (and hence current), such as is common in x-ray tube filament heater circuits. (a) Circuit schematic. (b) Details of the type of resistor employed.

3.7 ELECTRICAL ENERGY

Readers not conversant with the specific meanings of energy, work, and power may at this point profitably reread Section 2.3. When we talk about the electrical aspects of these concepts, we assume that the reader has a working knowledge of their specific meanings as employed in physics.

Energy

To express energy in electrical terms, we refer to Eq. (2.5) and express the work done by an electric field in transporting a charge q through a potential difference V as

$$W = Vq.$$

Now, substituting for the charge q in terms of current I, using Eq. (3.1), we get, in words

Work (or energy) = (potential difference)(current)(time);

or, in symbols:

$$W = VIt \qquad (3.9)$$

If the units for V are volts, the units for I are amperes, and the units for t are seconds, then W is in joules. We can readily see this by rewriting the right-hand side of Eq. (3.9) in terms of these units:

$$(\text{volt})(\text{amp})(\text{sec}) = \left(\frac{\text{joule}}{\text{coul}}\right)\left(\frac{\text{coul}}{\text{sec}}\right)(\text{sec}) = \text{joule}.$$

Question

How much energy is consumed by an electric heater operating at 100 volts and 15 amp for one hour?

Before we employ numbers, let us recapitulate the physical situation. Electrical energy is supplied by some source of EMF. This energy is employed to drive charges through the heater element, that is, to produce a current. The energy thus supplied, and which is used to overcome the electrical resistance of the heater element, ultimately appears in the form of heat. Now the numbers:

$$W = VIt = (100 \text{ volts}) \, (15 \text{ amp}) \, (60 \times 60 \text{ sec}) = 5.4 \times 10^6 \text{ joules.}$$

In terms of the power unit *watt*, defined in Section 2.3, we could write the above answer

$$W = 5.4 \times 10^6 \text{ watt-sec,}$$

or

$$W = \frac{5.4 \times 10^6}{3600} \text{ watt-hours,}$$

or

$$W = \frac{5.4 \times 10^6}{3600 \times 10^3} \text{ kilowatt-hours.}$$

Power

Since power is work (or energy) per unit time, we get, in electrical terms:

$$P = \frac{W}{t} = \frac{VIt}{t},$$

hence

$$P = VI, \qquad (3.10)$$

where P is in watts if V is in volts and I is in amperes. A quick unit check verifies this:

$$\text{watt} = \frac{\text{joule}}{\text{sec}} = \left(\frac{\text{joule}}{\text{coul}}\right)\left(\frac{\text{coul}}{\text{sec}}\right) = (\text{volt}) \, (\text{amp}).$$

Question

What is the power supplied to the heater discussed in the previous example?

Answer

$$P = VI = (100 \text{ volts})(15 \text{ amp}) = 1500 \text{ watts} = 1.5 \text{ kW} \qquad (\text{kW} \equiv \text{kilowatts}).$$

I^2R Losses

Note that, when we use Ohm's law, we may rewrite Eq. (3.10) in the following manner:

$$P = VI, \qquad P = (IR)I,$$
$$P = I^2R. \tag{3.11}$$

From this equation we may see that the power consumed by a circuit element, in heating it, varies as the square of the current. The energy consumption, W, during the time t would consequently be

$$W = I^2Rt. \tag{3.12}$$

This expression is, of course, simply another way of stating what we have previously expressed in Eq. (3.9).

In many cases this consumption of power, and consequently energy, is undesirable. For example, power is lost because of the heating-up of the conducting wires which carry current from the generating station to the hospital, and this is most undesirable. Since power is given by Eq. (3.11), one refers to this power loss as the I^2R loss. To reduce the I^2R loss, one provides conducting wires with a low R (e.g., copper) and, even more significant, transmits the power at the lowest feasible current.

A glance back at Eq. (3.10) shows that if the power transmitted to the user is to be kept constant and yet the current is to be low, then the voltage of the transmission system must be high: many thousands of volts. Therein lies the reason for high-voltage transmission lines. And yet in our homes and in the hospital, largely for reasons of safety, we use power at a relatively low voltage. This implies that there must be a system for stepping up and stepping down voltages. A discussion of this matter will be found in Section 6.4.

DC Circuit: A Further Example

Let us conclude this chapter by working stepwise through an example problem which touches particularly on the quantitative aspects of the present chapter. All the questions refer to the circuit of Fig. 3.19.

1. What is the total resistance of the parallel resistor group?

$$\frac{1}{R} = \frac{1}{12 \ \Omega} + \frac{1}{6 \ \Omega};$$

hence

$$R = 4 \ \Omega.$$

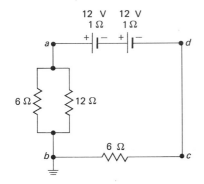

FIG. 3.19. A circuit with series and parallel connections.

2. What is the total circuit resistance, including the internal resistance of the two batteries?

$$R = 4\ \Omega + 6\ \Omega + 2\ \Omega = 12\ \Omega.$$

3. What is the total EMF?

$$\mathscr{E} = 12 \text{ volts} + 12 \text{ volts} = 24 \text{ volts}.$$

4. What is the current in the circuit?

At this point, it is worth reiterating that Ohm's law can be applied to the entire circuit, as well as to any part thereof. If we consider the total resistance, including the internal resistance of the batteries, then the total voltage to be employed is the EMF, $\mathscr{E}$.

$$I = \frac{V}{R} = \frac{24 \text{ volts}}{12\ \Omega} = 2 \text{ amp.}$$

5. What is the voltage (or voltage drop, or potential drop, or *IR* drop, or potential difference) across the parallel resistors?

$$V = IR = (2 \text{ amp})(4\ \Omega) = 8 \text{ volts.}$$

6. What is the current in each of the parallel resistors?

Consider the 6-Ω resistor:

$$I = \frac{V}{R} = \frac{8 \text{ volts}}{6\ \Omega} = 1.33 \text{ amp.}$$

Since 1.33 amp is the current in the 6-Ω resistor of the parallel group, and 2 amp go through the two parallel resistors combined, then the current through the 12-Ω resistor must be 0.67 amp. Let us check this result using Ohm's law again:

$$I = \frac{V}{R} = \frac{8 \text{ volts}}{12\ \Omega} = 0.67 \text{ amp.}$$

7. What is the *IR* drop across the resistor to the right of point *b*?

$$V = IR = (2 \text{ amp})(6 \ \Omega) = 12 \text{ volts.}$$

8. What is the internal *IR* drop across the battery combination, that is, the voltage drop due to the internal resistance of the batteries?

$$V = IR = (2 \text{ amp})(2 \ \Omega) = 4 \text{ volts.}$$

9. What is the terminal voltage of the battery combination?

By *terminal voltage* is meant the external voltage across the source of EMF when current is being drawn, as contrasted to the voltage across the source on open circuit. In the latter case the voltage is simply the EMF, $\mathscr{E}$.

$$\text{Terminal voltage} = \mathscr{E} - \text{internal } IR \text{ drop}$$

(see Question 8). Therefore

$$V = 24 \text{ volts} - 4 \text{ volts} = 20 \text{ volts.}$$

10. What is the current through the battery; through the resistor between *b* and *c*; through the parallel resistor group?

In all these cases, it is simply the current in the circuit; that is, 2 amp.

11. What is the current from *b* to the ground?

Zero.

12. What are the absolute potentials at points *a*, *b*, *c*, and *d*? Graph these voltages as a function of position in the circuit.

By definition the absolute potential at point *b* is zero. Hence, employing the results of Questions 5 and 7, we get

$$V_a = + 8 \text{ volts,}$$
$$V_b = 0,$$
$$V_c = -12 \text{ volts,}$$
$$V_d = -12 \text{ volts.}$$

For the graphical presentation, see Fig. 3.20. Note that the potential at the positive side of the battery of cells has the highest positive value. We therefore speak of the positive terminal of a source of EMF as being on the high potential side. Current in the external part of the circuit is said to be from positive to negative, or from high potential to low potential.

13. What is the power consumed in the 12-Ω resistor?

$$P = VI = (8 \text{ volts})(0.67 \text{ amp}) = 5.4 \text{ watts.}$$

14. How much heat energy is developed in the 6-Ω resistor between *b* and *c* in 5 sec?

$$W = VIt = (12 \text{ volts})(2 \text{ amp})(5 \text{ sec}) = 120 \text{ joules} \qquad \text{(or watt-sec)}$$

or

$$W = I^2Rt = (2 \text{ amp})^2(6 \ \Omega)(5 \text{ sec}) = 120 \text{ joules} \qquad \text{(or watt-sec)}$$

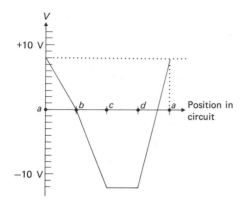

FIG. 3.20. Voltages at different points in the circuit of Fig. 3.19.

15. What is the efficiency of this combination of batteries?

By efficiency is meant the work output compared with work input. In this case, the work output per unit charge is the terminal voltage (see Question 9), and the work input is the total energy per unit charge which the chemical reactions in the batteries provide; that is, the EMF. Hence

$$\text{Efficiency} = \frac{20 \text{ volts}}{24 \text{ volts}} = 0.83 \quad \text{or } 83\%.$$

QUESTIONS

1. Determine the number of electrons required to yield one coulomb of electric charge.

2. Calculate the charge (in coulombs) passing through an x-ray tube during a one-fifth-second exposure at 100 mA.

3. Arrange the following materials in order, starting with the best conductor and ending with the best insulator: copper, silver, salt water, oil, aluminum, tungsten, glass.

4. What is the direction of electron drift (not conventional current direction): from high to low potential, or from low to high potential?

5. a) Do temperature changes affect conductors, semiconductors and insulators?
   b) State the effect, if any, on the resistivity of each of the three types of materials mentioned in (a) above.

6. In general, would you expect that elements which have negative valence would be insulators or conductors? Explain. (*Hint:* Refer to Section 1.8.)

7. State Ohm's law, and use it to solve this problem: What is the current through a 12-ohm resistance if the potential drop across it is 4.8 volts?

8. Employ the concept of potential difference to explain why two dry cells of equal EMF, when connected in parallel, provide simply an EMF equal to that of each cell alone, rather than extra voltage, that is, a higher EMF.

9. Calculate the total resistance of three resistances in parallel if they are 8 ohms, 4 ohms, and 24 ohms, respectively.

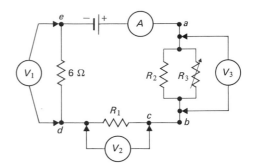

FIG. 3.21. DC circuit.

10. The following questions refer to Fig. 3.21. The voltmeter V_1 reads 12 volts, V_2 reads 4 volts, and the total resistance of the two parallel resistors is 4 ohms.

a)   What assumption are you making about the meters?
b)   What assumption are you making about the source of EMF?
c)   What assumption are you making about the connecting wires?
d)   Is the conventional current direction clockwise or counterclockwise?
e)   How large is the EMF?
f)   How large is the resistance of the resistor R_1?
g)   What is the reading of the ammeter A?
h)   What is the reading of the voltmeter V_3?
i)   If the resistor R_2 has a resistance of 8 ohms, what is the resistance set on the rheostat R_3?
j)   What is the current through R_3?
k)   What is the potential difference between points a and b?
l)   Which point, a or b, is at the higher potential?
m) What is the potential (absolute potential) of point d if point e is grounded?
n)   What is the potential difference between points c and b?
o)   What would happen to the total current in the circuit if the rheostat R_3 were turned to a lower resistance?
p)   What could be said about the respective currents through R_2 and R_3 in the case of (o) above?
q)   What would you do to "short circuit" this circuit?
r)   What danger is inherent in a "short circuit"?
s)   On the basis of the assumptions you made, what would happen to the total current in the circuit if voltmeter V_2 were removed?
t)   What would happen to the total current if the rheostat were disconnected?
u)   What would happen to the total circuit current if a source of EMF identical to the one in Fig. 3.21 were placed in a series connection with it, with the positive terminal of one connected to the negative terminal of the other?
v)   What would happen to the total circuit current if a source of EMF such as in (u) above were in series as in (u), but the positive terminal of one were connected to the positive terminal of the other?
w) What would happen to the total circuit current if a source of EMF identical to the one in Fig. 3.21 were added in a standard parallel connection to the original one (that is, positive terminal of one to positive terminal of the other, etc.)?

x) Does the answer to Question (w) above depend on the assumption stated in Question (b) above? Explain.

y) Is there any significance in the fact that the voltmeter V_1 is connected with wires at an angle and V_2 is connected with wires in a rectilinear configuration?

11. Sketch a circuit of a resistor connected to a source of EMF and include the proper meters required to experimentally determine the resistance of the resistor.

12. a) State what is meant by "line voltage drop."

b) Explain what causes this effect.

c) Assume for the purpose of this question that the power supply to the x-ray unit is steady DC. It is observed that before making an exposure the input voltage to the x-ray unit is 240 volts, but this voltage drops to 230 volts during an exposure that consumes 4.6 kilowatts. Calculate the resistance of the conducting cables between the x-ray unit and the power sourse. [Note: Students might return to this problem after studying alternating currents. One could drop the assumption of the first sentence, provided that one employs RMS values of current and voltage.]

13. Describe the construction and working principle of a rheostat.

14. a) Write an expression for the power consumed in an electric circuit as a function of the current and the circuit's resistance, and use the expression to find the power, in watts, if there is a current of 5 amperes and the circuit resistance is 10 ohms.

b) How much energy (in joules) is received by the circuit resistance if the current is on for five minutes?

SUGGESTED READING

EFRON, ALEXANDER, *Magnetic and Electrical Fundamentals.* New York: John F. Rider Publisher, Inc., 1959. For beginning physics students. Chapter 5 may provide useful additional examples relating to DC circuits.

HALLIDAY, DAVID, and ROBERT RESNICK, *Physics for Students of Science and Engineering.* New York: John Wiley, 1962 (second edition). Chapter 32 is for the more advanced student seeking examples in DC circuits.

HOLDEN, ALAN, *The Nature of Solids.* New York: Columbia University Press, 1965. A nonmathematical treatment of the concepts of modern physics as applied to the behavior of solids. Chapter XIII (Electrical Conduction) and Chapter XIV (Semiconductors) are excellent presentations of electrical conduction in quantum-mechanical terms. Many diagrams and exceedingly lucid explanations.

WHITE, HARVEY E., *Modern College Physics.* Princeton, N.J.: D. Van Nostrand, 1966 (fifth edition). Chapters 27 and 28 can well be handled by a beginning student wishing a little more practice with Ohm's law and a look at Kirchhoff's laws.

CHAPTER 4

Magnetism

The close relationship between this chapter and Chapter 3 will in due course become obvious. The key to this chapter lies in the fact that magnetism is more or less a manifestation of electrical charges in motion. A Danish physicist, who reputedly was once rejected for the University of Copenhagen's chair in physics because he was considered more a philosopher than a scientist, first put his fingers on this key. During the course of a lecture to a small group of advanced students in the spring of 1820, Hans Christian Oersted (1777–1851) observed a deflection of a magnetic compass needle when he happened to bring a wire carrying an electric current near it. According to some authorities, this was the only instance in the known history of science of a profound discovery having been made during a lecture demonstration.

Oersted's discovery first revealed the relationship between magnetism and electricity. But the credit for establishing a quantitative foundation for a theory which yields the equivalence of magnets with electrical circuits carrying currents, as far as magnetic effects are concerned, goes to Ampère, a French contemporary of Oersted. We first met Ampère in the previous chapter, where his name was applied to the unit for electric currents. Ampère's law, which states the quantitative relationship between current and magnetic field, along with an extension of this law as introduced by Maxwell (about whom we'll say a little more later), is one of the basic equations of electromagnetic theory.

Actually, the most complicated of magnetic phenomena—that is, the magnet, or more precisely the permanent magnet—has been around for a long time; but there was no understanding of the phenomenon such as we have today.

Certainly magnetite, or lodestone, a kind of rock which is naturally magnetic, was known to the Greeks in the seventh century B.C. It has not been definitely established how much earlier than this the properties of lodestone were known to man.

The first European treatise on magnetic behavior was also probably the first formally reported piece of experimental work in physics in Europe. The author of this work, which was carried out in the thirteenth century, was Pierre Pelerin de Maricourt, usually known by the name Petrus Peregrinus. Included in the discourse of Peregrinus were several suggestions regarding improvements to the mariner's compass, which at that time employed lodestone.

At this point we refer back to Dr. Gilbert, Queen Elizabeth's court physician, whose publication, *de Magnete* (1600) was cited in Chapter 2. Among other points that Gilbert made, he deduced that the earth itself was an immense permanent magnet.

Our present-day understanding of the magnetic behavior of strongly magnetic materials, such as iron, culminated in the domain theory of magnetism (which theory is heavily indebted to quantum mechanics) developed in the first half of the twentieth century. This theory, like most of modern physics, owes much to many contributors. If one name is to be singled out in connection with this theory of ferromagnetism, it is probably that of the French physicist, Pierre Weiss (1865–1940), who proposed the concept of magnetic domains in 1907.

Studying the symmetry of the interaction between a current and a magnet led Michael Faraday to the discovery of the effect which constitutes the basis of many electrical measuring instruments and the electric motor. And this within a year of Oersted's report of electromagnetism!

Finally, somewhere in this book, we should mention the achievements of James Clerk Maxwell (1831–1879). Perhaps now is the time, although reference to Maxwell fits in anywhere in a discussion of electricity, magnetism, and electromagnetic radiations, such as light and x-rays. Why? Because, almost magically, he synthesized all that was known about electricity, magnetism, and optics in his day in four succinct equations. These Maxwell equations are the hub of classical electromagnetic theory as employed today. Inherent in Maxwell's electromagnetic theory were predictions which, on purely theoretical grounds, ultimately led, among other things, to radio communication.

4.1 ELECTRIC CURRENTS AND MAGNETISM

Magnetic Field

Assuming that the reader is familiar with some of the elementary aspects of magnetism, we now define a magnetic field in qualitative terms entirely analogous to the ones we used to treat the electric field E in Chapter 2. By a magnetic field B we mean a region in space in which a magnet, such as an ordinary compass needle, experiences a force. The direction of B is the direction in which the north pole of a compass needle points. Since like magnetic poles repel and unlike poles attract, we arrive at the conclusion that the direction of the magnetic field of the earth is more or less from the earth's south pole to its north pole, and that actually the earth's north pole is a magnetic south pole! (See Fig. 4.1.)

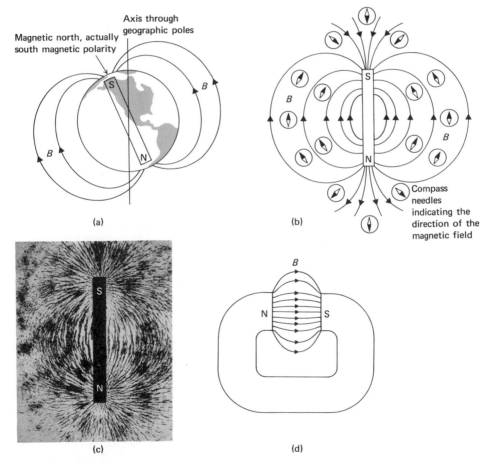

FIG. 4.1. Various types of magnetic fields. (a) Approximation of earth's magnetic field. (b) A bar magnet, showing how compass needles may be used to determine the direction of B. (c) Magnetic field of a bar magnet, indicated by iron filings on a glass plate. (d) The magnetic field in the gap of a horseshoe-type magnet.

The magnetic field, like the electric field, may be schematically represented by a series of lines, the direction of which indicates the direction of B, and how close the lines are together is representative of the strength of B. The closer these magnetic lines of force (or magnetic flux lines), the stronger the magnetic field B the lines purport to represent.

Figure 4.1(b, c, d) shows, in two of their three dimensions, some magnetic fields associated with common magnets. No doubt many readers, sometime during their earlier schooling, have seen how one may plot such magnetic fields: Some iron filings sprinkled on a glass plate over a bar magnet yield the result shown in Fig. 4.1(c). The reason these iron filings line up this way is that, in the presence of the magnetic field due to the magnet, the filings themselves become temporary magnets and thus line up along the direction of B like little compass needles.

We said earlier that the stronger the magnetic field B, the closer together the magnetic flux lines used to represent B. Thus B may be expressed as a density of these flux lines; B is therefore sometimes also referred to as the *magnetic flux density,* as well as the *magnetic induction,* or the *magnetic field intensity,* or simply the *magnetic field.* Suppose now that we wanted a measure, not of the magnetic flux density, but of the total magnetic flux in a given region (this concept will be important in the next chapter on induced EMF). What we are now talking about is schematically represented by the total number of lines of magnetic flux. Mathematically we could arrive at this quantity by multiplying the value of B by the area, perpendicular to B, through which B acts; that is,

$$\Phi = B \perp A \qquad (4.1)$$

where Φ is the magnetic flux, B is the flux density, and A is the total area having a flux density of B. The $\perp$ sign between B and A indicates that the surface A is perpendicular to the direction of B (see Fig. 4.2). The units (mks system) of the quantities in Eq. (4.1) are: B in weber/m², A in m², Φ in webers (the weber will be defined in terms of force, charge, and velocity in Section 4.3). We can see then that actually one could conceive a certain

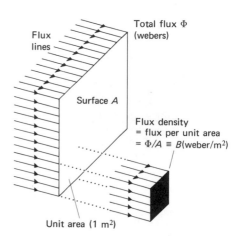

FIG. 4.2. The relation between total magnetic flux Φ and the flux density B.

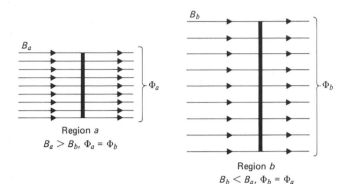

FIG. 4.3. Two regions with the same total number of magnetic flux lines, i.e., same Φ, but with different values of B.

number of flux lines as being equivalent to a weber and then so many lines per meter² would be equivalent to weber/m², the unit for B. Not infrequently magnetic fields, or flux densities, are also quoted in a much smaller unit, the *gauss*, where 1 weber/m² = 10^4 gauss. To clarify this distinction between Φ and B, refer to Fig. 4.3. Here we have two different B's shown, but the Φ in each case is the same.

Perhaps some numbers related to magnetic fields encountered in real life might be of interest. The earth's magnetic field has a value of B of approximately 5×10^{-5} weber/m² (or 0.5 gauss). An ordinary six-inch bar magnet such as is often used in school would have $B \approx 0.02$ weber/m² near one end. A small horseshoe magnet may have $B \approx 0.15$ W/m² in the gap. A so-called giant magnet used in ophthalmology to remove iron splinters from eyes may have $B \approx 0.5$ W/m², while the large magnet of a cyclotron might have $B = 1.8$ W/m². This last magnetic field is large enough so that, if a worker were holding an iron tool, such as a heavy wrench, in his hand near the magnet and someone inadvertently turned the energizing current of the magnet on, the unfortunate worker would be likely to appear in an x-ray department with a crushed hand to be radiographed.

Oersted's Discovery

Employing the concept of the magnetic field B, we can state Oersted's discovery as follows: With an electric current there is associated a magnetic field. (See Fig. 4.4)

The magnitude and direction of the magnetic field associated with a current depend on the magnitude and direction of the current. In the case of a long straight cylindrical wire, the magnetic field is cylindrically symmetrical, with the wire as a central axis. The strength of B varies inversely as the distance from the center of the wire (see Fig. 4.4). Now, it seems intuitively obvious that B should be less as one gets farther from the wire. Most people have seen that B gets less the farther one gets from an ordinary bar magnet. But the variation of B with the distance from the source of the

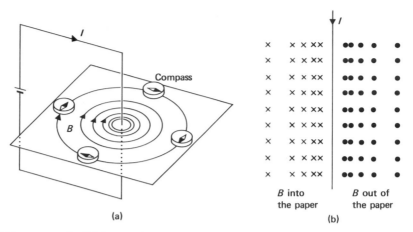

FIG. 4.4. (a) The magnetic field around a current-carrying conductor. The value of B is greater closer to the wire. (b) A representation of a similar field, looking perpendicularly at the upright wire.

magnetic field, although it is always one of decrease, is not always a simple reciprocal relationship. Rather, the variation depends on the geometry of the electric current causing B. Much more simple is the effect of the current on B: The larger the value of I, the larger B; a simple direct relationship.

A Right-Hand Rule

In both Chapters 2 and 3, we have pointed out that convention in the electrical world bases definitions and rules on what the relevant effects are with positive charges. Keeping in mind that we therefore speak of conventional current direction, or positive charge motion, real or imaginary, we can evolve a number of right-hand rules. Were we to consider electron flow, as a few elementary physics texts do, then the right-hand rules would have to be translated into left-hand rules.

The right-hand rule that concerns us here is the one which yields the direction of the magnetic field B associated with a current-carrying wire. Grasp the wire in the right hand with the thumb in the direction of the current I, and then the fingers will point in the direction of B. See Fig. 4.5, and for practice see also whether the rule checks with Figs. 4.4, 4.6, and 4.11. In the case of the latter figure, note that the indicated motion is that of an electron; that is, a negative charge.

FIG. 4.5. The right-hand rule employed to determine the direction of B associated with I in a current-carrying wire.

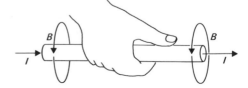

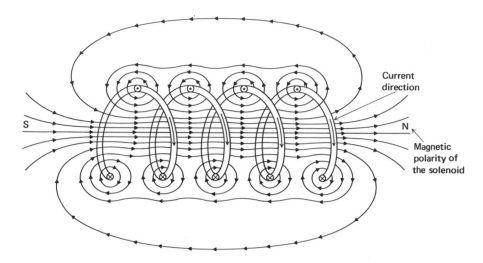

FIG. 4.6. Solenoid, with windings abnormally extended to permit indication of the various flux lines, that is, B in various places.

Electromagnets

Since the magnetic field intensity B produced by a current I depends on the current, two avenues for increasing B suggest themselves. One is simply to increase I in the wire. The other is not to increase I itself but to place two or more wires, each carrying the same I, adjacent to one another. In other words, to use a coil of wire. Such a coil is called a solenoid. Looking at the solenoid in Fig. 4.6 and applying the right-hand rule to each turn, one can see that the magnetic fields of adjacent turns in a solenoid of finite length tend to cancel each other between the turns, pronouncedly enhance each other through the inside of the cylindrical coil, and to some extent enhance each other along the outside length of the solenoid. In the limit of the individual solenoid wire turns (or loops, or windings) being very close together, the solenoid behaves rather like a cylindrical sheet of current.

Now look at the direction of the net magnetic field of our solenoid. It looks much like the magnetic field associated with a cylindrical magnet, or even a bar magnet. And where are the north and south poles? We have actually already located them by deducing the direction of the net magnetic field by means of employing our first right-hand rule to each solenoid turn. At this point, we suggest a second right-hand rule, which is merely a short cut for the case of a solenoid. Grasp the solenoid in the right hand with the fingers in the direction of the current and then the thumb points in the direction of the north pole of the "solenoid magnet" (see Fig. 4.7).

We reiterate then that when current is passed through a solenoid there is set up a magnetic field similar to that of a bar magnet. One can enhance this magnetic effect in actual practice by winding the wire around a core made of some ferromagnetic material such as iron. Without this

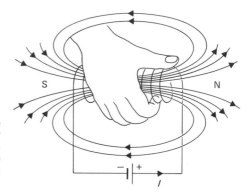

FIG. 4.7. Magnetic field of a solenoid. The right-hand rule indicates the north polarity of the solenoid. The relatively slight magnetic field due to the wires connecting the solenoid to the source of EMF has been neglected.

iron core there is, of course, a magnetic field B as soon as the solenoid current is turned on. However, there is additional magnetic flux when a ferromagnetic core is present, due to the atomic currents around individual nuclei of the core, or more precisely, due to the alignment of the magnetic moments of the electrons. One might say that the total magnetic field intensity at any point in space is the sum of two contributors: the flux density carried by empty space (air is almost like vacuum with respect to magnetic effects); and the flux density carried by the magnetized matter (iron in this case). Introduction of a suitable ferromagnetic core may increase the value of B within the solenoid by a factor of many thousands. In the language of physics, one says that the magnetic permeability of a ferromagnetic material is many thousand times greater than the permeability of air. Some explanation of this ferromagnetic behavior follows in Section 4.2.

In summary: Electromagnets may be made by winding several turns of an insulated conducting wire around a ferromagnetic core. The strength of the electromagnet will depend on the number of turns per unit length of core, the current, and the nature of the core.

Before we go on to look at some of the applications of electromagnets, we should perhaps point out that just as there are all kinds of shapes possible for ordinary permanent magnets, such as bar magnets, horseshoe magnets, disk magnets, etc., it is also possible to have all kinds of shapes of electromagnets simply by shaping the core appropriately. The windings do not need to cover all the core, since it is characteristic of a ferromagnetic core that, because of its high magnetic permeability relative to air, the magnetic flux lines—that is, the magnetic field—follow the shape of the core. Figure 4.8 shows a ring magnet of the electromagnetic type.

Electromagnetic Circuit Breakers and Relays

There is a considerable variety in the uses to which electromagnets may be put in the field of medicine. As we said earlier, one example of the use of a special electromagnet is to remove ferromagnetic metal splinters from

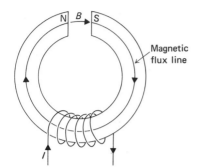

FIG. 4.8. Ring magnet, showing by means of a single representative magnetic flux line how the magnetic field produced by the windings is shaped by the ferromagnetic core.

eyes. In the x-ray department, electromagnets are used in various parts of the x-ray machine circuitry.

Consider, for instance, the protection required against excessive surges of currents from the mains through the autotransformer, which is the first main component of the x-ray unit relative to the incoming power supply. What is required here is essentially the same as what is required in the home. Somewhere between the lights and the incoming wires from the electrical company supplying the power is a panel containing either fuses or circuit breakers, the latter usually of the electromagnetic type. Figure 4.9 shows the principle of operation of an electromagnetic circuit breaker. As we pointed out earlier, the basic rationale is that the larger the current I, the stronger the associated magnetic field B.

When the current I becomes larger than the value wanted in the circuit, then the electromagnet becomes sufficiently strong to attract the latch. Thus the arm, under spring action, separates the contact points and thereby opens the circuit. To reset the breaker—that is, to close the circuit —there is usually a trigger of insulated material which can be used to push the arm back into place, closing the contacts.

The type of circuit breaker we have just described is an *overload circuit breaker,* in that it protects electrical circuits against excessive currents. It is also possible to design an electromagnetic circuit breaker

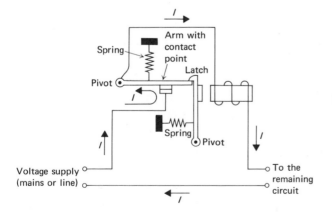

FIG. 4.9. Overload circuit breaker.

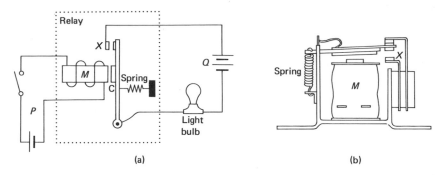

FIG. 4.10. Electromagnetic relay. (a) Schematic of a simple relay. (b) A commercially produced relay.

which would open the circuit if the current dropped below a certain prescribed value. Such *underload circuit breakers* are used in conjunction with relays, such as we shall discuss below, to trigger fire-alarm systems.

Using an electromagnetic device to open and close switches serves another exceedingly useful purpose: Circuitry becomes possible in which current changes in one circuit can be used to open and close the switch in a second, entirely separate, circuit. Such a device is called an *electromagnetic relay*.

Electromagnetic relays are found in x-ray circuits in a number of places: for example, the exposure switch, the tube selector for radiography or fluoroscopy, the meter selector for mA or mAs, and the tube overload breaker. The latter relay is designed to open the low-voltage primary circuit when the tube current in the high-voltage secondary circuit approaches a value high enough to damage the x-ray tube.

When we look at Fig. 4.10(a), we see how an electromagnetic relay works. When the switch in circuit P is closed, the electromagnet M is energized; thereupon the piece of ferromagnetic material C on the switching arm is moved to the left sufficiently far to close the contacts at X. This completes circuit Q and the light goes on. That is, by closing circuit P we are able to close circuit Q. In x-ray circuitry this particular setup is approximated by the exposure switch circuit (circuit P) and the primary circuit of the high-voltage transformer (circuit Q). Students may wish to relate this situation even more closely to the actual x-ray circuitry after studying Chapter 8. It will then be apparent that the EMF in circuit Q is the voltage supplied by the autotransformer and the load represented in Fig. 4.10(a) by the light bulb is the load on the primary of the high-voltage transformer. This particular use of relays permits the operator to control circuits with fairly high voltages and currents by manipulating simple low-voltage circuitry.

What we have shown in Fig. 4.10(a) is, of course, an oversimplification with respect to the present state of technological sophistication. But the principles employed are quite correct, and the relay as shown really would work. Figure 4.10(b) shows what a commercially produced electromagnetic relay might look like.

4.2 THE NATURE OF MAGNETIC MATERIALS

Atoms, Electricity, and Magnetism

To explain the various magnetic behaviors of different materials, it is useful to employ the Bohr concept of the atom. Visualizing electrons revolving about a nucleus as well as rotating about their own axes suggests that, quite in accord with Oersted's observations, one might expect to find an atomic magnetic effect. After all, charges in motion result in an associated magnetic field. There are, indeed, two such magnetic effects: one due to orbital motion, and one due to spin. Both effects are usually expressed in terms of quantities, the precise definitions of which serve no real purpose in our qualitative analysis. However, we should know a little about these quantities, and certainly their names: *orbital magnetic moment* and *spin magnetic moment*.

These quantities, the magnetic moments, may be related to the magnetic intensity B with which we are already familiar; roughly we can say that these magnetic moments, in direction and magnitude, indicate the nature of B. We may perhaps get a little more definite idea of what is implied by the term magnetic moment by considering a familiar object such as a small compass needle. Let us characterize the magnetic behavior of this compass needle by introducing a quantity, having both a magnitude and a specified direction. This quantity we shall call the magnetic moment of the compass needle, illustrated by the arrow in Fig. 4.11(a). Then we can say that, in an externally applied magnetic field B, there is a torque exerted by B on the magnetic moment of the compass needle which tends to line up the magnetic moment (and hence the compass needle) with B. Also the magnetic moment itself sets up at all points in space a magnetic field similar to that indicated by the magnetic flux lines shown in Fig. 4.1(c).

Now it can be shown that the magnetic effects of a current loop are correctly given by associating with it a magnetic moment as described above, where the direction of the magnetic moment is perpendicular to the loop, as is shown in Fig. 4.11(b). The overall magnetic behavior of a given material is thus conceived as being the result of the magnitudes and directions of all the various electron orbital and spin magnetic moments (see Fig. 4.11).

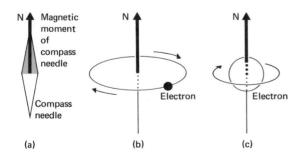

FIG. 4.11. Magnetic moments. The heavy arrows indicate their directions. (a) Compass needle magnetic moment. (b) Orbital magnetic moment of an electron. (c) Spin magnetic moment of an electron.

In any one atom these electron magnetic moments may cancel each other (oppositely directed and of equal magnitude) or not cancel each other. Hence each atom may behave like a magnet or not. In iron, for example, the electron swarm, or cloud, of the atom has a net magnetic moment. The iron atom behaves like a magnet. In a way, then, we may think of a bar of iron as consisting of many, many individual atomic magnets. Bismuth, on the other hand, has nonmagnetic atoms because the net magnetic moment of each bismuth atom is zero. Bismuth is said to be diamagnetic.

Domain Theory

Materials which are thought to have many individual atomic magnets do not necessarily exhibit strong magnetic behavior. An example is sodium. If such materials are only weakly attracted by magnets, they are said to be *paramagnetic*.

Of most interest to us are the materials which are strongly attracted by magnets, in which large values of B can be achieved by the application of an external magnetic field; in other words, those materials which have a high magnetic permeability. These materials, known as *ferromagnetic materials*, may not have net atomic magnetic moments any greater than those of paramagnetic materials. However, in these ferromagnetic materials there exists a local alignment of magnetic moments even in the absence of an externally applied magnetic field. This characteristically ferromagnetic effect is known as *spontaneous magnetization*. Since thermal agitation tends to result in random orientation of atoms, it is not surprising to find that with increasing temperature the pronounced magnetic effect of ferromagnetic materials decreases.

This grouping of atoms with similarly aligned magnetic moments is known as a *domain*, shown in Fig. 4.12. There may be about 10^{15} atoms in a domain. Although many of the atomic magnetic moments within each domain are aligned, the net effect is still zero in an unmagnetized piece of ferromagnetic material because of the random alignment of the domains' magnetization. However, when such a material is subjected to an exter-

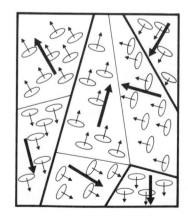

FIG. 4.12. Representation of the domains in a polycrystalline ferromagnetic material. The heavy lines represent crystal boundaries, while the lighter ones are magnetic domain boundaries. In each domain the atomic current loops indicate alignment of magnetic moments within the domain. The heavy arrows indicate the net magnetic moment of the respective domains.

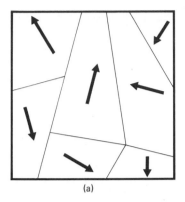
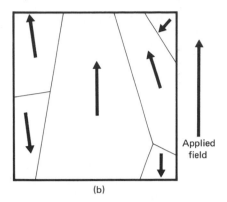

(a)

(b)

Applied
field

FIG. 4.13. Magnetization of a ferromagnetic specimen. Domain walls shift and domains rotate to produce alignment with the applied field. If the applied field is sufficiently strong, these processes continue until complete alignment is achieved. The material is then magnetically saturated. (a) Unmagnetized. (b) Magnetized, but not to saturation.

nally applied magnetic field, the domain walls move, to the extent that those domains aligned with the applied field grow at the expense of the other domains; and some unaligned domains may actually be caused to rotate, lining up with the applied field. Thus the end result is a considerable enhancement of the applied magnetic field (see Fig. 4.13). We say that the material is strongly magnetic. The most important of the strongly magnetic, or ferromagnetic materials, iron, was known for this magnetic property probably in prehistoric times. However, ferromagnetism being a relatively rare property, thousands of years passed before G. Brandt in 1733 uncovered this property on the part of another element, cobalt. Although iron, cobalt, nickel, gadolinium, terbium, dysprosium and holmium are the ferromagnetic elements, many alloys with ferromagnetic properties are now also known. Some of these alloys, strangely enough, contain no ferromagnetic elements.

To conclude our brief excursion into the realm of modern magnetic theory, let us point out some of the observed phenomena for which the present theory can give account. First of all, breaking a magnet, laterally, into two parts yields two magnets. Breaking one of these parts again yields two more still smaller magnets, and so on. Presumably one could carry this fragmentation on down to the atomic level and still end up with magnets, each a dipole; that is, each displaying a north-and-south polarity. In fact, to date no one has been able to isolate a single magnetic pole; the present electrical theory of magnetism is in this respect upheld. (In fact there are strong reasons to believe that magnetic monopoles do not exist.) Then there are the following facts: One can magnetize a piece of iron by stroking it with a magnet, which really just means placing all parts of it in the strongest part of a magnet's field. Magnetization in the presence of a field can be helped by mechanical agitation to aid alignment. Conversely, one can demagnetize a specimen by agitating it by thermal or mechanical means in the absence of an external field. These observations all fit the theory.

The above points must not, of course, be taken as a proof that the theory is the absolute truth. In fact, this theory of ferromagnetism is, in essence, one that involves crystalline structures. Thus we may have difficulty in accommodating the "glassy," noncrystalline magnet recently produced at the California Institute of Technology. Investigators there apparently were able to produce paper-thin samples of an iron-rich alloy with a microscopic structure more like glass or a liquid, yet which had strong ferromagnetic properties.

In any event, any set of observations cannot so much prove a theory as support the theory by not disproving it. That is, after all, possibly the best that science can do! Perhaps one should not even delve into the matter of absolute truth. With respect to a theory, probably the most sensible question is whether or not it is successful and at the same time reasonably succinct.

Magnetic Materials

Ferromagnetic materials may be separated into two main classes according to characteristics which lend themselves to two distinct applications. On the one hand, there are the magnetically "soft" materials, which are of little use in making permanent magnets, and, on the other hand, there are the magnetically "hard" materials, which make good permanent magnets.

A magnetically "soft" material is characterized by the fact that, although it is readily magnetized when an external field is applied, its own magnetic field collapses as soon as the externally applied field is removed, thus leaving the material in much (but not quite) the same magnetic state it was in before (see Fig. 4.14). These materials are known as *magnetic-core materials* and, as their name implies, they find extensive use as core materials for electromagnets and transformers. In both these applications the core material should greatly enhance the magnetic effect of a current-carrying coil, but also the effect of the core should closely follow the magnetic field applied via the electric current. After all, an electromagnetic relay, for example, would be of little use if it only worked once because the core had become permanently magnetized when the circuit was first closed. Examples of good core materials are high-purity iron and various alloys, such as Permalloy and Mumetal.

Magnetically "hard" materials are known as *permanent-magnet materials*. They are harder to magnetize than core materials but, on the other hand, they retain a considerable residual magnetism after the externally applied magnetizing field has been removed (see Fig. 4.14). We have already encountered a permanent-magnet material of sorts—an iron oxide, Fe_3O_4, known as lodestone—which sparked early investigations of magnetism. Modern steels and alloys are, of course, much more effective for producing permanent magnets. Examples are certain chromium or tungsten steels, and alloys such as Alnico.

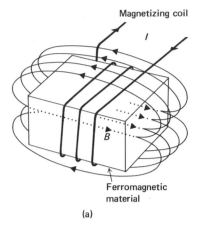

Magnetizing coil

(a)

Ferromagnetic
material

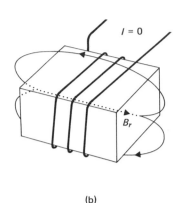

(b)

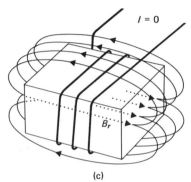

(c)

FIG. 4.14. The two classes of ferromagnetic materials. (a) Current in the magnetizing coil induces a magnetic flux density B in the material. (b) Magnetic core materials. When magnetizing current stops, that is, when $I = 0$, the magnetic field collapses, leaving very small residual flux density, or retentivity, B_r. The material is only very slightly magnetized. (c) Permanent magnet material. When $I = 0$, there remains a large residual flux density, B_r. The material is a strong magnet. Its retentivity is high.

Making a Magnet

If you have never made a magnet you might try the following experiment to see that our theoretical discussion is actually borne out in practice. We want to make a permanent magnet, so we choose a magnetically hard material like a steel darning needle. (If we were going to make an electromagnet—that is, one which works only when the magnetizing current is on—we would choose a "softer" material, such as an ordinary nail.) Check to see that the needle is not already magnetized by testing it with iron filings, tacks, or paper clips. Assuming that the needle is not magnetized, now wrap a few turns, say about 20, of insulated copper wire, such as used in the electric bell circuits of homes, around the needle. Fasten one end of the wire (with insulation removed!) to a dry cell, as shown in Fig. 4.15. Now momentarily connect the other end of the wire to the other dry-cell terminal, and you have made yourself a magnet: the needle. If you want to squeeze more physics out of this simple experiment, you might use the appropriate right-hand rule to predict which is the north end of the needle and then test this conclusion by using an ordinary pocket compass.

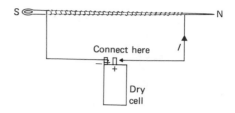

FIG. 4.15. Magnetizing a darning needle.

Now let us retrace our steps in order to look more closely at what happens during the course of such an experiment. We are going to introduce the necessary measuring devices to measure the magnetic field strength of the darning needle as the magnetizing current through the copper wire is increased from zero to its maximum value by means of some variable souce of EMF. In practice, one usually performs such experiments with the ferromagnetic material in the shape of a ring, for reasons which need not concern us now; no difference in physical principles is involved.

Figure 4.16 shows the observed relationship between the magnetizing current I on the abscissa and the magnetic field strength B of the darning needle on the ordinate. First of all, we see that the needle is originally unmagnetized and that, as the magnetizing current and hence the externally applied magnetic field increases, the magnetic field of the needle grows larger. Note that finally it appears that further increases in the externally applied magnetization yield no further increase in the magnetic effect of the needle. At this stage, all the domains in the needle have become aligned with the externally applied field; the needle is as magnetized as it can become. This value for the B of the needle is indicated on the graph by B_s, and is called the *magnetic saturation*.

Now, since our discussion arose out of the making of a permanent magnet, the really important point to note is that when we let the magnetizing current I die out, that is, when the externally applied field is removed, the value of B for the needle does not return to zero. The needle is now truly an independent, permanent magnet. The value of B retained is designated B_r, and referred to as the *retentivity*. A good permanent magnet has a high retentivity, while a good core material should have a low retentivity. Ideally, of course, the retentivity of a core material is zero. But that situation is not fulfilled in practice. Why not? It appears

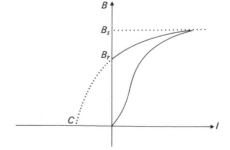

FIG. 4.16. How an externally applied magnetic field, expressed in terms of the magnetizing current I, affects the magnetic field B of a piece of magnetic material (such as a darning needle).

that crystallographic imperfections in a ferromagnetic material (and there always are some such imperfections as impurities, strains, etc.) hinder the shift in domain walls.

Admitting some lack of rigor in favor of simplification, we might describe what is involved here as follows. Work has to be done during the magnetization process to shift the domain walls, and the energy required ultimately shows up as heat. The energy is no longer available to completely rearrange domains as they were before magnetization. In other words, the magnetization process is not completely reversible. To get our needle back to zero B, we actually have to do more work. We have to apply an external field in the opposite direction to the one we originally used to magnetize the needle. The reverse current required to achieve this result is marked on the graph as C. That characteristic of a magnetic material which means that the material requires considerable expenditure of energy to demagnetize it is called its *coercivity*.

Obviously a good permanent magnet should have a large coercivity, because then it will not readily lose its magnetism when subject to stray magnetic fields, or heating, or mechanical shock. A good core material, on the other hand, should require as little energy as possible to demagnetize it. Low coercivity is the most important characteristic of core materials. A good core material may even have a high retentivity and be saved by the compensating grace of a low coercivity which permits removal of the residual magnetism with little expenditure of energy. The coercivity of a core material may be as little as one one-thousandth of that of a permanent-magnet material.

Hysteresis

Looking again at Fig. 4.16, we now note the fact that for values of the externally applied magnetizing field, as represented by the magnetizing current I, there are in general two values of the magnetic field B induced in our ferromagnetic sample. In other words, the magnetic behavior of the sample depends on its magnetic history. The sample, as we noted before, still has a magnetic field even after the external magnetizing field has been removed. The B of the sample lags the external magnetizing field. This lagging is referred to as *hysteresis* (to lag behind).

What would the situation be if we performed an experiment in which we did not just magnetize a sample but actually demagnetized it, magnetized it with the polarity in the opposite direction, demagnetized it, and then remagnetized it as originally? The result could be shown on a graph such as Fig. 4.17, which is known as a *hysteresis loop*. The practical implication of this hysteresis loop is that, since most of our present-day electrical devices operate with alternating currents, changing directions many times a second, the ferromagnetic materials employed are often processed through such hysteresis cycles. This means we are using energy to magnetize some piece of iron, to demagnetize it, and to remagnetize it with opposite polarity many times a second. This process is using up energy, which appears in the material as heat. . The energy loss is known as *hysteresis loss*. We shall have cause to refer to this hysteresis loss again in

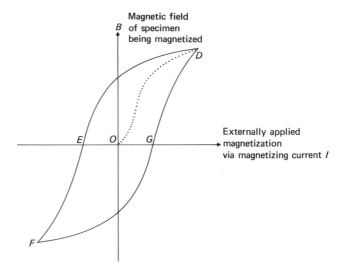

FIG. 4.17. Hysteresis loop. Original magnetization from O to D; demagnetization (involving some oppositely directed magnetizing field) from D to E; magnetization with polarity opposite to original polarity, from E to F; again demagnetization from F to G; back to original magnetization, from G to D.

Chapter 6, when we discuss transformers. It can be shown that the area inside a hysteresis loop is directly proportional to the energy expended in taking the magnetic material through the complete magnetization cycle.

We may thus also describe core materials and permanent-magnet materials in terms of their hysteresis loops (see Fig. 4.18). Core materials should, of course, have the narrowest possible hysteresis loop, implying

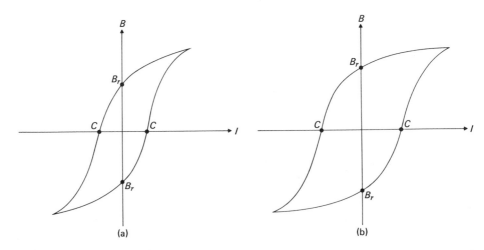

FIG. 4.18. Types of hysteresis loops. (a) Magnetic-core material: small coercivity and small loop area. (b) Permanent-magnet material: large coercivity and large loop area.

that the least possible energy is lost in unnecessary, and usually undesirable, heating of the core material.

Magnetic Shielding

Since much of what we use in everyday life (your watch, for example) is made of ferromagnetic materials, and since external magnetizing fields seem everywhere (wherever electrical currents occur), how can one prevent unmagnetized materials from becoming magnetized, and magnetized materials from becoming demagnetized, by these stray external magnetic fields? Would the best way to shield something from magnetic effects be by using a sheet of glass, or a sheet of copper, or a sheet of iron? The answer is: iron. Because a magnetic insulator as such is not known, the most effective way to shield something from magnetic effects is to provide a magnetically permeable material which would cause the field to be deflected through it, rather than through the air to the object being shielded. (Refer again to Fig. 4.8.) Hence a core-type material of high magnetic permeability in a watch casing will, to a considerable extent, keep the working parts of the watch from becoming magnetized.

4.3 MAGNETIC FIELDS AND ELECTRIC CHARGES

We are, from early schooling, familiar with the fact that a magnet can be used to lift another magnet, the north pole of one magnet being adjacent to the south pole of the other. That is, we are accustomed to the interaction between two sources of magnetic fields, although it is extremely unlikely that we ever thought of such a commonly known fact in such sophisticated terms. The merit of the more sophisticated expression of a simple phenomenon lies in the fact that it may widen our horizons by describing a specific situation in more general terms. In this particular case, since we are no strangers to the interaction between two bar magnets, the realization that we have here simply the interaction between two magnetic fields should make it readily acceptable that there should be an interaction, a force, between an electrical charge in motion (a current) and a magnetic field. Why? Because with the electric charge in motion there is also associated a magnetic field (Oersted effect), and hence we have basically the same ingredients as in the case of the two magnets.

The Motor Effect: Another Right-Hand Rule

The above ideas seem simple enough in retrospect. But, though magnetic behavior of ferromagnetic materials was known to the ancients, the extrapolation to the idea that there is a force exerted on electric charges moving through a magnetic field was not known until its discovery by Michael Faraday on Christmas Day in 1821.

This effect—that is, the force on electric charges moving through a magnetic field—can easily be demonstrated (see Section 4.5, Question 11), and visualized in terms of a straight current-carrying wire placed between the poles of a magnet (see Fig. 4.19).

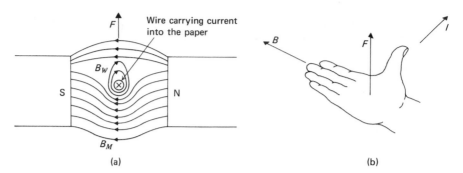

FIG. 4.19. The force on a current-carrying conductor in a magnetic field. (a) Schematic showing the interaction between the magnetic field B_W of the wire carrying current I and the magnetic field B_M of the magnets. This representation shows why frequently the magnetic-flux lines are imagined to be elastic. (b) The right-hand rule which yields the direction of the force on the wire in (a).

Note the relative directions involved. The directions may be expressed in another right-hand rule [see Fig. 4.19(b)]. If the fingers of the right hand point in the direction of the magnetic field B, the thumb in the direction of the current I, then the force on the current is perpendicular to, and out of, the palm. In other words, the important quantities, B, I, and F must be mutually perpendicular. (It is this interesting effect, not encountered before in this text, of a force being exerted directly perpendicular to the force field involved, that makes it relatively easy to design an electrical motor, as we shall shortly see.) In the event that B and I are not perpendicular, then the force depends only on those components of B and I which *are* perpendicular. If I is parallel to B then, of course, it is impossible to conceive of a component of B perpendicular to I, and the force is consequently zero. And this is what is observed in fact (see Fig. 4.20).

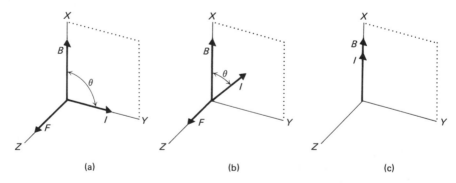

Fig. 4.20. The relationship between B, I, and F, where F is the force experienced by a conductor carrying I, while in a magnetic field B. (X, Y, Z, are mutually perpendicular axes.) (a) Here $\theta = 90°$, and hence F has maximum value. (If $B = 1$ Wb/m^2, the length of the conductor is 1 m, and $I = 1$ A, then $F = 1$ N.) (b) $\theta < 90°$, and hence F is smaller than in part (a). (c) $\theta = 0°$, B and I are parallel, and hence $F = 0$.

The quantitative relationship (which is, however, meaningless in the absence of the restrictions regarding directions as discussed above) expressing this motor effect is

$$F = B \perp Il, \tag{4.2}$$

where F is the force (newton) exerted on a wire of length l (meter), carrying a current I (ampere), in a magnetic field B (weber/m²). As in previous usage, the sign $\perp$ indicates B and I (that is, in effect, the wire length l, which carries I) are perpendicular.

Rearranging this equation in the form

$$B = \frac{F}{Il}$$

(still keeping in mind the mutual perpendicularity requirements of B, F, and Il), we see that the equation explicitly defines B in terms of force, current, and length. Also the unit for B is now defined as

$$\frac{\text{weber}}{\text{meter}^2} = \frac{\text{newton}}{\text{ampere-meter}},$$

and hence the unit of magnetic flux Φ is also defined

$$\text{weber} = \left(\frac{\text{weber}}{\text{m}^2}\right)\text{m}^2 = \left(\frac{\text{newton}}{\text{ampere-m}}\right)\text{m}^2 = \frac{\text{newton-m}}{\text{amp}}.$$

Now what, really, does all this mean? Let's take the case of the unit for B. If a wire one meter long carrying a current of one ampere across a magnetic field experiences a force of one newton, then, by definition, we say that the magnetic field has a strength of one weber/meter² [see Fig. 4.20(a)].

An equivalent way of expressing Eq. (4.2) is

$$F = qB \perp v, \tag{4.3}$$

where F is the force on a positive charge q moving at right angles to a magnetic field B with a speed v.

This equation may be used, for example, to determine the deflections of the electron stream heading for a television screen (Fig. 4.21). A practical application in radiography is in the design of closed-circuit television re-

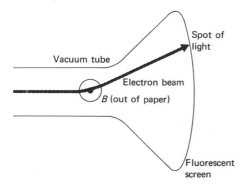

Vacuum tube

Spot of light

Electron beam

B (out of paper)

Fluorescent screen

FIG. 4.21. Television picture tube, showing the deflection of the electron beam due to a magnetic field perpendicular to and out of the paper. This schematic could represent looking down on the picture tube, that is, looking down on the horizontal deflection coils causing the B.

ceivers as employed in conjunction with image intensifiers in fluoroscopy (see Section 12.5).

Note that the right-hand rule related to Eq. (4.2) applies also to Eq. (4.3). When you use this right-hand rule to check Fig. 4.21, remember that, since this refers to a television receiver, what is shown is a stream of electrons, not positive charges. The deflection of electrons should, of course, be opposite to the deflection predicted for positive charges.

Definition of the Ampere

We have previously defined the coulomb, the unit of electric charge, in terms of the ampere. And we have also in this section used the ampere to define the unit of magnetic flux. Earlier (Section 2.1) we pointed out that we were taking the ampere as the undefined, fundamental unit of electricity, and that we would define it only in terms of an operational definition, a cookbook rule telling how it is measured. We are finally arriving at the proper stage for this cookbook rule.

Refer to Fig. 4.22. What is the magnetic field at point P due to the current carried by a straight wire into the paper? Down, yes, according to the right-hand rule associated with the Oersted effect. Now suppose that we were to place a second straight current-carrying wire through point P; then, according to Eq. (4.2), this second wire would experience a force to the right if the current direction is directed oppositely to that of the first wire, according to the right-hand rule associated with the motor effect.

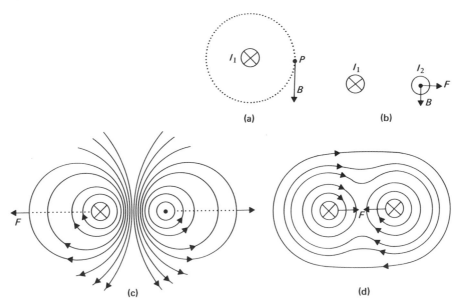

FIG. 4.22. The effect of one current-carrying conductor on another. (a) The direction of the magnetic field at P due to I_1. (b) The force on I_2 at P due to magnetic field of I_1. (c) Schematic showing how wires are forced away from each other when currents are oppositely directed. The wires are forced away from the region of the strongest magnetic field. (d) The case of attraction: currents in the same direction.

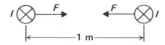

FIG. 4.23. The ampere. If $F = 2 \times 10^{-7}$ newton for each meter length of wire carrying the current I, then $I = 1$ ampere.

A similar argument shows immediately that the first wire now, due to the presence of the second, also experiences a force. Measurements of the force between two current-carrying conductors can be made in practice. Since this force will depend on the current carried by the wires and the distance between them, it has been internationally agreed to define the ampere as follows:

> *One ampere* is that unvarying current which, if present in each of two parallel conductors of infinite length and one meter apart in empty space, causes each conductor to experience a force of exactly 2×10^{-7} newton per meter of length (see Fig. 4.23).

4.4 DC METERS AND MOTORS

Let us now use our ideas about the force on electric charges in motion to describe the operation of some basic electrical devices: electric meters and electric motors.

The Galvanometer

The *galvanometer* is the basic current-detecting and current-measuring device. We shall restrict our discussion to a particular type of galvanometer, the d'Arsonval moving-coil galvanometer (named after the French physician and physicist, Arsene d'Arsonval, 1851–1940, who was a pioneer in electrotherapy). This instrument is shown in simplified form in Fig. 4.24.

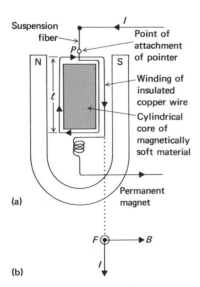

FIG. 4.24. D'Arsonval moving-coil galvanometer. (a) Schematic of the meter. (b) The direction of the force on the longitudinal part of the winding on the right, employing the directions associated with Eq. (4.2).

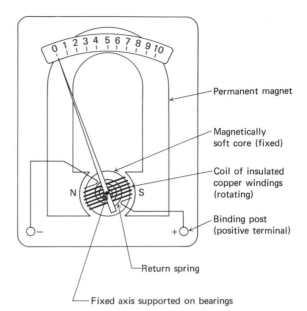

FIG. 4.25. Galvanometer with the moving coil attached to an axis supported on bearings.

Permanent magnet

Magnetically soft core (fixed)

Coil of insulated copper windings (rotating)

Binding post (positive terminal)

Return spring

Fixed axis supported on bearings

What happens when a current flows in the direction shown? First of all, let us consider that part of the wire winding in which the current is going down at the right. Using the right-hand rule associated with Eq. (4.2), we see that there is a force on that wire out of the paper. Now the part on the left in which the current is shown going up: The right-hand rule shows that there is a force on this wire into the paper. Hence there is a twisting effect, or torque, on the winding, tending to turn it about a vertical axis. How much the torque is, of course, depends on the force on each longitudinal wire. From Eq. (4.2) we see that, since both the length l of the wire and the magnetic field B of the permanent horseshoe magnet are constant, the force is dependent only on the current through the winding, providing, of course, that the angle through which the coil twists is small. The latter restriction follows from the perpendicularity require- ment of Eq. (4.2). Now then, the larger the current, the larger the force on each longitudinal wire, and hence the greater the torque. The greater the torque the further the winding will twist about the vertical axis. How far it will twist with a given current depends on the nature of the suspension fiber. It seems, therefore, altogether likely that one could attach a pointer to the winding, sticking out of the paper at P. Then one could calibrate the instrument so that a given current would be indicated by a certain rotation of the pointer relative to some affixed scale. Note that the direction of rotation depends on the current direction. Consequently, some galvano- meters have a scale with the pointer at zero at the center of the scale. Whichever way the needle goes in this case indicates the current direction.

If, on the other hand, the instrument is arranged in the manner shown in Fig. 4.25, one must be careful to pass the current only in the proper direction. For this reason, such instruments have a plus and a minus sign on the respective terminals or binding posts. The plus terminal must be connected to the high-potential side of the circuit.

Finally, analysis based on Eq. (4.2) (as well as on the elastic properties of the suspension fiber) reveals that the deflection shown on a circular scale is directly proportional to the current I. By "directly proportional" is meant, of course, that as the current gets twice as large as some previous value, so does the deflection of the galvanometer pointer needle as shown on the scale. Such a linear relation between current and size of deflection is also approximately true for small deflections on a flat scale.

At this point we should note that we have concerned ourselves only with the wires up and down, but not with the part of the wire winding which is horizontal at the bottom and at the top of the winding. What forces act on these as the result of a current going through the winding? In the equilibrium position there is no force, because I and B are parallel. Once the current is out of the equilibrium position, our knowledge of the directions involved in Eq. (4.2) indicates that there is a force up on one end and down on the other. This effect, however, does not disturb the rotation about the vertical axis.

In actual practice, instead of one winding several windings are used, that is, a moving coil is employed to increase the torque, and thus the movement of the pointer. Such a galvanometer is an exceedingly sensitive instrument and must consequently not be subject to any sizable currents, which would heat up and burn out the coil.

It is, of course, not necessary to have the coil freely suspended vertically. Figure 4.25 shows a different arrangement, which was invented by an American scientist, Edward Weston. The coil in this galvanometer is firmly supported on a fixed axis supported by bearings. The opposition to the torque produced by current going through the coil is supplied by a hairspring. This version of the moving-coil galvanometer finds wide use as the chief constituent of DC voltmeters and ammeters.

Note that in this type of galvanometer, as in the d'Arsonval one, permanent magnets are used. It is naturally possible to replace these permanent magnets with electromagnets energized by the same current that goes through the moving coil. Instruments operating in this manner are known as *dynamometers*.

The Ammeter

Galvanometers, as we stated before, are delicate, sensitive, low-resistance instruments. With a little modification they may serve as ammeters or as voltmeters. Let us first consider an ammeter.

The purpose of the ammeter is to measure the current through a circuit. This meter can in this sense be visualized as a flow meter such as is employed to measure the water flow through a pipe. In the latter case, the pipe has to be cut or separated somehow to permit the insertion of the flow meter; in the former case, the circuit has to be broken to insert the ammeter. Now the insertion of a meter introduces a new resistance into the circuit: the resistance of the meter. One way to minimize this resistance

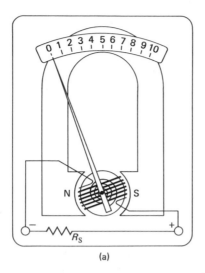

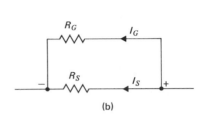

(a)   (b)

FIG. 4.26. Ammeter. (a) Schematic showing the moving-coil galvanometer connected in parallel with the very low resistance shunt, R_S. (b) Circuit diagram of the arrangement shown in (a).

is to use a galvanometer in parallel with a very-low-resistance shunt, combining the galvanometer and the shunt into one instrument, the *ammeter* (see Fig. 4.26). This arrangement achieves the desired result because, as we discovered earlier in connection with Ohm's law, the total resistance of two resistances in parallel is less than the smaller of the two resistances in the combination. Thus the disturbance introduced in the circuit is minimized. Another aim is also achieved by this combination: We can now measure a sizable current without damaging the galvanometer because most of the current will go through the low-resistance shunt and just a little of it will go through the galvanometer itself to give us a reading.

How then does the ammeter give a reading of the current if most of the current does not go through the galvanometer, the very mechanism which causes the needle to move along the scale? We can obtain the answer to this question by the following analysis, which refers to Fig. 4.26(b). Using our knowledge of the addition of parallel resistances (Eq. 3.8), we get

$$\frac{1}{R_G} + \frac{1}{R_S} = \frac{R_G + R_S}{R_G R_S}.$$

Therefore the total meter resistance (galvanometer and shunt) is

$$\frac{R_G R_S}{R_G + R_S}.$$

Now, Ohm's law (Eq. 3.5) applied to the entire meter gives

$$V = \left(\frac{R_G R_S}{R_G + R_S}\right) I,$$

while Ohm's law applied to the galvanometer part of the meter alone yields

$$V_G = R_G I_G.$$

But $V = V_G$ (potential difference between the same two points in the circuit), and hence, if we equate the above two expressions for V, we have

$$\left(\frac{R_G R_S}{R_G + R_S}\right) I = R_G I_G \quad \text{or} \quad I = I_G\left(\frac{R_G + R_S}{R_S}\right). \tag{4.4}$$

Equation (4.4) shows that the current I in the circuit is equal to the current I_G through the galvanometer times a constant determined by the galvanometer resistance R_G and the shunt resistance R_S. This means one could calibrate—that is, adjust the numbers—on the galvanometer scale to read directly the circuit current I. We have an ammeter.

Ammeters of the type described above in conjunction with rectifiers to change the alternating current of the x-ray machine to DC, are used in the x-ray circuit as mA meters, which are calibrated to read average values of the current through the x-ray tube.

The Voltmeter

To measure the voltage across some resistance, one would want to connect the galvanometer across the resistance being investigated. This move would, however, do two unfortunate things: (1) It would grossly reduce the total circuit resistance, because, compared with the resistance of most circuit elements, the galvanometer resistance is very low, and one thus has a parallel-resistance group with one very low resistance. (2) It would cause a surge of current through the galvanometer, burning out its coil. For these reasons, the *voltmeter* consists of a galvanometer in series with a very high resistance (see Fig. 4.27). Using simple algebra, along with

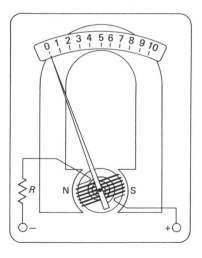

FIG. 4.27. Voltmeter composed of a moving-coil galvanometer connected in series with a high resistance R.

Ohm's law and the theorems on the addition of resistances, we may show that this instrument can be calibrated so that the deflection of the needle of the galvanometer part of it indicates the voltage between the two points to which the voltmeter is connected. Since we find no such DC voltmeter in x-ray equipment, we shall not indulge in the analysis here. But we recommend this analysis to those students wishing to increase their facility with Ohm's law.

To reiterate: the voltmeter measures potential difference between two points in a circuit, that is, across some circuit element. Unlike the ammeter, which must be inserted directly into the circuit by first breaking the circuit somewhere, the voltmeter is connected across the circuit element in question.

The Electric Motor

As a further example of the practical application of the physical principle embodied in Eq. (4.2), we now look at a DC motor.

We have already shown in the case of the galvanometer that the force experienced by a current-carrying conductor may be employed to cause rotation. Consequently, if the twisting suspension fiber of the galvanometer in Fig. 4.24 were replaced by a longitudinal axis and bearings, we might expect continuous motion as long as the current were on and the magnetic field were present. What kind of motion? Note that the force on the wire at the right is originally out of the paper. If this wire is now rotated into the left position, the current direction relative to the magnetic field would again cause a force out of the paper. Similarly, the wire originally at the left will always experience a force into the paper. The best that can be hoped for is an oscillatory motion, that is, the wire loop swinging back and forth through half a turn.

On the other hand, if, just at the moment when the two vertical wires of the loop have completed a quarter turn, it were possible to have some device switch the polarity of the connections to the loop, then we could get rotation. Thus, just as the right vertical wire of the loop swung past the center position between the magnetic poles, we would have the current going up instead of down, so that the force on the wire would be into the paper. Similarly, the left wire, which first had a force into the paper, would now be on the right and would have a force out of the paper. Rotation would be established. In actual practice, the function of the change-over device is carried out by means of a split-ring commutator (see Fig. 4.28). Just at the right moment the brush, which makes the sliding contact with the commutator, switches from one half to the other half, thus changing polarity. (Note that in Fig. 4.28 at the crucial changeover point the battery is temporarily disconnected from the rotating loop; the brushes touch neither commutator segment. Although this arrangement is workable and simple to comprehend, in actual practice the brushes usually span the gap, thereby briefly short-circuiting the battery. At this instant only a negligible current flows through the loop and hence the effect on the rotating loop is the same as we have indicated in Fig. 4.28.)

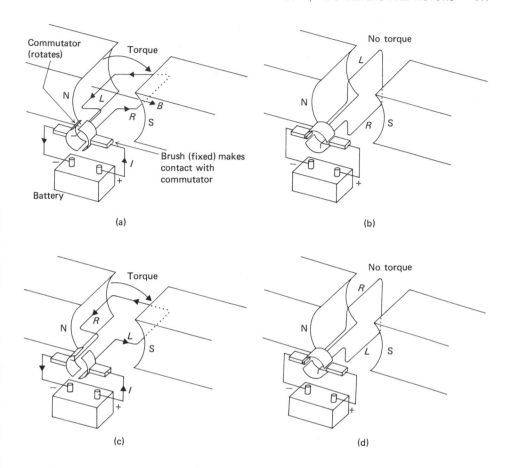

FIG. 4.28. DC motor. Schematic showing the basic elements. Parts (a), (b), (c), and (d) show successive positions involved in a complete rotation. In each case R and L are the parts of the winding in the right and left positions, respectively, in case (a).

Students who are already familiar with the notion of alternating current may suggest that this feat of changing current directions in order to get rotation could be achieved by using an alternating current instead of direct current. And that thought is correct. However, the motor would be condemned to rotate at one speed only: the speed of the frequency of the alternations of the alternating current.

In x-ray machines, the most common use for an electric motor is to rotate the anode in a rotating-anode x-ray tube. However, the motor employed for this purpose works on a different principle from the DC motor described above. This other type of motor, an induction motor, will be described in Section 6.6. Motors similar to the type discussed in the current chapter, however, may find use in the tilting of x-ray tables, in rapid film changers, and in the operation of tomographic equipment.

QUESTIONS

1. Define the following terms:
   a) lodestone
   b) magnetic field
   c) permanent magnet
   d) electromagnet

2. Suppose that two quite strong bar magnets were placed, one on top of the other, in a cradle which prevented them from moving any way other than up and down. What might be observed? Would the observed effect depend on the relative positions of the magnets' north and south poles? Explain.

3. Distinguish between the magnetic field B and the magnetic flux Φ.

4. Sketch the magnetic field you would expect in the region between two bar magnets with their north poles adjacent. [*Hint:* Recall the nature of the electric field between two like charges.]

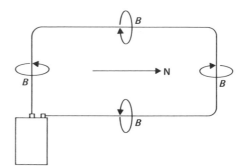

FIG. 4.29. The magnetic effect associated with a current-carrying wire.

5. Refer to Fig. 4.29, and answer the following questions:
   a) Indicate the direction of the current.
   b) Describe what would happen to a compass needle freely suspended under the bottom wire (the wire lies along a north-south line).
   c) Give the name of the scientist who discovered the effect concerned.

6. Figure 4.30 shows three different cases of the magnetic field of a current-carrying solenoid: vacuum core, paramagnetic core, ferromagnetic core. Which is which?

7. Indicate some components of the x-ray machine which depend heavily on ferromagnetic materials.

8. The magnets used in ophthalmology for the removal of ferromagnetic splinters from eyes generally fall into two classes: a small magnet, called the hand magnet, and a large so-called giant magnet.
   a) Both these magnets are electromagnets, rather than permanent magnets. Why?
   b) Even the hand magnet is quite heavy. Why?
   c) Figure 4.31 shows the magnetic field around the probe of a hand magnet. Where is the field greatest? Does the field drop off significantly in a small distance from the point of the probe?

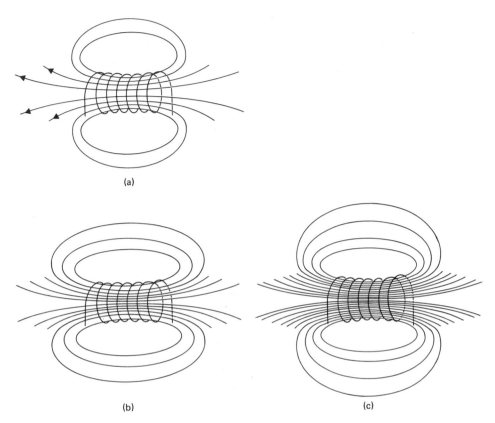

FIG. 4.30. The effects of different cores on the magnetic field of a solenoid carrying the same current.

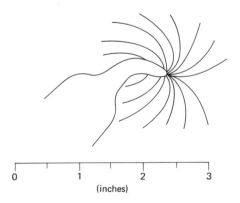

FIG. 4.31. Probe of an ophthalmological hand magnet. An approximate indication of the magnetic field is given.

9. Outline briefly the essentials of the domain theory of ferromagnetism.

10. On the same axes sketch the hysteresis curves of a material suitable for the core of an electromagnet and one suitable for making permanent magnets. With reference to your graph, comment on the important characteristics such as coercivity and retentivity.

11. Sketch a circuit showing the operation of an electromagnetic relay.

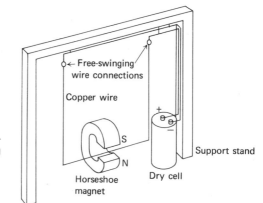

FIG. 4.32. Experimental setup demonstrating the force on a current-carrying conductor in a magnetic field.

12. What is the direction of the motion of the wire in Fig. 4.32 when the switch S is closed?

13. Figure 4.33 shows the essential features of a moving-coil galvanometer. Give the current direction which would cause the rotation indicated.

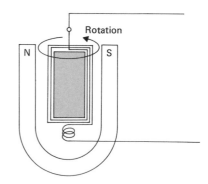

FIG. 4.33. A moving-coil galvanometer. What is the current direction?

14. a) Describe the construction of a moving-coil ammeter.
    b) How would this instrument have to be modified to serve as a voltmeter?

15. What are the functions of the split-ring commutators in an electric motor? Explain fully.

16. Describe qualitatively the manner in which the ampere is defined.

SUGGESTED READING

BITTER, FRANCIS, *Currents, Fields and Particles*. New York: Technology Press of Massachusetts Institute of Technology, and John Wiley, 1956. The author is a foremost authority on magnetism. (Bitter and H. J. Williams of the Bell Telephone Laboratories developed a method for outlining domains in an actual ferromagnetic sample by applying a colloidal suspension of iron oxide powder to the sample's surface.) Chapter 5 on magnetic fields is highly recommended to the advanced student. Diamagnetism is discussed in Chapter 6. Calculus is required for the quantitative part of the discussion, but a valuable insight into magnetic behavior may be gained without rigorously following the mathematical analysis.

EFRON, ALEXANDER, *Magnetic and Electrical Fundamentals*. New York: John F. Rider, Inc., 1959. Chapters 1 and 3 provide excellent brief supplementary reading for beginning physics students. The introduction of the left-hand motor rule on page 66, although quite correct, may be misleading to students of our text. The rule is equivalent to the right-hand rule stated in our Section 4.3.

LEMON, HARVEY B., *What We Know and Don't Know About Magnetism*. Chicago: Museum of Science and Industry, 1946. This 60-page booklet is an excellent, thorough treatment of the nature of magnetic materials. Can be understood by anyone who has a basic idea of atomic structure such as outlined in our Chapter 1.

MARCUS, ABRAHAM, *Basic Electricity*. Englewood Cliffs, N.J.: Prentice-Hall, 1958. Chapter 6 is a detailed but elementary, nonmathematical treatment of DC meters. Chapter 17 on electrical motors provides extra reading for those students who wish to look at this topic in more detail than provided in our Section 4.4.

STOUT, MELVILLE B., *Basic Electrical Measurements*, Englewood Cliffs, N.J.: Prentice-Hall, 1960. A reference for those students wishing to consult an authoritative treatise on various electrical meters. Chapter 17, Electrical Indicating Instruments, provides an excellent, largely descriptive summary of meters for both DC and AC. For example, from the discussion of the limitations of the different types of meters it may readily be understood why, in x-ray circuits, the mA meter is composed of a DC meter with a rectifying bridge, and why the mA meter is calibrated in average values of the current.

CHAPTER 5

Induced Currents

In Chapter 4, we talked about the fact that Oersted's discovery of the close connection between electricity and magnetism was the key to many electric and magnetic phenomena.

Many investigators, when they realized that electric currents result in magnetic fields, began to ponder about turning Oersted's key the other way: Could magnets be used to produce electric currents?

As we know, the answer to this question is yes. And upon this answer depends the production of the electric current employed in x-ray machines.

The discovery that electric currents could be induced in a circuit subjected by some means to a changing magnetic flux was made independently by Joseph Henry in the United States and Michael Faraday in England.

Joseph Henry (1797–1878), a professor of mathematics and physics at the Albany Academy, apparently discovered the phenomenon of induced currents a year before Faraday; but Faraday is the acknowledged discoverer of the phenomenon because he published his results first. However, in his paper of 1832, Henry not only corroborated Faraday's findings but added a major discovery not previously reported: that of self-induced currents, that is, currents induced by a circuit within itself when the circuit is opened or closed.

Faraday, whom we first met in this book in connection with the concept of the electric field, spent most of his working life in the Royal Institution in London, where he started as a laboratory assistant and ended as director. In addition to his fundamental discovery of the fact that magnetic effects could be employed to produce electric currents, he is also credited with inventing the first real electric generator, or dynamo, which consisted of a copper disk revolving between the poles of a permanent magnet.

While all this activity was going on in England and the United States, similar investigations were being pursued in Russia by H. F. E. Lenz (1804–1865), who made a further contribution to the subject. In fact, just a few years after Faraday's first paper on induced currents, Lenz reported a basic principle which apparently had escaped both Henry and Faraday. This principle permits the prediction of the direction of the induced current in any situation. As we shall shortly see, the names of Lenz and Faraday are now given to the main physical principles which form the basis of this chapter.

At this point, now that we have enunciated the basic physics, the engineers and inventors rightly enter the picture. First comes the German electrical engineer, E. W. von Siemens (1816–1892), who modified the generator in the modern direction by replacing the permanent magnets by electromagnets, energized by the current produced by the generator itself.

Finally, the credit for making the dynamo efficient enough to supply electricity at commercially acceptable costs goes to the great American inventor, Thomas Alva Edison (1847–1931) who is probably better known for achieving a similar practical success with the incandescent light bulb.

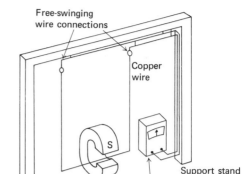

FIG. 5.1. Experimental setup to demon-strate the electric circuit induced in a conductor moving across a magnetic field.

5.1   INDUCED EMF

We shall shortly describe some simple experiments to show how a current might be produced in a circuit by means of magnetism. But before we do so, it is well to point out that, although the ideas involved seem simple and somewhat obvious in retrospect, they were not readily revealed at first. After Oersted's discovery that magnetism was produced by electricity, many investigators placed conductors and magnets together, but without success. What was lacking was some motion or change of the magnet relative to the wire. It was this discovery of the notion of change of the magnetic flux which represents the genius of Faraday. Let us see.

Some Simple Experiments

First we employ an apparatus consisting basically of a wire and a horse-shoe magnet as shown in Fig. 5.1. This arrangement is similar to that of Fig. 4.32, but with this difference: In place of a source of EMF (dry cell), we now have a galvanometer. This time, instead of causing the wire to swing when the circuit with the dry cell is closed, we shall swing the wire by hand and so hope to get an EMF which will set up a current through the galvanometer. Such an EMF is called an induced EMF.

Already it seems apparent that an electric motor which converts electrical energy into mechanical energy is but a dynamo, which con-verts mechanical energy into electrical energy, run in reverse. There is, in fact, a quantitative equivalence between motors and generators which is not trivial. This equivalence follows from one of the cornerstones of physics: the law of the conservation of energy.

Enough of this. On with our experiment, which we hope will show that we have a simple generator. What do we see when the wire is hanging still? We note no deflection on the galvanometer. Now let us effect some change in the situation. Let us swing the wire out of the jaws, or poles, of the magnet. A deflection appears on the galvanometer! Moreover, swing-ing the wire into the jaws of the magnet again produces a deflection, but in the opposite direction.

One more thing we could try: swinging the wire more quickly than before. Doing this, we note that the galvanometer deflection is increased, implying that we have a larger current, which in turn implies that we have induced a larger EMF.

Apparently what is required is motion of the wire relative to the magnet. What is more, the direction of the induced EMF depends on the direction of the motion, and the size of the EMF depends on the speed of the motion. Surprising as it may seem, we could have predicted these results from Eq. (4.3). Moving electric charges (electrons in the wire) more or less perpendicularly through the magnetic field B (of the horseshoe magnet) with a speed v, we would get a force on the electrons either to the right or the left according to

$$F = qB \perp v. \qquad (4.3)$$

This sideways force on the electrons pushes the electrons along the horizontal wire. But why do electrons in the rest of the circuit move and ultimately cause a galvanometer deflection? Coulomb's law. The electrons which are caused to move by the magnetic force push on the others with electric repulsion which we quite expect according to Coulomb's law.

We might try the right-hand rule associated with Eqs. (4.2) and (4.3) to predict the direction of the induced current. Assume that the wire is swinging into the jaws of the magnet, as shown in Fig. 5.2. From the polarity of the magnet, we see that the direction of B is upward between the jaws or poles of the magnet. Thus the indicated direction of v, which is into the page, shows that the force on a positive charge would be toward the right. Since conventional current direction is the direction positive charges would travel, this means that the conventional current in the moving wire is to the right, as shown. The electrons in the wire are then, of course, actually experiencing a force in the opposite direction, which causes them to drift toward the left.

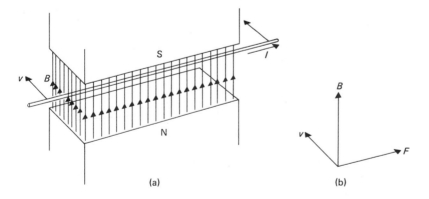

(a)   (b)

FIG. 5.2. The direction of the induced current when a wire moves across a magnetic field. (a) Closeup of the poles of the magnet of Fig. 5.1, showing the direction of the induced current I. (b) The directions associated with Eq. (4.3) show a force on positive charges in the direction of F, thereby indicating the expected direction of the current I.

Well, if moving a wire across a magnetic field causes an EMF to be induced in it, we might rightly ask what would happen if the wire were kept steady and the magnet were moved instead. We could get the answer from a relativity argument. But we shall use Faraday's magnetic flux lines instead. Moving the wire with the magnet kept still caused the wire to cut magnetic flux lines. Now keeping the wire still and moving the magnet will also cause the wire to cut magnetic flux lines. Thus we might expect to find an EMF in this case also. And we do. The easiest way to demonstrate this effect is by moving a magnet into or out of a coil, as shown in Fig. 5.3.

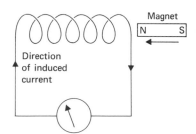

FIG. 5.3. Inducing an EMF, and consequently a current, in a stationary circuit by moving a magnet.

Using a coil instead of a single loop, as in the circuit of Fig. 5.1, has an advantage in that an EMF is induced in each winding, or loop. The windings, since they are part of a continuous wire, may then be considered as a number of sources of EMF connected in series, so that the total induced EMF is the sum of the EMF's induced in each winding.

The magnet in the above instance could, of course, be replaced by a current-carrying coil. This is no surprise, since after all a current-carrying coil is simply a way of providing a magnetic field, just as is the magnet.

Now let us think about what is going on when one moves a magnet near a coil in order to induce an EMF in the coil. When the magnet is far away from the coil, the coil "sees" hardly any magnetic field. In fact, if the magnet is far enough away, to all intents and purposes the value of the magnetic field, or flux density B, at the position of the coil, due to the magnet, may be considered zero. Another way of stating this fact is to employ the notion of magnetic flux discussed in Section 4.1. In this case, the magnetic flux Φ through the coil is zero. Bringing the magnet closer increases the value of B near the coil. In Fig. 5.4 we see more and more flux lines pass through the coil as the magnet comes closer. In short, the total flux Φ through the coil is changing. And it is while Φ is changing that the induced EMF is noted. As soon as we stop moving the magnet the value of Φ through the coil, although no longer zero, stays constant, and the galvanometer indicates no more induced EMF, since apparently there is no longer any current through the galvanometer.

This latter viewpoint is of the utmost significance. It suggests that if by some means the flux Φ through the coil changes, there is induced an EMF in the coil. And the significance lies in the fact that we might change

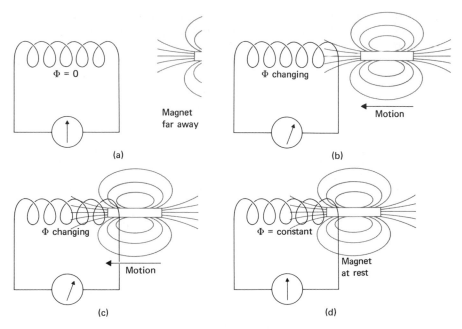

FIG. 5.4. Current is induced in the coil when the flux through the coil is changing.

the flux through the coil by simply having a second coil near it, as shown in Fig. 5.5, and closing the circuit of the second coil, thereby causing the flux to increase in the region of the first. This is the profound discovery that Faraday made. Opening and closing the circuit in the one coil causes

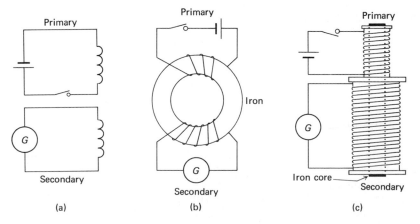

FIG. 5.5. Varying Φ through the secondary by opening and closing the primary circuit induces an EMF in the secondary as noted by the galvanometer G. (a) The basic requirements. (b) Arrangement such as used by Faraday. (c) Setup as often used in physics experiments. In both (b) and (c) the induced EMF is increased by using a ferromagnetic core common to the primary and the secondary.

an EMF in the other. We call the coil which provides the original current the *primary coil* and the one in which the EMF and current is induced the *secondary coil*.

As is to be expected, once the current of the primary coil has reached its maximum value, there is no more change in the flux Φ through the secondary, and therefore the current in the secondary disappears, re-appearing again momentarily when the primary circuit is opened.

Faraday's Law

The simple experiments described above demonstrate the essence of Faraday's discovery: that EMF's may be induced in a conductor in three seemingly different ways. One, by moving a conductor near a magnet; two, by moving the magnet instead of the conductor; and three, by chang-ing the current in a nearby conductor.

In summarizing Faraday's discoveries, we said that EMF's could be induced in three *seemingly* different ways. The emphasis is on seemingly. Because, as we hope we have made clear in our discussion of the simple experiments, the different ways seem to have this in common: that an EMF is induced in a circuit whenever the flux through the circuit varies with time. This statement is known as *Faraday's law*. It may be stated suc-cinctly in the form of an equation:

$$\mathscr{E} = -\frac{\Delta\Phi}{\Delta t} \, , \tag{5.1}$$

where $\mathscr{E}$ is the induced EMF. Actually $\mathscr{E}$ refers to the EMF induced in a simple circuit, by which we mean a single loop or winding. If a coil of N number of windings, or turns, is involved, then the magnitude of the total EMF induced would be $N(\Delta\Phi/\Delta t)$. The symbol $\Delta\Phi$ refers to the change in total magnetic flux through the circuit in the time interval Δt, which change in flux may be effected either by changing B or by changing the effective area of the circuit, as one would expect from the definition of Φ in Eq. (4.1). The minus sign is usually introduced to signify the fact that the direction of the induced EMF and the current resulting from it is in opposition to the flux change which produced it. However, before we em-bark on a discussion of this latter point, known as *Lenz's law*, it behooves us to consider a few other relevant matters.

First let us point out that if, as in the practical case, the rate of change of magnetic flux is not constant, then to get the instantaneous value of $\mathscr{E}$ at a given time, it is necessary to let the time interval shrink: to take the limiting value of $\Delta\Phi/\Delta t$ as Δt goes to zero. This is exactly the same idea as that presented in Section 1.6 on radioactive decay, and that of the instantaneous value of electric current dealt with in Section 3.1. (Students familiar with calculus will realize that Faraday's law should really be written

$$\mathscr{E} = -\frac{d\Phi}{dt} \, ;$$

that is, $\mathscr{E}$ is the first derivative of flux with respect to time.)

At this point it might also be well to review the relevant units: If Φ is in webers and t in seconds, then $\mathscr{E}$ is in volts.

Then we might draw on what we discussed in the last chapter on solenoids and core materials to predict that if the primary coil and the secondary coil of Fig. 5.5(a) were both wound on the same ferromagnetic core, as shown in Fig. 5.5(b) and (c), the induced EMF would be greatly enhanced. This is found to be so. After all, using a ferromagnetic coil greatly increases the value of B and hence of Φ through the core. This idea, coupled with Faraday's law, indeed predicts such an increase in $\mathscr{E}$, because when the primary circuit is closed the current rises and B accordingly grows. Hence Φ grows; that is, changes: we have a $\Delta\Phi$. Now if, in the same time interval Δt, the growth is to a large Φ, as opposed to a small Φ without the core, then this means a larger $\Delta\Phi$. Now we are full circle: If $\Delta\Phi$ gets larger while Δt stays the same, then Eq. (5.1) shows that the magnitude of $\mathscr{E}$ is increased, because $\Delta\Phi/\Delta t$ has been increased.

Finally, we would detract somewhat from the generality of Faraday's law, Eq. (5.1). Perhaps some students, noting how an induced EMF explained via Faraday's law, Eq. (5.1), can also be explained directly using Eq. (4.3) will wonder if there is such a thing as an induced EMF which may be explained by Eq. (4.3), but not by means of Faraday's flux changes. Yes, there is. However, we do not want to delve into electromagnetic theory to the extent of discussing all the possible complications. [Students wishing to see how one can use Eq. (4.3), the force on a moving charge, to explain an induced EMF in the case in which there is no reasonable way of equating the situation to a magnetic flux change within the circuit involved are referred to page 17-3 of the volume by Feynman listed at the end of this chapter.]

Lenz's Law

The basic idea of Lenz's law has already been expressed in an earlier paragraph. Let us now demonstrate how this law, which specifies the direction of induced EMF's, is but a consequence of that fundamental principle: the conservation of energy.

Referring to Fig. 5.3, in which the N-pole of a bar magnet is moved toward a coil, we ask, "What would be the magnetic polarity of this solenoid due to the induced current?" Remember that prior to the motion of the magnet there was no current in the solenoid. When current appears in the solenoid there must be energy supplied from somewhere. The "somewhere" is whoever is moving the magnet toward the coil. Now if the direction of the induced current were such as to produce an S-pole at the right end of the coil, facing the magnet, then the magnetic attraction would cause the magnet to move further toward the coil. That is, the current induced by the magnet's motion would itself cause the magnet to continue the same motion and thus cause more current. No outside source of energy would be required to produce the induced EMF which causes the current in the coil. Perpetual motion! The conservation-of-energy principle would be violated because we would be getting energy in the solenoid spontaneously. Consequently we must conclude that, in

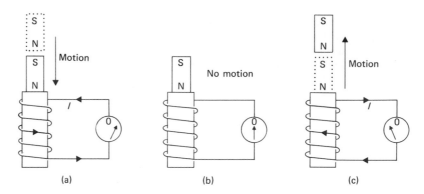

FIG. 5.6. Lenz's law, along with the right-hand rule shown in Fig. 4.7, yields the directions of the induced currents *I*. In (b) there is no flux change and hence no induced current.

the case described, the induced EMF direction and the resulting induced current direction is such as to produce an N-pole facing the magnet. Then whoever is moving the magnet has to expend energy to keep the magnet moving against the magnetic repulsion. And this is the observation made experimentally.

What if one were to create a flux change by moving the bar magnet away from the coil? Then the induced current would be in the direction to yield an S-pole at the end facing the magnet. Again, whoever is moving the magnet has to supply energy; this time to do work against magnetic attraction. This is the energy which then appears in the coil in the form of an induced EMF.

Lenz observed these results and formulated the following principle, now known by his name: An induced EMF is in such a direction as to tend to set up a current whose own magnetic field will oppose the original action which produced the induced current. It is this opposition which is implied by the minus sign in Faraday's law.

We could abbreviate the above statement by saying simply: The induced EMF opposes any flux change (see Fig. 5.6). Whether the flux change in the coil is caused by moving a magnet near it or by opening and closing a primary circuit near it is, of course, irrelevant. Both situations involve flux changes.

5.2 GENERATORS

Electric generators, or dynamos, in the conventionally employed sense differ from the devices employed in the simple experiments we have just discussed only in that they are engineered to provide a continuous EMF as efficiently as possible. This fact generally implies some kind of a rotating device.

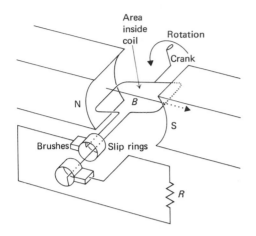

Area inside coil

Rotation

Crank

N

B

S

Brushes Slip rings

R

FIG. 5.7. Simple generator. Turning the crank causes an alternating EMF at the slip rings. The brushes make connection to an external circuit, giving an alternating current through *R*.

A Simple Generator

In examining a simplified form of a rotating generator capable of producing an EMF, we turn again to the notion that a generator is like a motor. Students should note the similarity between Fig. 5.7, which shows a generator, and Fig. 4.28 of the motor shown in the previous chapter. (The difference between the commutator arrangements has nothing to do with the fact that one is a motor and the other a generator. This difference is due to the fact that the motor is for DC and the generator shown produces alternating current.)

The generator, of course, requires some nonelectrical energy input. Let us assume simply that we have someone to turn a crank which will cause the wire coil (or loop, or turn, or winding) to rotate. In actual practice, of course, the mechanical energy is usually supplied either by water falling, or by some internal combustion engine, or by a steam engine.

We now apply Faraday's law to show why an EMF is induced in the generator's winding and how this EMF varies during the course of the rotation of the winding.

In the following discussion, we shall make reference throughout to Fig. 5.8. We employ the concepts of B, the magnetic field, or flux density; Φ, the total magnetic flux; and, of course, Faraday's law. Let us proceed with these tools.

At position P the coil is at right angles to the magnetic field B, represented by equally spaced flux lines to indicate a uniform magnetic field. In this position, the inside area A of the coil is perpendicular to the flux lines and the total flux through the coil is equal to BA, which is the maximum value of the flux through the coil. On the other hand, at position S the coil is oriented parallel to B and hence the effective area of the coil —that is, that component of A which is perpendicular to B — is zero. There is no flux through the coil. When we consider these two extremes, we realize that when the coil rotates from P to S there is a change in flux

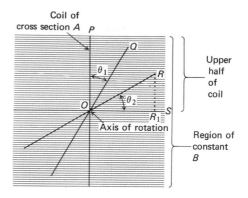

Coil of cross section A

Upper half of coil

Region of constant B

FIG. 5.8. Looking endwise at the coil of the simple generator of Fig. 5.7. The single-loop coil is shown in four successive positions: P, Q, R, and S. The total magnetic flux Φ through the coil at any time is $B \perp A$, which may be represented by the number of flux lines crossing the coil.

through A; that is, there exists a $\Delta\Phi$ in a time interval Δt, which in turn depends on the speed of rotation. Now a $\Delta\Phi/\Delta t$ means that there is an EMF induced in the coil, according to Faraday's law.

Next we show that although there is an EMF induced in the coil, this EMF is not constant. Consider the motion from P to Q. This is case 1: It involves angular motion through an angle θ_1. Note that fewer flux lines are going through the coil after rotation through θ_1 than before. So there is an induced EMF. But what about case 2, the motion from R to S? If $\theta_1 = \theta_2$, then the time interval Δt for each case is the same, assuming a uniform rotational speed. But in case 2 the reduction of flux lines from R to S is much greater than in case 1: The $\Delta\Phi$ is much greater. Since, as we just mentioned, Δt is the same but $\Delta\Phi$ is larger, this means that the ratio $\Delta\Phi/\Delta t$ is larger, which means that $\mathscr{E}$, the induced EMF in case 2, is larger than in case 1.

Thus it appears that an EMF is induced in the coil, but that the EMF varies, depending on the position of rotation.

Another point to note is that for the instant the coil passes through position P the entire maximum area of the coil is presented perpendicularly to the field B. No change in Φ takes place as one takes the limit of making θ_1 very, very small. At this point there is, for an instant, zero induced EMF.

On the other hand, at position S, even the slightest displacement causes a significant change in Φ through the coil. Here the EMF is at its maximum.

To those who find this trafficking with vanishingly small intervals of time (and of space) somewhat disconcerting, we can offer little comfort other than trust. The alternative is to learn something about the calculus. It turns out that some of the answers one jumps to on the basis of so-called ordinary arithmetic are just not true in dealing with the limits of quantities as you let them become either infinitely small or infinitely large. A different way of calculation is required: the differential and integral calculus. Perhaps some readers have discovered this for themselves through the fact that ordinary arithmetic does not yield what everyone knows is the

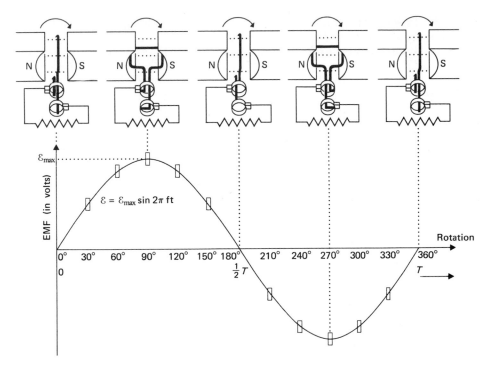

FIG. 5.9. Generation of a sinusoidal alternating EMF, showing a complete revolution of the armature (that is, one complete cycle). The abscissa shows how the degrees of rotation may be related to the period T, the time for a complete cycle.

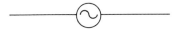

FIG. 5.10. Circuit symbol for a source of sinusoidal alternating EMF.

right answer to the problem of Achilles and the tortoise. (If you are not familiar with this story, see Appendix A.)

Now we have gone far afield! Back to generators and one more issue before stating the final result. Note that on the right of position P the upper end of the coil is moving downward relative to the magnetic field B. This relative motion we know yields the direction of the induced EMF, either by application of the right-hand rule associated with Eq. (4.2), or of Lenz's law. Now visualize this originally upper end of the coil after it has turned through half a cycle, 180° or π radians. This end is now moving through B in an upward direction. Consequently we would expect (and we do find) an EMF induced in the opposite direction. Figure 5.9 shows the situation for a complete cycle.

The EMF of Fig. 5.9 is termed an alternating EMF, the symbol for which is shown in Fig. 5.10. Discussion of alternating EMF's and currents forms the basis of the following chapter, since alternating currents, that is AC, play a major role in the x-ray machine.

The shape of the curve representing the EMF as shown in Fig. 5.9 is sinusoidal. That is to say, the EMF varies with time as a sine function. The term sine refers to a trigonometric expression often related to a right-angled triangle, in which case the sine of an angle is the ratio of the side opposite the angle to the hypotenuse of the triangle. (See Appendix A.) That such a seemingly peculiar relationship should enter our discussion of a generator derives from the definition of Φ. Recall that Φ is the product of A, the inside area of the coil, and B, the magnetic field, where B is perpendicular to A. Now look again at Fig. 5.8, position R. Here the B is not perpendicular to A. But B is perpendicular only to an area represented by the edge view RR_1. Now since

$$\sin \theta_2 = RR_1/OR$$

where OR represents the area A, we find that RR_1, which we call the effective area, A_2, is given by

$$RR_1 = A_2 = A \sin \theta_2.$$

Consequently, the flux through the coil in this position is

$$\Phi = BA_2 = BA \sin \theta_2.$$

But the EMF is given by

$$\mathscr{E} = - \Delta\Phi/\Delta t. \tag{5.1}$$

Hence it appears that substitution for Φ will introduce a trigonometric function such as $\sin \theta$, or sometimes $\cos \theta$, depending on which angle is labeled θ.

This is as far as we want to go. We simply want to show that the EMF varies, and make plausible why it might vary sinusoidally, that is, why the EMF of a rotating generator may be expressed by a sine function:

$$\mathscr{E} = \mathscr{E}_{max} \sin 2 \pi f t, \tag{5.2}$$

where $\mathscr{E}_{max}$ is the maximum EMF in volts (position S in Fig. 5.8), f is the frequency of rotation of the coil in revolutions/second, and t is the time in question in seconds, as shown on the abscissa of the graph in Fig. 5.9. Note that the frequency f is the reciprocal of the time required for a complete cycle. This time interval is known as the *period, T*. For example, if the frequency is 50 cycles/second, then T would be $\frac{1}{50}$ second.

The input voltage to x-ray machines, since it depends on conventional generating plants, is of the form of Eq. (5.2). It is essentially a sinusoidal alternating voltage, which yields sinusoidal alternating current or simply sinusoidal AC. We say "essentially sinusoidal" because in practice the voltage supplied by the generating station may vary slightly from a perfect sinusoidal form. Incidentally, the reader should note that whereas AC is an abbreviation for alternating current, it is common practice to call an alternating voltage an AC voltage, and the source of this voltage an AC

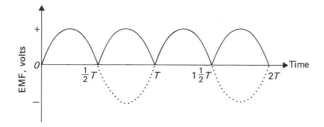

FIG. 5.11. Output voltage of a DC generator. The dotted lines show the alternating EMF as produced by the rotating coil, while the upper solid lines show the pulsating direct voltage appearing at the split-ring commutators. The time axis shows the time in fractions of periods, T.

generator, or an alternator. Even an alternating current itself is often in practice redundantly referred to as an AC current.

Of course, it is possible to lead the induced current from the generator via a split-ring commutator, as employed in the DC motor of Fig. 4.28. In this case, although the generator still generates an AC voltage, the externally connected load now receives pulsating DC voltage, as shown in Fig. 5.11.

Practical Generators

Let us review the essential ingredients of a simple AC generator and then enlarge on these ingredients to give some indication of what is involved in practical generators.

The basic ingredients: a coil of wire (rotor) rotating in a constant magnetic field (produced by the stator), and a system of sliding contacts, as discussed in Section 4.4 for motors, to lead off the induced current.

The induced EMF is, of course, increased by having a coil consisting not of a single loop but of many, and by increasing the speed of rotation; also, having the coil wound on a ferromagnetic core helps. This arrangement of wire wound on a core is referred to as the *armature*.

In practice it is advantageous to achieve both a larger EMF and a higher frequency than is possible with a single coil rotating at a reasonable speed between a single pair of magnetic poles. One can achieve these ends by connecting several coils in series and providing additional pairs of magnetic poles. Figure 5.12 shows the situation of two coils at right angles (each coil represented by one turn only) rotating between two pairs of magnetic poles. Notice what happens to the frequency of the alternations of the EMF in this case. Since a complete cycle of alternating EMF involves a coil passing by an N-pole to an S-pole and back to an N-pole again, we see that in this case a complete EMF cycle is achieved with only half a revolution of the armature. To obtain a 60-cycle voltage, such as is employed in North America, this particular generator would have to rotate at only 30 revolutions per second. Obviously it is an advantage to reduce the speed of the rotating machinery as far as possible. Consequently, even more than four magnetic poles may often be employed.

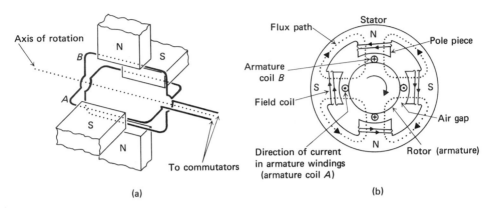

FIG. 5.12. Four-pole AC generator. (a) Simplified version showing two coils, A and B, in series and at right angles. (b) Schematic of a four-pole commercial generator.

Then, as Siemens first proposed, it is advantageous to replace the various permanent magnetic poles by electromagnets energized by current produced by the generator itself. You might ask how a generator can ever get started under these conditions. The answer lies in what was discussed in Section 4.2. The ferromagnetic cores of the electromagnets, although magnetically soft, still have a little residual magnetism. Their retentivity is not quite zero, so that once some outside exciter current has been employed to start the generator in the first place, it is quite possible to restart it later without any outside current source.

Finally, it is pointed out that armature winding is more complicated than the winding of the electromagnet, or field windings; and also the armature windings need better insulation than the field windings. Consequently, the usual practice is to keep the armature stationary and to rotate the electromagnets, or as is commonly said, *rotate the field*. Such an arrangement is shown in Fig. 5.13. In this case, since the armature does not move, it is called the *stator*, and the rotating field coils are termed the *rotor*.

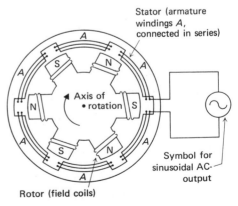

FIG. 5.13. Six-pole AC generator with the field coils as rotor. Direct current to energize the field coils is supplied through brushes and a split-ring commutator (not shown). The AC output comes directly from the ends of the armature windings.

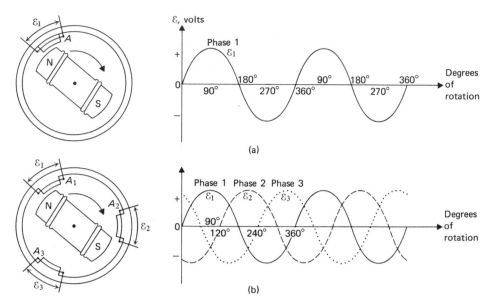

FIG. 5.14. Comparison of single and three-phase generators and their voltage outputs. (a) Two-pole, single-armature, single-phase generator of the type shown in Fig. 5.13. (b) Two-pole, three-armature, three-phase generator.

Multiphase Generators

The generators discussed so far all have this in common: the armatures, in the cases of more than one armature, were connected in series. The result is that any of these generators produces a single EMF, as given by Eq. (5.2), between its terminals. These generators are termed single-phase generators. They produce single-phase AC.

Now consider the case of the generator shown in Fig. 5.14(b). The three armature windings each have their own connections to the world outside the generator. The armatures are independent; they each produce their own EMF, as given by Eq. (5.2). But with this important difference, which may readily be seen by reference to Fig. 5.14: The maximum EMF in armature A_2 is induced one-third of a rotation, that is 120°, after the maximum in armature A_1. We say that the voltages induced in armatures A_1 and A_2 are out of phase by 120°. Similar considerations applied to armatures A_2 and A_3 and then to A_3 and A_1 show that there are three separate voltages, each of the same form, but differing in phase, that is, reaching their respective maxima and minima at different times.

This type of generator is called a *multiphase* or *polyphase generator*. Figure 5.14 shows a particular polyphase generator, that is, a three-phase generator in comparison with a single-phase one. Polyphase generators offer certain advantages, and consequently most of the electrical energy supplied in the world today is originated in three-phase systems. We shall discuss three-phase AC further in Section 6.7.

5.3   INDUCED CURRENTS AND MOTORS

At the outset we should note that although the term "induced currents" has been used in our heading above, and is common in much of the literature of electrical engineering, this term is not rigorously correct. What is more correct is to speak of induced EMF's. Such an EMF may give rise to currents. And such currents are often referred to as induced currents.

Those readers who may consider all this as pedantic quibbling should realize that EMF's may be induced without giving rise to currents (if there is no complete circuit). Now with the record straight we proceed.

Back EMF

We now refer the reader back to the discussion of motors in Section 4.4. Since we have noted the equivalence of the electric motor and the electric generator, it must seem reasonable to expect a motor, which like a generator has a conducting armature moving relative to a magnetic field, to produce an EMF itself. This is indeed so.

The EMF generated by a motor is called the *back EMF* since, according to Lenz's law, it is in such a direction as to oppose the very EMF which drives the motor. Obviously there can be no back EMF until the motor is actually running. Moreover, the back EMF is bound to reach its maximum value only when the motor is operating at its full speed. This all means that, since there is little opposition to current when the external EMF is first applied to start the motor, the current drawn by the motor on starting is much greater than it is after the motor is running at its full speed. The actual variation between current on starting and current on normal full-speed operation is generally so large that special account has to be taken of this fact in the design of electric motors.

Eddy Currents

Now turn back to Fig. 5.7, which shows a simple generator. Let us briefly analyze this generator directly, employing the principle of the force on a charge moving through a magnetic field, Eq. (4.3), rather than Faraday's law. As the right-hand part of the loop is moving up across the magnetic field, Eq. (4.3) indicates that a current will be set up toward the back, toward the handle. By the same token, in the left-hand part of the loop the current is out toward the slip rings; in short, there is a current explained in terms of the force expressed in Eq. (4.3). We actually covered the details of the application of Eq. (4.3) to this case in Section 5.1, with particular reference to Fig. 5.2.

There is then no question that in a loop of conducting material rotating in a magnetic field there would be set up an induced current. Now imagine a great number of such metal loops of various sizes, without insulation, all fitted together to form a solid cylinder. Next imagine this cylinder rotating in a magnetic field, as shown in Fig. 5.15. We might expect that all kinds of current loops would develop in the cylinder as it is rotated. And this is found in practice.

These current loops induced in any conducting material subjected to a changing magnetic field are called *eddy currents*. Moreover, according

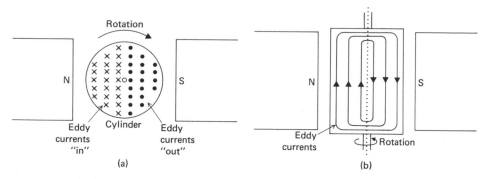

FIG. 5.15. Eddy currents: solid metal cylinder rotating in a magnetic field. (a) Cross section showing the direction of the eddy currents whose paths are indicated in the longitudinal top view (b). View (a) is looking up from bottom of view (b).

to Lenz's law, the direction of the eddy currents will be such as to oppose the cause which produced them. In the case of the rotating cylinder, the direction of the eddy currents is such as to produce magnetic effects which oppose the rotation.

Eddy currents are sometimes useful and sometimes undesirable. They are useful for producing magnetic damping in many electrical measuring instruments. This means that eddy currents are employed to stop a pointer from swinging wildly past its final indicating position. The idea of damping is well demonstrated by the braking of the pendulum in Fig. 5.16. Eddy currents are also very useful in that they are the basis of the induction motor which we shall discuss shortly.

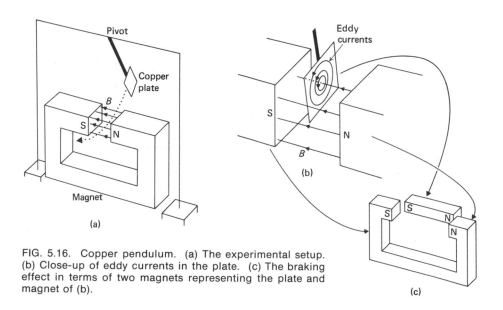

FIG. 5.16. Copper pendulum. (a) The experimental setup. (b) Close-up of eddy currents in the plate. (c) The braking effect in terms of two magnets representing the plate and magnet of (b).

They are undesirable in that they are a source of unwanted heating and energy loss in many electrical components subjected to rapid magnetic flux changes. We shall return to this aspect of eddy currents when we discuss transformer losses in Section 6.4.

The Induction Motor

Pursuing the concept of the braking of the pendulum of Fig. 5.16 can lead to the simplest of AC motors. In this type of motor, unlike the motors discussed in Chapter 4, the energy is fed not to the rotor via brushes, but to the stator. Such a motor is called an *induction motor.* It is the kind used to drive the rotating anode in an x-ray tube. Figure 7.23 shows how the rotor and stator are arranged with respect to the rest of the parts of a rotating anode tube.

Induction motors also find use in some x-ray table-tilting equipment and, in fact, in any machinery in which variable speed control is not an important factor. Although variable speed control is possible with induction motors, DC motors, as described in Section 4.4, are more frequently employed when variable speed is desired.

How does the induction motor work? Recall that the copper plate of Fig. 5.16 was braked by the magnet. In other words, because of eddy currents one would have to employ energy to drag the plate through the gap of the magnet. Or another way of looking at it: if we moved the magnet while the plate was in the gap, again because of eddy currents, we would drag the plate along. By exactly the same process, if we rotated the magnet just above and not touching a freely suspended plate, we would rotate the plate as shown in Fig. 5.17. One can readily perform this experiment at home with a reasonably strong horseshoe magnet and a thin aluminum foil disk, as shown in the figure.

Now the effect of a rotating magnet may be created without, however, actually rotating a magnet. An arrangement of coils as shown in Fig. 5.18 does the trick. If, as in part (a) of the figure, current is passed through windings (1) and (4), the direction of the magnetic field B will be as shown. If the current is then successively switched from one set of opposite windings to the next and the process is repeated continuously, we get a complete sequence of changes in the direction of B from the condition in part (a), through part (f), back to part (a). Further, if this sequence of events is carried out smoothly, we have a rotating magnetic field but, as stated

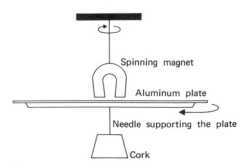

FIG. 5.17. A simple eddy current, or induction motor.

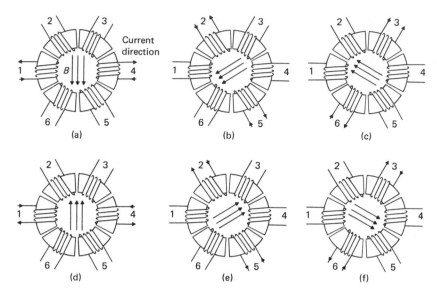

FIG. 5.18. A rotating magnetic field: the essence of the induction motor.

before, without any actual mechanical rotation involved. This smooth rotation of currents, and consequently of B, can be achieved most simply by connecting the three pairs of opposite coils to a three-phase electrical power supply.

In the event that an x-ray unit is connected to a single-phase electrical supply (which is most frequently the case in fact), then special circuits which achieve one or more phase shifts are employed to energize the stator of the anode motor.

So far, of course, we have just reached the point of having a rotating magnetic field. But the rest should by now be obvious. If a copper cylinder were placed inside the ring shown in Fig. 5.18, then from our previous discussion of eddy currents we would expect eddy currents to be induced in the cylinder in such a direction that the cylinder would be dragged around by the rotating magnetic field. And that is essentially what happens in the case of the rotating anode motor. The copper cylinder is the rotor.

Note the advantage of this motor with respect to the x-ray tube. We can get the anode to rotate inside a completely sealed-off tube without requiring any direct connections, electrical or mechanical, to the outside of the vacuum x-ray tube. We shall recall these matters in Section 7.5 when we discuss x-ray tube targets.

5.4 MUTUAL INDUCTION

In our previous discussion of electric generators, we talked about the current being induced in the armature by means of a magnetic flux change through the armature windings brought about by motion of the armature relative to the magnetic field. Earlier, in our first discussion of Faraday's law, we pointed out that an EMF may be induced in any coil, called the *secondary*, by flux changes brought about simply by changing the current in some adjacent coil, called the *primary*. The phenomenon is that of *mutual induction*. We look at it a little more closely now.

DC Behavior

Essentially, mutual induction may be considered a vehicle for the transfer of energy from one coil to another via the medium of a changing magnetic field. Let us look at Fig. 5.19. When the primary circuit is closed, a magnetic field will build up in the region of both the primary and the adjacent secondary circuit. That is, the secondary circuit experiences a change in magnetic flux, an EMF $\mathscr{E}$, and consequently a current, is induced in each turn, or winding, of the secondary coil in accord with Faraday's law,

$$\mathscr{E} = -\,\Delta\Phi/\Delta t. \tag{5.1}$$

Before the primary circuit was closed, there was no magnetic field. But, when the primary current flows there is a magnetic field with S-polarity at the bottom of the primary coil. Thus, in accord with Lenz's law, the induced current in the secondary should yield an S-pole at its top end. In that way, the magnetic field of the secondary opposes and tends to cancel the magnetic field of the primary in the region between the two coils. All this is indicated in part (a) of Fig. 5.19.

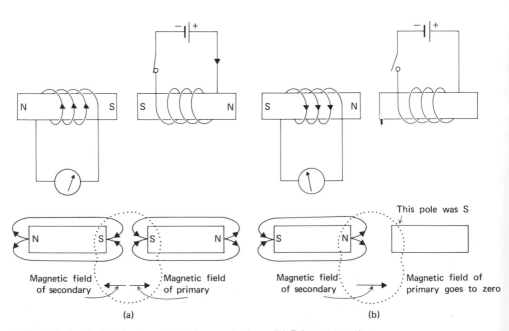

FIG. 5.19. Mutual induction. (a) Primary closing. (b) Primary opening.

As soon as the primary current has reached its final steady value, although there is then still a magnetic field associated with the primary, this field is no longer changing. There is no changing B, therefore no changing Φ, and hence the secondary no longer experiences a $\Delta\Phi/\Delta t$. The induced current dies out.

The only way we can now get another current pulse in the secondary is to open the primary, as in part (b) of Fig. 5.19. Now the primary current is dying out; the B is going to zero. There is now again a change in Φ experienced by the secondary. And since the primary magnetic field is collapsing, the induced current in the secondary will now be in the opposite direction to that of part (a), in order to oppose the collapse of the magnetic field formerly maintained by the primary.

As soon as the primary current has completely died out there will, of course, no longer be any induced current in the secondary.

Although the preceding discussion of mutual induction in the case of DC serves to illuminate the essence of the physics involved, practical applications of interest to us lie in the related behavior with AC.

AC Behavior

From our previous considerations, we can certainly say that the magnitude of the induced EMF and hence the magnitude of the induced current in the secondary will depend on a number of items: the magnitude and rapidity of the current change in the primary; the relative numbers of turns on the primary and secondary windings; the magnetic permeability of the region in which the process is taking place, that is, the type of core (if any) employed; the proximity of the two coils. All these factors influencing the magnitude of the induced EMF are usually expressed succinctly in the equation

$$\mathscr{E}_2 = -M\frac{\Delta i_1}{\Delta t}, \tag{5.3}$$

where $\mathscr{E}_2$ is the EMF induced in the secondary, $\Delta i_1/\Delta t$ refers to the current change in the primary and M is a constant, called the mutual inductance, which depends on all the remaining items enumerated above.

In practical applications, to make the most of the magnetic permeability and the proximity of the two coils, the primary and the secondary are usually wound on the same ferromagnetic core, and sometimes one coil is wound right on top of the other. Such an arrangement, for example, is used in a metal locator devised for the localization of metallic foreign bodies in surgery, both preoperatively and during the actual removal procedure. This metal locator, in a way, is an adjunct to x-rays; it does not supplant them but rather provides instant and, in the case of ferromagnetic materials, highly precise localization which can be of great value during the progress of an operation.

In the diagnostic x-ray field, the most important application of mutual induction is the *transformer*, in which continuous voltage changes in the primary cause a continuous, variable voltage to be induced in the secondary. Transformers will be more fully discussed in Section 6.4.

Circuit symbols relevant to mutual induction are shown in Fig. 5.20.

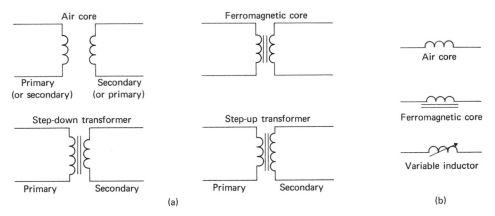

FIG. 5.20. Induction circuit symbols. (a) Mutual induction. (b) Self-induction.

5.5 SELF INDUCTION

In the case of mutual induction, we accept the fact that a varying current in the primary coil resulted in a magnetic flux change in the region, thus, in accord with Faraday's law, inducing an EMF in a nearby coil, the secondary. But the primary itself is, of course, in the same region of changing magnetic flux. In other words, since the primary is also in a region of changing magnetic flux, it should itself have induced in it an EMF opposing this changing flux. It does. The process is called *self induction* and it means: While a current is increasing in a coil, an opposing EMF, and hence an opposite but smaller current, is induced in this very same coil. Conversely, when the main or primary current in the coil is decreasing, a small current is induced in the same direction as the primary current. In both these cases the direction of the induced current is, as stated in Lenz's law, in opposition to the change in the main or primary current.

Self induction is a process characteristic of a circuit component having self inductance. Self inductance may be viewed as analogous to the inertia of matter. Just as the inertia of a mobile x-ray unit opposes any change in the unit's velocity, so the self inductance of an electrical circuit opposes any change in the circuit's current.

The circuit symbol for self inductance is as shown in Fig. 5.20. The circuit component which pronouncedly exhibits self inductance is called an *inductor*. This use of terminology is like the usage of resistor and resistance and capacitor and capacitance which we encountered earlier.

DC Behavior: A Transient Phenomenon

Let us view the phenomenon of self induction in a simple circuit. Reference in the following discussion is to Fig. 5.21. We close the switch, as in part (a) of the figure. The induced EMF opposes the EMF $\mathscr{E}$ of the battery and thereby impedes the rise of the current to its full value. We may also view the situation from the standpoint of current: The battery causes a primary current, i_p; the self-induced EMF causes a smaller but opposing

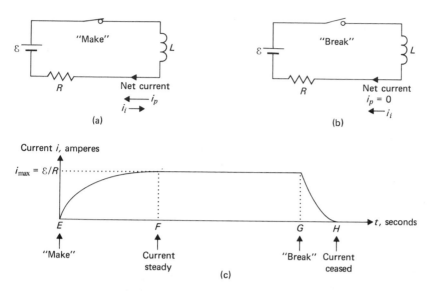

FIG. 5.21. The effect of self inductance on a simple DC circuit. (a) Circuit switch just closed. (b) Circuit switch just opened. (c) Graph of the current for cases (a), (b), and the time in between.

induced current, i_i. The net current in the circuit is the difference between these two currents. Either viewpoint leads to the fact that the current does not rise instantaneously to its full, or steady state Ohm's law value ($i_{max} = \mathcal{E}/R$) when the switch is closed. The amount of delay depends on the inductance L of the circuit as well as the circuit resistance R. If the inductance (that is, self inductance) of the circuit is large, then the time for the current to reach its maximum steady-state value will be large. Since, until the current does reach its maximum value, there is a change taking place in the current, we call this changing a *transient phenomenon*. The changing current is called a *transient current*. And, to reiterate, this transience is due to the inductance L.

The magnitude of the inductance L is primarily dependent on the number of turns of the inductance coil, or inductor, as well as on the nature of its core. If the core is ferromagnetic, then obviously the magnetic flux changes will be more pronounced and hence the induced EMF more pronounced; that is, the inductance L is said to be larger. None of these points, however, is meant to imply that a coil, either with or without ferromagnetic core, is necessary in order for some self-induced EMF to be generated in a circuit. After all, a complete circuit composed of only a single wire loop would itself be subjected to a changing flux when the circuit were opened or closed. There is therefore a certain inductive effect associated with any circuit, even if no special inductance coil forms part of the circuit. The situation is analogous to that of resistance: Since there is no resistanceless conducting wire, there is always some R associated with any circuit, just as there is always some L.

When the current of Fig. 5.21 has reached its maximum value, point F on the graph of part (c), then there is, of course, no further change in magnetic flux and hence no induced EMF.

Now what if the switch is opened, as shown in part (b) of the figure? The energy that has been stored in the magnetic field associated with the circuit will now act to maintain the status quo, that is, to keep the current going. This means that the induced EMF this time, quite in accord with Lenz's law, acts to prolong the current for a short time. The primary current, to all intents and purposes, is zero as soon as the switch is opened, but the induced current is not, and therefore we have, for a short interval, some current in spite of the open switch; and sometimes this current is seen to arc across the air gap between the switch contact points as they separate.

In the case of both increasing and decreasing primary current, the self-induced EMF is given by the expression

$$\mathscr{E} = - L \frac{\Delta i}{\Delta t}, \tag{5.4}$$

where $\mathscr{E}$ is the self-induced EMF, L is the inductance of the circuit, and $\Delta i/\Delta t$ is the rate of change of the primary current.

Note the similarity between Eqs. (5.3) and (5.4). What we want to reemphasize by drawing the reader's attention to this similarity is that in any induced EMF the really crucial element is the $\Delta i/\Delta t$ (or for those versed in calculus, the limiting value of this ratio, that is, the di/dt). And again we further emphasize: This is quite as we would expect, given Faraday's law.

Although the growth curve of the current, from E to F in Fig. 5.21(c), is quite simple to calculate if we know R, L, and $\mathscr{E}$, the decay curve, from G to H, poses greater problems. This is so because a new and indeterminate circuit resistance is added in series when the switch is open. After all, one way of looking at an opening in a circuit, when no arcing is going on, is to consider the resistance as infinite. The situation is quite complicated. For example, there will be momentary dielectric breakdown, sparking, current oscillations, and electromagnetic radiation. However, although it is not possible to determine the precise nature of the current decay curve, we can say (see Fig. 5.21) that the decay curve is much steeper than the current growth curve.

The fact that arcing across a switch gap does take place in many instances points to an interesting fact, and one which is quite in accordance with the appropriate theoretical analysis: The potential difference across the switch immediately upon "break" is considerably higher than the EMF $\mathscr{E}$. You may recall, for example, that in our earlier discussion of the spark or sphere gap voltmeter (Section 2.4) we noted that a very high voltage was required to produce even a very short spark in air. Well, this high voltage across the opening switch is the momentarily self-induced EMF which appears as the magnetic field of the circuit collapses. In many electrical circuits special by-pass arrangements are provided when the switch is opened so that the energy of the magnetic field is absorbed in a resistor in the form of heat rather than in a high-voltage arc, which is not only possibly dangerous but certainly results in the melting or pitting of the switch contacts.

This way of producing a high voltage by making and breaking a low-voltage circuit has been used by the automobile industry for years in the ignition coil that provides the high voltage which makes spark plugs in the engine spark. And, of course, the induction coil was the chief source of high voltage in the early x-ray days. The gas-filled x-ray tube shown in operation on the frontispiece of this book is operated by this means. In fact, if you look carefully at the picture you will see the actual induction coil.

AC Behavior

If we refer again to the graph in Fig. 5.21(c), we see that two steady-state conditions exist: steady current, i_{max}, from F to G, and steady zero current from H onward. In the two regions described there is therefore no further concern with self induction. Suppose, however, that we had a system in which the switch was continually being opened and closed; or that instead of a battery (that is, a DC source of EMF) we had an AC source of EMF. Then we could never neglect the matter of inductance. That is, in AC circuits the inductance of the circuit is continually impeding the change in the current impressed by the source of EMF. For this reason, in AC circuit analysis, the inductance of the circuit, just like the resistance, needs always to be considered.

The actual quantity of "opposition" due to an inductance L is called the *inductive reactance* and is noted by X_L. Both the resistance R and the inductive reactance X_L of an AC circuit are part of the overall opposition to current change in AC known as the *impedance, Z*. We shall discuss this matter further in Chapter 6.

QUESTIONS

1. a) State Faraday's law of electro-magnetic induction.
    b) Describe any simple experiment which illustrates the above principle.

2. Refer to Fig. 5.22.
    a) If the conductor is moved as shown, is there a current induced? If so, in what direction through the galvanometer, from x to y, or y to x?
    b) If the conductor is moved horizontally parallel to the magnetic flux lines, is there a current induced? If so, in what direction?

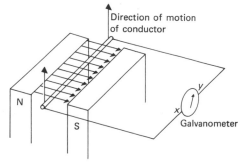

FIG. 5.22. An experimental setup, similar to that of Fig. 5.1, for producing an induced EMF.

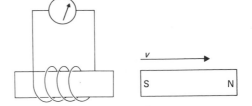

FIG. 5.23. Bar magnet being moved away at speed *v* from a coil with a ferromagnetic core.

    c) If the conductor is moved in the direction exactly opposite to that shown, is there a current induced? If so, in what direction?

3. Refer to Fig. 5.23.
    a) What is the direction of the current induced in the coil?
    b) What principle or law did you employ to arrive at the answer for (a) above?
    c) What is the magnetic polarity at the left end of the coil?
    d) What would happen to the induced current if the ferromagnetic core were removed?
    e) What would happen to the induced current if the speed of motion of the bar magnet were increased?
    f) What would happen to the EMF induced in the coil if the number of windings were doubled?
    g) What would happen to the induced current if the magnet were kept at rest and the coil were moved to the left with the same speed *v*?

4. For the case of mutual induction between two coils, indicate any two means by which the EMF induced in the secondary might be increased.

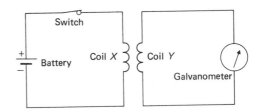

FIG. 5.24. Mutual induction.

5. Refer to Fig. 5.24.
    a) Which coil is the primary and which is the secondary?
    b) What is the direction of the current in the primary when the switch is closed?
    c) What is the direction of the current in the secondary just after the switch is closed?

6. Refer to Fig. 5.25.
    a) Is this device, as shown, a motor or a generator?
    b) Is this a DC or an AC device?

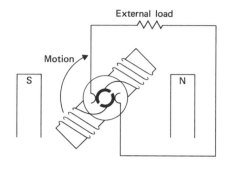

FIG. 5.25. A device such as is often employed in elementary physics experiments.

    c) At the instant shown, with the motion indicated, what is the direction of the current through the external load?

7. What is the frequency of the AC generated by the alternator of Fig. 5.13 if it rotates at 1200 rpm (revolutions per minute)?

8. Sketch a waveform diagram (voltage as a function of time) for the case of an AC generator producing a single-phase sinusoidal EMF of maximum 120 volts and frequency of 60 cycles per second. Place the appropriate numerical values on the axes.

9. a) Describe what is meant by eddy currents.
    b) Would eddy currents be more readily produced in iron or in copper? Explain.

10. Distinguish between the terms self induction and mutual induction. Employ diagrams.

11. What type of motor is employed to rotate the anode in an x-ray machine? Explain how this motor works.

12. What important component of x-ray circuitry depends on mutual induction?

13. a) Sketch the circuit, and a graph of the current as a function of time, when the switch on a simple DC circuit, containing a resistor, is closed.
    b) Repeat (a) for the case in which an inductance coil is added in series to the resistor. On the graph, use the same scale for current and for time as in case (a).

14. If the speed of rotation of a generator were increased, what, if anything, would happen to (a) the maximum EMF produced; (b) the frequency of the EMF?
    c) What fundamental physical principle or principles is/are employed to arrive at the answers above?

15. Sketch the graph of a sinusoidal voltage as a function of time for: (a) single-phase AC; (b) two-phase AC; (c) three-phase AC.
    d) With one pair of magnetic poles, how many separate armature coils are required to produce three-phase AC? How would these armature coils be oriented?
    e) Which of the above types of AC find use in x-ray equipment?

SUGGESTED READING

BEISER, ARTHUR, *Modern Technical Physics*. Reading, Mass.: Addison-Wesley, 1966. Chapter 27 on Electromagnetic Induction provides brief supplementary reading on the matter of induced EMF's. The expression for AC varying periodically as a sine or cosine function is derived from the concept of the force on electric charges moving through a magnetic field. No calculus required.

FEYNMAN, RICHARD P., ROBERT B. LEIGHTON, and MATTHEW SANDS, *The Feynman Lectures on Physics*, Volume II. Reading, Mass.: Addison-Wesley, 1964. The ten pages comprising Chapter 16 of these lectures by one of the foremost theoretical physicists of our time present an exceedingly lucid, nonmathematical treatment of induced currents, including the induction motor. Although mathematically the rest of this book is considerably beyond the level used in our text, this one chapter is well worth reading by anyone at any level of physics.

MARCUS, ABRAHAM, *Basic Electricity*. Englewood Cliffs, N.J.: Prentice-Hall, 1958. Chapter 11 on Mechanical Generators offers much more detail than the discussion in our text. Practically no mathematics is employed, but nevertheless excellent descriptive passages and figures give a valuable insight into the generation of electric current.

RICHARDS, J. A., JR., F. W. SEARS, M. R. WEHR, and M. W. ZEMANSKY, *Modern University Physics*. Reading, Mass.: Addison-Wesley, 1960. Chapter 27 presents some of the topics of our chapter at a higher level. Calculus is used. Recommended for the advanced student.

CHAPTER 6

Pulsating and Alternating Currents

Now that we have looked at the more basic elements of electricity—that is, static electricity, direct currents, magnetic effects, and induced currents—let us turn to that more complicated development which presently predominates in the generation, transmission, distribution, and ultimate use of electricity: alternating currents, or AC.

In these days, the power supplied to the hospital and ultimately to the x-ray machine is almost invariably AC power, and it is likely to remain so for many years to come. In fact, even if DC appears more and more in the future, its use will probably be for long-range transmission, while the advantages of easy voltage changes, up or down, of AC seem to mark it as generally the more suitable way to distribute power to the users.

Not that AC was the first to be employed in commercial power distribution. This distinction goes to DC, which was employed by the great American inventor, Edison (whom we mentioned earlier in connection with the development of the electric generator), who put electric lighting on the map when he arranged to light the main street of Menlo Park, New Jersey, on New Year's Eve, 1879.

The great difficulty facing the electrical industry in the late nineteenth century was the considerable loss they encountered when they had to transport the electricity over wires. Since it was found that electricity could be transported more efficiently at high voltages, as we noted in Section 3.7, Nikola Tesla

(1856–1943), a Croatian-American electrical engineer, developed transformers which could boost electricity to high voltages for transmission and then lower the voltage for relatively safe usage. Transformers, of course, as we can gather from the discussion in Chapter 5, do not work on steady DC; they are AC devices. Hence there actually developed a bitter personal struggle between Edison and Tesla on the subject of DC versus AC. In the final analysis, the telling point was transport efficiency and AC won out. A rather sad sidelight of this whole issue is that in 1912 the Nobel prize committee intended to award the Nobel prize in physics jointly to Edison and Tesla, but the latter refused to be associated with Edison. Consequently in the end the prize went to a Swedish inventor.

Next we must mention Steinmetz. In the early 1920's there was a common saying, half joke and half serious, that only seven people in the world understood Einstein's theory of special relativity. Charles Proteus Steinmetz (1865–1923), a European who emigrated to the United States, was one of the seven. Steinmetz, a phenomenal electrical genius, worked out in detail the theory of AC circuitry, using complex numbers (a system in which appears that seemingly mysterious number, $\sqrt{-1}$). This work firmly established the victory of AC over DC.

Although for the x-ray machine we like to get the high voltages available through AC, ultimately we prefer a direct current through the actual x-ray tube.

This process of changing AC to DC is called *rectification.* The important figure in this area is the Englishman, Sir John A. Fleming (1849–1945), who at one time served as a consultant to Edison. Fleming's valve tube of 1904, based on an earlier discovery by Edison, is a device which, roughly speaking, allows AC to enter but permits only DC to leave. We shall discuss this rectifying tube in some detail in Section 7.6.

Certain solid materials, certain crystals, for example, have long been known to perform rectification functions similar to those of Fleming's valve. Barrier layer rectifiers, such as copper–copper oxide and iron–selenium, have been developed. And more recently the work of W. B. Shockley, J. Bardeen, and W. H. Brattain of the Bell Telephone Laboratories showed that germanium crystals containing traces of certain impurities are better rectifiers than many of the crystals earlier employed. These three physicists were awarded the Nobel Prize in physics in 1956 for their discovery that certain combinations of these new solid-state rectifiers could do all that a radio tube could do. That is, they discovered what is now called a *transistor.*

However, for the moment we shall not be concerned with transistors. In this chapter our main interest lies in the fact that solid-state rectifiers are more and more replacing valves, or tubes as they are known in North America, even in the high-voltage rectifying circuitry of some x-ray machines.

6.1 SOME BASIC IDEAS OF VARYING CURRENTS

In the previous chapter we touched on some of the basic ideas of AC. Let us briefly review some of the pertinent basics and add to them. We shall consider the "why" of AC.

Advantages of AC

We discussed I^2R losses in conducting cables in Section 3.7, where we pointed out that it was advantageous to transmit power at high voltages. With step-up transformers, one can achieve this advantage of reducing I^2R heating losses in the cables. However, transformers do not work with DC, but rather with AC. Therein lies the major advantage of AC.

Another point in favor of AC hinges on the induction motor that we talked about in Section 5.3. This motor requires AC. In general, it may also be said that AC motors are probably cheaper, and less subject to maintenance troubles, than DC motors.

Finally, we should add that AC, albeit at much higher frequency than for normal power requirements, is imperative for modern communication. Radio waves, for example, are generated by a rapidly alternating current in a transmission antenna.

AC Terminology

By now it should be amply clear to the reader that AC refers to a current which is periodically changing direction. It therefore makes no sense to assign a current direction in AC circuits, such as we have done earlier in connection with DC circuits.

Although in the true sense AC refers to alternating currents in general, without restriction as to how the current varies, we shall use the term AC to refer to a sinusoidally varying current. In other words, we refer not to currents represented by the waveforms (b) and (c) of Fig. 6.1, but only to that labeled (a). We are concerned with sinusoidally varying current because, as our previous discussions on the generation of electricity have made plausible, the voltage supplied by the electric power company

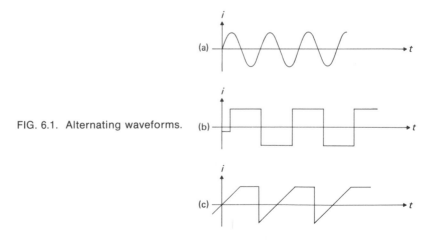

FIG. 6.1. Alternating waveforms.

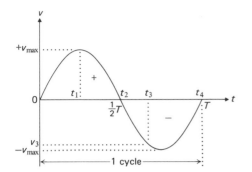

FIG. 6.2. Sinusoidally varying alternating voltage of the form $v = v_{max} \sin 2\pi\, ft$. The total time for one cycle is the period T.

is essentially sinusoidal; the voltage is of the form

$$v = v_{max} \sin 2\pi\, ft. \tag{6.1}$$

In Fig. 6.2 we show such a voltage. Let us now consider some of the relevant terms with reference to this figure. First of all, the figure shows the value of the voltage at certain instants after an arbitrarily assigned time zero. For example, at t_1, the voltage has its maximum value v_{max}; at t_2 the voltage is zero; at t_3 the voltage is some negative value v_3; at t_4 the voltage is again zero.

The value of the voltage at t_1, that is, its maximum or peak value, is also known as the *amplitude* of the voltage. In general, the maximum value of any periodic waveform is called the amplitude.

As we implied in Section 5.2, the total time taken for the voltage to go from any given value to the succeeding same value, that is, the time required for one complete cycle of voltages, is called the *period T*. We have also mentioned before that there is a definite relationship between the frequency f and the period T. In the case of the 60-cycle voltage common in North America, the period for one complete cycle is $\frac{1}{60}$ sec. A common European frequency is 50 sec^{-1}. The period in this case is $\frac{1}{50}$ sec. In general, the relationship between frequency and period is

$$f = \frac{1}{T}, \tag{6.2}$$

where f is the frequency (expressed per second, that is, with the unit sec^{-1}) and T is the period (expressed in seconds).

An AC voltage or current waveform may also be graphically displayed by using the abscissa to indicate angle rather than time, as shown in Fig. 6.3. This is not surprising because, after all, a quantity that is a sine function (that is, a quantity that varies sinusoidally) must vary as some reference angle changes because the value of the sine of an angle naturally depends on the angle. If we look at Eq. (6.1) and write

$$\sin \theta = \sin 2\pi\, ft,$$

then

$$\theta = 2\pi\, ft. \tag{6.3}$$

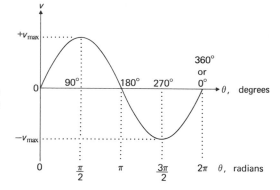

FIG. 6.3. Voltage as a function of the angle θ, where $v = v_{max} \sin \theta$; or, since $\theta = 2\pi ft$, $v = v_{max} \sin 2\pi ft$.

Since 2, π, and f are constants, we can readily see that when the value of t is changed, the value of θ changes in accordance with t. In other words, an abscissa in terms of θ rather than in terms of t makes good sense.

Now compare Fig. 6.3 with Fig. 6.2. When $t = 0$, then, from Eq. 6.3, $\theta = 0$. And the sine of zero degrees is zero; hence we note that $v = 0$ at $t = 0$ and at $\theta = 0$. Next we must draw on our knowledge of trigonometry to the extent of realizing that the maximum possible value of sine is one, and this maximum value is reached when $\theta = 90°$ (or $\pi/2$ radians). Now when $t = \frac{1}{4}T$, we note, again from Eq. (6.3):

$$\theta = 2\pi f \tfrac{1}{4}T = (\pi/2)fT.$$

But from Eq. (6.2) we have $f = 1/T$; hence

$$\theta = \pi/2.$$

In other words, we expect $v = v_{max}$ when $t = \frac{1}{4}T$ or $\theta = \pi/2$, as shown in the two figures concerned. In electricity, this angle θ is sometimes referred to as the *electrical angle*, or *phase angle*. Pursuing the same type of discussion for the second half of the period T will yield the appropriate voltage, time, and electrical angle relationship for the negative alternation of the cycle.

In the case of the simple generator of Fig. 5.9, this electrical angle may, of course, be directly considered as the angle of rotation of the loop between the magnetic poles.

At this point, you might ask why all this fuss about angles. The fact is that in AC it turns out that the current may not be at its maximum value through some circuit element when the voltage is at its maximum. This important fact is expressed in terms of the electrical angle by saying that the voltage and the current are out of phase by so many degrees, or radians. In Fig. 6.4, we see the AC case of the voltage across, and current through, an inductance coil (see Section 6.2). Note that the voltage and current are out of phase by 90° ($\pi/2$ radians). Since the current reaches its highest value after the voltage, we say that the current lags the voltage by 90°, where 90° is the phase angle.

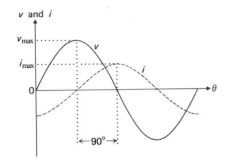

FIG. 6.4. Voltage and current phase relationship in a purely inductive circuit. The current lags the voltage by 90° ($\pi/2$ radians).

Recall also that the concept of phase and phase difference in voltages was encountered in the discussion of the induction motor in Section 5.3.

Average Voltage and Current Values

We have just noted a peculiar fact regarding AC. Unlike DC voltages and currents, AC voltages and currents can be out of phase. Another problem of AC, of course (of no concern in steady DC), is the fact that the question arises as to what is meant by a given current, or voltage value. After all, over a cycle this value might be anything from zero to its maximum positive value to its maximum negative value and back to zero. Since there is an infinity of instantaneous current values between $-i_{max}$ and $+i_{max}$, the instantaneous value of a current is obviously of little general use. Take an average value, you say. Over what time interval? A complete cycle. Good. That makes sense. Now let us take this average over a complete cycle. A moment's reflection on the nature of the sine wave form indicates that for each positive value of the current there exists in a cycle a negative value of equal magnitude. This means that the average over the cycle is zero. Thus the average in this case is hardly very informative.

Now it is possible to employ some special averages which might serve some purpose. For example, if we took the average of the absolute values of the current—that is, the magnitudes only, without concerning ourselves with the concept of positive and negative—then we would get a nonzero average. But there is a more significant average. It is called the *effective value*, and it is this average that is most generally employed.

The effective value of an alternating current is that value which would produce heat in a resistor at the same rate as a direct current of the same numerical value. In other words, an AC current of 15 amp, effective value, would give the same heat in a toaster as would a DC current of 15 amp applied to the same toaster for the same period of time. Now it turns out that this effective value is a special kind of average of the alternating current. We recall the troublesome aspect of averaging over an AC cycle because of equal positive and negative values. Well, one way of obviating this difficulty is to square the current; then there are no negative values. Then we could take the average of the squared values of the current through one cycle, and then take the square root of this average. What have we done? Taken the square root of the average, or mean, value of the square

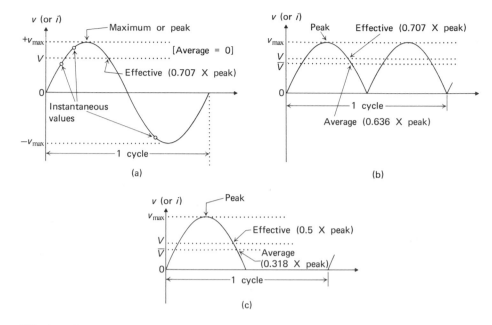

FIG. 6.5. Peak, average, and effective (RMS) values of voltage (or current) for sinusoidal AC (a), and pulsating DC (b) and (c). (a) AC. (b) Full-wave rectified AC. (c) Half-wave rectified AC.

of the current. We call this value the *RMS value*, or the root-mean-square value. This special average, the RMS value, is also the effective value of the alternating current.

What the RMS, or effective, value of an alternating current is in terms of its maximum value, of course, depends on the waveform. In the case of sinusoidally varying AC, we find that the effective value, which we shall simply label I, is given by

$$I_{\text{RMS}} \equiv I_{\text{eff}} \equiv I = 0.707 \, i_{\text{max}}.$$

(A derivation of this relationship can be found in the book by Beiser, listed in the Suggested Reading at the end of this chapter.)

If we employ a certain type of average of current values, then it seems reasonable that we ought to employ the same type of average value of voltage. We refer to the effective (or RMS) voltage V, given by

$$V_{\text{RMS}} \equiv V_{\text{eff}} \equiv V = 0.707 \, v_{\text{max}}. \tag{6.4}$$

This means that the voltage at an outlet, if quoted at 120 volts, is 120 volts RMS. In other words, the actual maximum voltage appearing across the outlet is

$$v_{\text{max}} = \frac{V}{0.707} = \left(\frac{120}{0.707}\right) \text{ volts} = 170 \text{ volts.}$$

Now it is almost safe to say that, except in the x-ray world, whenever one deals with AC one always implies that the voltages and currents given are effective, or RMS, values. We shall shortly encounter the exceptions in the x-ray department especially when we note what is meant by kV and mA. But before we do, let us summarize the peak, average, and effective values for sinusoidal waveforms in Fig. 6.5. Note the nonzero ordinary average in the case of rectified AC, which is then really no longer AC but pulsating DC.

kV and mA Values

Let us briefly review some of the symbols for current and voltage used to this point, and then deal with the usage of these terms and symbols in medical x-ray work. First of all, we recall that I and V were used in the early discussions of DC, at which time we were considering only the steady-state situation.

When we discussed transient behavior in Section 5.5, then we had to distinguish the steady-state current I from the instantaneous value of the current. At that point we introduced i, in accordance with general practice in the electrical field, where the lower-case letters apply to instantaneous values.

Then when we dealt with AC we used i and v for instantaneous values, and I and V for effective, or RMS, values. Sometimes one writes I_{eff} or I_{RMS} to emphasize that the RMS value is meant; $\bar{I}$ and $\bar{V}$ are the symbols generally used for average values.

Now in the x-ray department, it is common practice to speak of kV. However, by this is not meant the RMS value of the kilovoltage, but rather the peak value. This practice follows from the fact that the peak, or maximum, voltage is of considerable interest in that it sets the upper limit of the energy of the x-rays produced. Sometimes, instead of kV, the symbol kVp is employed. In either case, the meaning, unless specified otherwise, is the same: the peak value of the voltage, in kilovolts.

Not only does kV *not* refer to RMS values, but neither does mA. By mA one means the average value, in milliamperes, of a pulsating DC, as shown in Fig. 6.5 (b and c). The reason for this lies essentially in the type of meter employed to indicate the current through the x-ray tube. This meter, the mA meter, responds to the average value of a pulsating DC. Thus an exposure at 100 mA and 70 kV means that the maximum voltage across the x-ray tube is 70 kilovolts, and the average of the pulsating DC current through the tube is 100 milliamperes.

Other than kV and mA, however, voltages and currents quoted elsewhere in the x-ray department, and the hospital in general, will be RMS values. For example, if a fuse needs replacing, one needs to know the current for which the fuse is designed. Say it is 15 amp. This means 15 amp RMS. Then, as stated before, if an outlet is marked 120 volts, this means 120 volts RMS. And if a 240-volt outlet is required to operate a large mobile x-ray machine, this means 240 volts RMS.

6.2   AC AND OHM'S LAW

We shall consider here a series AC circuit, as shown in Fig. 6.6(a). Thorough analysis of such a circuit, and more complicated ones, is beyond the scope of this book. But we do want to indicate a few notions about AC circuits so that we can draw on these notions in subsequent discussions of x-ray tubes and circuits. In this perusal of AC circuits, we shall draw heavily on earlier discussions of DC (Chapter 3), of capacitors (Section 2.6), and of self induction (Section 5.5).

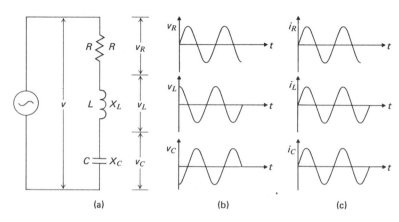

FIG. 6.6.   AC series circuit.   (a) The circuit consisting of a resistance R, an inductance L, and a capacitance C. The impeding effect on the current is given by the resistance R, the inductive reactance X_L, and the capacitive reactance X_C.   (b) Voltage-time graph, showing the phase differences among the voltages across R, L, and C.   (c) The current is the same throughout the circuit and is in phase with the voltage across R.

The complications of AC, as implied earlier, arise from the continuous variation of the applied EMF. A knowledge of calculus and complex numbers (recall the reference to Steinmetz and $\sqrt{-1}$ in the introduction to the present chapter) is required for a rigorous analysis of AC. However, readers who wish to obtain more insight into AC circuit analysis than we shall provide here can do so to a degree without these mathematical sophistications by consulting the book by Beiser listed at the end of this chapter.

Inductive Reactance

Unlike the case with steady DC, opposition to AC current does not depend on the circuit resistance alone. Although a resistor impedes the flow of alternating current and thereby dissipates, in the form of heat, some of the electrical energy which passes through it, an inductor, while also impeding the current flow, does not consume any electrical energy.

As stated in Section 5.5, the opposition to an AC current offered by an inductor stems from the self-induced back EMF produced by the very current itself, quite in accord with Faraday's law. This self-induced back EMF is what constitutes the voltage drop across an inductor, which is given by

$$V_L = IX_L,\qquad(6.5)$$

where V_L is the RMS voltage across the inductor, of inductance L, I is the RMS current through the inductor, and X_L is the inductive reactance, the opposition to current flow analogous to R in the case of a resistor, and like R, measured in ohms.

The inductive reactance in turn is given by

$$X_L = 2\pi f L,\qquad(6.6)$$

where f is the frequency of the AC and L is the inductance of the inductor. The unit for L is the henry.

As we pointed out earlier in Section 5.5, increasing the number of turns of the induction coil increases L, and using a ferromagnetic core vastly increases L over its value with an air core. Since such a coil significantly impedes alternating current, the term *choke* or *choke coil* is sometimes employed, in the sense that the inductor "chokes" the current. (See Section 8.3 for the use of a choke in an x-ray machine.)

Further, since the opposition to current flow depends on magnetic flux changes, it seems reasonable to expect the back EMF, and hence the opposition—that is, the inductive reactance—to increase with increased current frequency, as is shown by Eq. (6.6). Readers who don't find this comment rather obvious at this point might do well to reread Section 5.1.

So the inductor opposes an AC current. But why does it not consume energy as a resistor does? In the first place, we must make clear that here we are talking about an ideal inductor, that is, one which has no resistance whatsoever. (In practice this is obviously not quite the case, since even copper wire, as we have noted earlier, has some electrical resistance.) Now what happens in the case of the inductor is that as the current in the circuit is growing, energy is taken up by the inductor in establishing a magnetic field. But this energy is not dissipated in the form of heat, as in a resistor; rather the energy is stored in the magnetic field. Now when the current decays the magnetic field associated with the inductor collapses and the associated energy goes back into the circuit: the collapsing magnetic field opposes the decay of the current by inducing a current in the same direction as the decaying current. Thus ideally no energy is consumed by the inductor, or the inductive component of a circuit, even though this inductive component impedes the current.

Inductors, as non-energy-consuming current limiters, are extensively employed in the starting circuits of present-day fluorescent lights.

Also the fact that the inductive reactance, defined by Eq. (6.6), can be varied by changing the nature of the core of an inductor, has been employed in mA control in x-ray machines. Consider a circuit such as the one in Fig. 6.7. With a given input voltage, or EMF, the current in the

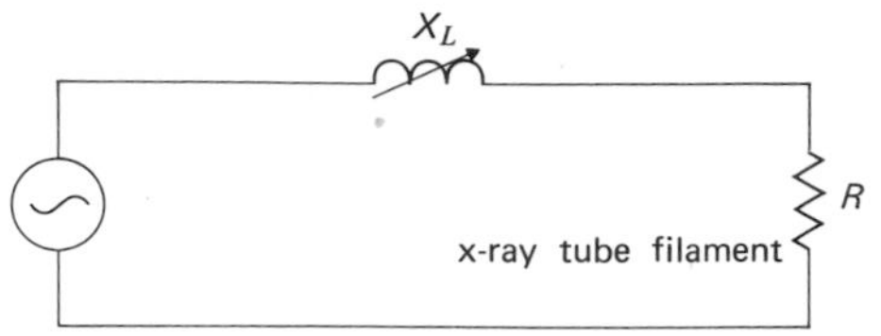

X_L

FIG. 6.7. Controlling the temperature of the x-ray tube filament by means of a variable inductor.

R

x-ray tube filament

circuit depends on all the current opposition, that is, both the resistance R, and the inductive reactance X_L. If X_L is decreased, the current in the circuit is increased; therefore the heating rate in the x-ray tube filament, resistance R, is increased and thus the filament temperature is increased. Since the x-ray tube mA depends on the filament temperature (we'll discuss this more fully in Section 7.2), decreasing X_L by turning a knob which slightly retracts the ferromagnetic core of the inductor has the effect of increasing the mA. It is thus possible to achieve a continuous mA control which itself consumes no energy.

Nowadays, however, it is more usual to find a stepwise mA control employing a rheostat, as discussed in Section 3.6. After all, the amount of energy consumed by the resistors involved is not exorbitant and resistors are smaller, more rugged, and probably cheaper to construct than inductors.

One other point regarding the inductance of an AC circuit has to do with phase difference. We have already alluded to this fact in Fig. 6.4, to which we now refer again. Recall that the voltage across an inductor is the self-induced or back EMF. This, as we know, is greatest when $\Delta\Phi/\Delta t$, the magnetic flux change, is greatest. The $\Delta\Phi/\Delta t$ is, of course, greatest when the magnetic field change $\Delta B/\Delta t$ is greatest, and this in turn is greatest when $\Delta i/\Delta t$ is greatest. Now a sinusoidally varying current has its greatest rate of change as the current is changing from positive to negative values, or vice versa; that is, $\Delta i/\Delta t$ is greatest when i is zero. This means that at the instant the current is zero the voltage across the inductor is already at a maximum, that v has reached its maximum ahead of i. And conversely, by the time the current is at its maximum, the voltage has dropped to zero. The current reaches its maximum a quarter of a period, or 90°, after the voltage. The current and voltage of Eq. (6.5) are out of phase.

Now the current and voltage in the case of a resistor are *in* phase. Furthermore, the current in the circuit is everywhere the same; that is, quite plausibly, the electric charge motion is the same throughout the circuit. This means that therefore the voltage across R and the voltage across L in Fig. 6.6 are out of phase. This is a new and different concept not encountered in our DC studies. And it means that voltages in an AC circuit cannot be added by the straightforward arithmetic approach we used in DC. However, we shall not go into the appropriate mathematical procedures for AC in this text. Students who want to acquaint themselves with some of the quantitative procedures for AC are referred again to the book by Beiser listed at the end of this chapter.

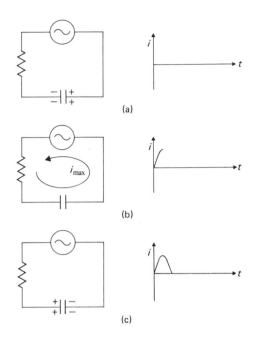

FIG. 6.8. The capacitor as an AC circuit element. (a) Capacitor charged, current at zero. (b) Capacitor fully discharged, current at maximum. (c) Capacitor now charged in opposite direction, current at zero, and about to start in direction opposite to that shown in (b).

Capacitive Reactance

What we said in our discussion of the capacitor in Section 2.6 points to the fact that, in the case of DC, once the capacitor is fully charged no more current flows. The capacitor then acts like an open circuit. But what if, before the capacitor is fully charged, the current direction were reversed? The situation would then be as shown in Fig. 6.8. In other words, for AC the capacitor does not yield the effect of an open circuit. AC can flow with a capacitor in the circuit, but the current is impeded to some extent by the capacitor.

The impeding effect of a capacitor on an alternating current is due to the reverse potential difference which appears across it as the electric charge builds up on the capacitor plates. This potential difference, or potential drop, affects the total circuit current just as the potential drop across a resistor does. The impeding effect of a capacitor on the current is called the *capacitive reactance*. The voltage across the capacitor is given by

$$V_C = IX_C, \tag{6.7}$$

where V_C is the RMS voltage across the capacitor, of capacitance C, I is the RMS current, and X_C is the capacitive reactance which, like the resistance and the inductive reactance, is measured in ohms.

The capacitive reactance in turn is given by

$$X_C = \frac{1}{2\pi fC}, \tag{6.8}$$

where f is the frequency of the AC and C is the capacitance in farads, as defined by

$$C = \frac{q}{v} \, . \tag{2.6}$$

(Note that the instantaneous voltage, applicable to a given charge q, has been designated now with a lower-case v in accordance with the symbol usage established in this AC discussion.)

   Let us see if the inverse dependence of X_C on f and C seems plausible. If C is large, then Eq. (2.6) shows that for a given charge q on the capacitor plates, the voltage is smaller than in the case of a small C.

   Further, if the frequency is large, or high, then the period is short, each cycle is brief, and less charge is deposited on the respective capacitor plates in each half of the cycle than if the frequency is low. Hence, according to Eq. (2.6), with a given capacitance the implication is that the current-impeding voltage is smaller, and the opposition to current is less. We say that capacitive reactance is less.

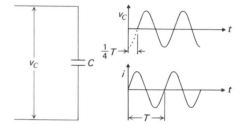

FIG. 6.9. The current into and out of a pure capacitor with an AC voltage applied leads the voltage across the capacitor by one-fourth of a period.

   Note that the reverse potential difference, the voltage opposing the current, is at a maximum when the capacitor has accumulated all the charge it will during the half cycle concerned. This is another point we can see by perusal of Eq. (2.6): The voltage has its maximum value when the charge q has its maximum value. But at the instant that q has reached its maximum value, the current reaches zero. The current was at its maximum or peak value earlier when the capacitor was uncharged and the voltage across the capacitor was consequently zero. In other words, the current is out of phase with the voltage across the capacitor. The current leads the voltage by a quarter of a period, or a phase angle of 90°, as shown in Fig. 6.9.

   Like the ideal inductor, the ideal capacitor consumes no energy. The energy stored in the electric field of the capacitor when it is fully charged is returned to the circuit during the discharging process.

Impedance

Since a resistor, an inductor, and a capacitor all oppose an alternating current, it is customary to speak of the combined current-impeding effects of these three types of circuit elements. The resistance R, the inductive reactance X_L, and the capacitive reactance X_C together form what is termed the *impedance*, Z, of the AC circuit.

In the series circuit of Fig. 6.6 the impedance is given by

$$Z = \sqrt{R^2 + (X_L - X_C)^2}, \tag{6.9}$$

where Z, on the basis of the units for R, X_L, and X_C, is given in ohms.

The apparently peculiar addition format for these three current-impeding effects arises from the fact that the voltages across R, L, and C are out of phase. The voltage across L leads the voltage across R by 90°, which is in phase with the current, and the voltage across C lags by 90°, as shown in Fig. 6.6(b).

Perusal of Eq. (6.9) shows that when the term $(X_L - X_C)$ is zero, either because neither an inductor nor a capacitor is in the circuit, or because the inductive reactance is equal to the capacitive reactance, the impedance is simply equal to R. The circuit is purely resistive.

Ohm's Law for AC

We are now able to write Ohm's law in the way it is applicable to AC:

$$V = IZ, \tag{6.10}$$

where V is the RMS voltage, I is the RMS current, and Z is the impedance, in ohms, of that part of the circuit to which the V refers. Note again that because of phase differences the voltages across various parts of an AC circuit do not add arithmetically to yield the total voltage. Moreover, it is possible to have a voltage across an inductor or a capacitor much higher than the EMF or input voltage to the circuit.

6.3 POWER IN AC CIRCUITS

In Section 3.7 we showed that for DC the power consumed by any circuit elements, or the circuit as a whole, is given by

$$P = VI. \tag{3.10}$$

This expression is inadequate for AC. Why?

Real and Apparent Power

Let us consider an inductor. It consumes no energy, and hence no power. Yet there is an AC voltage across the inductor and there is an AC current. That is, $VI \neq 0$ and yet $P = 0$.

How could we modify Eq. (3.10) to obtain one which gives reasonable results? What would make sense would be to multiply VI by some factor F, which factor would be equal to unity for a resistor and zero for an inductor and/or a capacitor. Because if we write

$$P = VIF,$$

this reduces to $P = VI$ for a resistor ($F = 1$) and $P = 0$ for an inductor and/or a capacitor ($F = 0$). And that seems to make sense.

What must F be? If

$$F = R/Z,$$

we have achieved our purpose. And it turns out that analysis from first principles does indeed yield such an expression for AC power. It is usually written

$$P = VI \cos \theta, \tag{6.11}$$

where P is the power in watts, V is the RMS voltage, and I the RMS current.

Power Factor

The expression $\cos \theta$ of Eq. (6.11) is what we called F before. It is the power factor, in which the angle θ refers to the electrical or phase angle between the voltage and the current. In other words,

$$\cos \theta = R/Z, \tag{6.12}$$

where R and Z are the resistance and the impedance of the circuit component or components involved. Let us just check. If the circuit is purely resistive, then in accord with Eq. (6.9), $Z = R$ and $\cos \theta = 1$, and hence $P = VI$; while if the circuit is, for example, purely capacitive, then $R = 0$ and $\cos \theta = 0$, and hence $P = 0$. Students familiar with trigonometry will see this point from the trigonometric viewpoint also. In a purely capacitive circuit the voltage and current are out of phase by 90°, that is, $\theta = 90°$, and hence $\cos \theta = \cos 90° = 0$. In practice the power factor may have any value between the limits of zero and 1, depending on the relative sizes of the resistance and the inductive and capacitive reactances.

Equation (3.10) is, however, also sometimes used in AC work. It is called the *apparent power,* in volt-amperes or kilovolt-amperes (kVA). The maximum power permissible with electrical devices is frequently stated in terms of kVA (see Section 6.4).

But of more import is the real power, in watts, as given by Eq. (6.11).

Although Eq. (3.10) is not generally applicable—that is, it does not yield the real power in both DC and AC cases—it is possible to rewrite this equation in a form that makes it generally applicable. We start with

$$P = VI \cos \theta, \tag{6.11}$$

where the power factor, $\cos \theta = R/Z$ (Eq. 6.12). Substituting this result in Eq. (6.11) yields

$$P = VI \frac{R}{Z}.$$

Now using Ohm's law for AC, Eq. (6.10), we can substitute for V in the above equation and obtain

$$P = (IZ)\, I\, \frac{R}{Z}$$

or

$$P = I^2 R. \tag{6.13}$$

This result is generally applicable for both AC and DC, providing that, in the case of AC, the RMS current value is employed. In fact, Eq. (6.13) is found to be identical in form to Eq. (3.11).

6.4 TRANSFORMERS

We shall see in Chapter 8, today's x-ray equipment is dependent on a considerable range of both fixed and variable voltages. The very process of delivering electrical energy to the hospital requires a variety of voltages, as we pointed out in the introduction to this chapter (see Fig. 6.10).

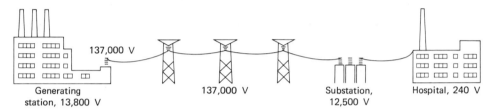

FIG. 6.10. Long-distance transmission of electrical energy. Transformers raise the voltage at the generator, lower it at city substations and again at residences or other points of usage. Large hospitals may have their own substations.

The devices that produce these ups and downs in voltages—that is, *transformers*—are probably the most widely used of all electro-magnetic apparatus. Quite sensibly, if the transformer steps up a voltage, it is called a *step-up transformer*. The transformer which provides the high voltage across the x-ray tube is a step-up transformer. Conversely, *step-down transformers* reduce the voltage. The transformer that provides the low voltage used in heating the x-ray tube filament is a step-down transformer. Most people nowadays have step-down transformers in the home to step down from 120 volts to the 6 or 12 volts employed in doorbell circuits.

Aside from stepping up or down a voltage, transformers may also be employed to insulate one circuit from another. This aspect is sometimes very useful in high-voltage circuitry, in that it permits one to insert a meter without directly connecting to the high-voltage part of the circuit.

Moreover, a device known as a *betatron*, which is finding common use in the production of x-rays for therapeutic purposes, may be described in terms of transformer action. However, we shall not discuss the betatron further in this text.

Transformer Operation

As we implied in our earlier discussion of mutual induction (Section 5.4), the transformer in its simplest form consists of two conductive coils wound on a common core of ferromagnetic material, as shown in Fig. 6.11.

Since the modern iron-core transformer is coming so close to perfection, we may analyze it, for many practical purposes, as though it were an

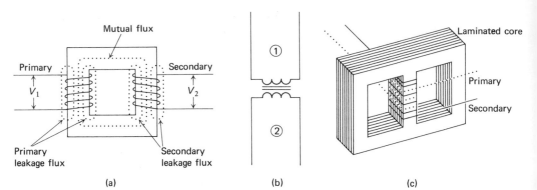

FIG. 6.11. Transformers. (a) Core-type transformer, showing magnetic flux leakage. (b) Circuit symbol for ferromagnetic core transformer. (See also Fig. 5.20.) (c) Shell-type transformer. Most transformers are of this type, having concentric windings to minimize flux leakage.

ideal transforming device. By *ideal*, we mean that essentially no energy losses occur.

Let us now consider the ideal transformer of Fig. 6.11(b), in the case in which the secondary circuit (2) is open; that is, there is no load.

On the primary side (1) we have, with AC applied, a $\Delta i_1/\Delta t$. This implies there is a $\Delta\Phi_1/\Delta t$, which in turn means an $\mathscr{E}_1$ in accordance with Faraday's law. $\mathscr{E}_1$ is the self-induced back EMF of the primary coil. Hence the terminal voltage, V_1, on the primary is given by

$$V_1 = \mathscr{E}_1 + I_1 R_1,$$

and if $R_1 \approx 0$, as we assume for the ideal transformer, then

$$V_1 = \mathscr{E}_1.$$

Using Eq. (5.1) for a coil of N_1 turns, we get

$$\mathscr{E}_1 = -N_1\,\Delta\Phi_1/\Delta t;$$

that is,

$$-\Delta\Phi_1/\Delta t = V_1/N_1. \tag{6.14}$$

Now we look at the secondary side. There is a flux change experienced by the secondary coil: We have a $\Delta\Phi_2/\Delta t$, that is, an $\mathscr{E}_2$, given for a coil of N_2 turns by

$$\mathscr{E}_2 = -N_2\,\Delta\Phi_2/\Delta t;$$

that is,

$$-\Delta\Phi_2/\Delta t = \mathscr{E}_2/N_2.$$

With no load on the secondary, of course, the EMF $\mathscr{E}_2$ induced in the coil is the same as V_2, the terminal voltage of the coil; that is,

$$\mathscr{E}_2 = V_2, \tag{6.15}$$

and hence

$$-\Delta\Phi_2/\Delta t = V_2/N_2. \tag{6.16}$$

Now since in an ideal transformer there is no flux leakage, the primary and the secondary coil both experience the same flux changes. We can equate the right-hand members of Eq. (6.14) and Eq. (6.16) because

$$\Delta\Phi_1/\Delta t = \Delta\Phi_2/\Delta t.$$

Thus we get

$$\frac{V_1}{N_1} = \frac{V_2}{N_2},$$

or, as is usually written,

$$\frac{V_1}{V_2} = \frac{N_1}{N_2}, \tag{6.17}$$

where (to review) V_1 and V_2 are the terminal voltages of the coils, that is, the voltages across the coils, and N_1 and N_2 are the number of turns in each. One should also add that the waveforms for V_1 and V_2 are identical.

We conclude the analysis by noting that the above result can be shown to be approximately true also if there is a load applied to the secondary, that is, if the secondary circuit is closed.

Note that Eq. (6.17) shows that the ratio of the primary to the secondary voltage is apparently independent of all parameters except the relative numbers of turns in the coils.

Continuing to lean on our proposition that transformers are very efficient, very close to ideal, we now say, therefore, that the power input to the primary must equal the power output of the secondary. Employing Eq. (6.11), the proper expression to use for AC, we see that there is the problem of the power factor to be considered. Fortunately it can be shown, by an analysis that is more thorough than ours, that the power factor for the secondary is the same as for the primary. This fact yields the convenient result that, since $P_1 = P_2$,

$$V_1 I_1 = V_2 I_2.$$

And since

$$V_1/V_2 = N_1/N_2,$$

we get

$$I_1/I_2 = N_2/N_1. \tag{6.18}$$

In other words, the currents are in inverse ratio to the respective numbers of turns.

So we see that the transformer is a sort of electrical "lever." With a lever, as you undoubtedly know, you can pry up a heavy weight for a short distance by applying a small force to the lever handle through a long distance. But the work (energy), and consequently power, that you get out of this procedure is the same as the work that you put into it.

Transformer Characteristics

An important characteristic of the transformer is that when the secondary circuit is open the primary carries a negligibly small current. This useful attribute derives from the fact that the large inductance of the primary chokes the current. However, because of the high permeability of the core, even the small primary gives sufficient flux. Hence the voltage of the secondary is not affected by the fact that the primary current is very small. The secondary terminals on open circuit are hence just like terminals of a battery on open circuit in the case of DC.

If the secondary is closed through a large impedance, little secondary current evolves. As the secondary impedance decreases, more secondary current appears. This means that more energy is taken by the secondary, a fact which is reflected by a proportionate increase in primary current. That is, the secondary current automatically regulates the primary current. But the two terminal voltages are not basically affected by these current changes. If an AC voltage of unvarying peak value is applied to the primary, the secondary will also maintain the "constant" AC output voltage; that is, except for the slight matter of the voltage or IR drop across the secondary winding. If the secondary current becomes sufficiently large, then obviously there will be a significant IR drop across the secondary coil; that is,

$$\mathscr{E}_2 = V_2 \tag{6.15}$$

no longer holds. The terminal voltage V_2 is now less than $\mathscr{E}_2$ by the amount of the IR drop across the secondary winding.

All this means that, even with a constant AC voltage input to the primary, the voltage output of the secondary will depend to some extent on the secondary current.

The above notion is referred to as *voltage regulation,* defined as

$$\text{Regulation} = \frac{\mathscr{E}_2 - V_2}{V_2}. \tag{6.19}$$

Usually the regulation is expressed in terms of percent. It is, as a rule, of the order of a few percent.

In radiography voltage regulation is important because we see that the kV across the tube will be less than that selected prior to the exposure. Moreover, the difference between selected and actual values will not remain constant, but will depend on the mA selected. With 50 mA the difference between $\mathscr{E}_2$ and V_2 ($\mathscr{E}_2$ being the open-circuit voltage, that is, the selected voltage, and V_2 being the terminal voltage, that is, the voltage across the tube on exposure) might well be negligible, but with 200 mA it would be significant.

As we mentioned in our discussion of line voltage drop (Section 3.5), most modern x-ray equipment is supplied with compensating circuitry such that, on exposure, one really obtains the actual kV intended, regardless of the mA selected. We shall discuss these considerations further in Section 8.2.

As we noted earlier, Eq. (6.17) shows that for an ideal transformer the voltage ratio is independent of the frequency of the AC. A good question to ask at this point is *why* that is so, because after all an induced EMF depends on a $\Delta\Phi/\Delta t$, which in turn is dependent on the frequency. One might consequently, on first thought, presume that therefore an increase in frequency would yield a larger secondary voltage. But this is not so; because if there is a fixed input voltage to the primary, then the back EMF induced in the primary must necessarily (except for the small IR drop across the primary) equal this input voltage. Certainly the back EMF of the primary cannot be larger than the input voltage. The principle of the conservation of energy suggests this. Therefore we sum up as follows: Increasing the frequency increases the impedance of the primary, thereby reducing the primary current, and hence the flux, sufficiently to balance the reduction of the time of the flux change. That is, although Δt decreases with increased frequency, $\Delta\Phi$ consequently also decreases so that $\Delta\Phi/\Delta t$ remains constant.

This analysis, of course, is based on the assumption that the transformer is an ideal transformer. It is quite true that, since actual transformers fall a little short of the ideal, there is indeed some change in the primary–secondary voltage ratio as the frequency changes. But the change is very small for the frequency variations of a few cycles/sec which one may get at a normal power outlet; negligibly small as far as x-ray machines are concerned.

Nevertheless, there is a so-called *frequency compensator* in the x-ray tube filament heating circuit. By now we realize, however, that this compensating component is not intended to compensate for voltage ratio changes in the filament heating transformer (see Section 8.3), but to keep the input voltage to this transformer constant by compensating for the impedance changes of circuit components preceding the filament transformer when frequency fluctuations occur.

Naturally we would expect every transformer to have some kind of limiting characteristics, depending on its construction. For example, a maximum voltage: Exceeding the specified voltage limits might result in a breakdown of the insulation or, more likely, in overheating which would ultimately cause the insulation to burn. These limits which specify the operating conditions a transformer is designed to meet are called its *rating*. The characteristics usually specified are frequency, primary and secondary voltages, and power in kVA. There are also different ratings depending on whether intermittent or continuous use is involved. When a transformer is to be used intermittently, the kVA rating can be much larger, because the specific heat of the metal parts is sufficient to provide the necessary short-term heat-absorbing capacity to prevent damagingly high temperatures. For example, a transformer rated to operate *continuously* at 100 kV and 25 mA may probably be safely employed for *momentary* use at 100 kV and 100 mA.

Finally let us consider efficiency. As we implied earlier, transformers may in practice achieve efficiencies of between 90–99%. Efficiency is here taken in the quite usual sense:

$$\text{Efficiency} = \left(\frac{\text{energy output}}{\text{energy input}}\right) 100\%. \tag{6.20}$$

Some Simple Calculations

Consider a step-up transformer in which the secondary has 1000 times as many turns as the primary.

If 10 mA are delivered by the secondary at 100 kV, what is the primary current? (Assume RMS values.)

Assuming 100% efficiency, we get

$$I_1/I_2 = N_2/N_1; \tag{6.18}$$

$$I_1 = I_2\frac{N_2}{N_1} = (10 \text{ mA})(1000) = 10^4 \text{ mA} \qquad \text{or} \qquad 10 \text{ amp.}$$

What is the primary voltage?

$$V_1/V_2 = N_1/N_2; \tag{6.17}$$

$$V_1 = V_2\frac{N_1}{N_2} = (100 \text{ kV})\left(\frac{1}{1000}\right) = 10^{-1} \text{ kV} \qquad \text{or} \qquad 100 \text{ volts.}$$

Or:

$$P_1 = P_2,$$

$$V_1 I_1 = V_2 I_2,$$

$$V_1 = \frac{V_2 I_2}{I_1} = \frac{(100 \text{ kV})(10 \text{ mA})}{10^4 \text{ mA}} = (100 \text{ kV})\,10^{-3}$$

$$= 10^{-1} \text{ kV} \qquad \text{or} \qquad 100 \text{ volts.}$$

Now let us suppose that the high-voltage transformer of a certain x-ray machine is 95% efficient. How many watts of power must be supplied to the primary to achieve an exposure of 70 kV, 50 mA? (Assume RMS values.) From Eq. (6.20):

$$\text{Efficiency} = \left(\frac{\text{power output}}{\text{power input}}\right) 100\%.$$

Hence, as a decimal fraction,

$$\text{Efficiency} = \frac{\text{power output}}{\text{power input}}.$$

Thus

$$\text{Power input} = \frac{\text{power output}}{\text{efficiency}}$$

$$= \frac{(70 \times 10^3 \text{ volts})(50 \times 10^{-3} \text{ amp})}{0.95}$$

$$= \left(\frac{70 \times 50}{0.95}\right) \text{ watts} = 3700 \text{ watts} \qquad \text{or} \qquad 3.7 \text{ kW.}$$

(Note that the power output is 3500 watts, or 3.5 kW.)

Transformer Losses

In spite of the high efficiency of transformers, as exemplified by the previous example, the losses which exist are nevertheless significant, particularly from the standpoint of long-term operation. What are these losses?

First there is the I^2R loss (see Section 3.7) in the windings. This loss is minimized by making the windings of as heavy a copper wire as is consistent with sound economical and structural considerations. Like the other losses to be discussed, this energy loss appears as heat energy, thus causing an undesirable temperature rise and consequent cooling problem in the transformer.

Then there are the core losses: hysteresis and eddy current. Hysteresis losses (see Section 4.2) refer to the energy required to continuously reorient the magnetic domains in the core which is subjected to continuously changing magnetizing current. This loss is minimized by employing a core material, such as silicon iron (SiFe) which has a low coercivity and a very narrow hysteresis loop.

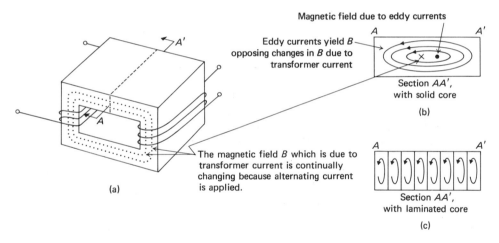

FIG. 6.12. Laminated transformer core reduces eddy currents. (a) Transformer. (b) Section of core, assuming core solid. (c) Section of laminated core, showing the net longer current paths effected.

Since the core, although it is insulated from the windings, is nevertheless subjected to a continuously varying magnetic field, and since the core is a metal, we would expect eddy currents in accord with the discussion of Section 5.3. To minimize eddy currents the transformer core is usually composed of laminations, as shown in Fig. 6.12, with the laminations insulated from each other. One result of the use of the laminations is longer total current paths. The consequent effect of a greater total resistance then leads to a decrease in total eddy currents in accord with Ohm's law.

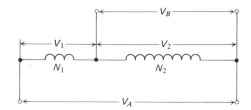

FIG. 6.13. Autotransformer with a turns ratio of $(N_1 + N_2)/N_2$.

Autotransformers

A special type of transformer in which the two windings are not electrically insulated from each other but are connected in series is known as an *autotransformer*. Analysis of an ideal device of this type, as shown in Fig. 6.13, yields

$$\frac{V_A}{V_B} = \frac{N_1 + N_2}{N_2}, \tag{6.21}$$

where $V_A = V_1 + V_2$, the voltages across coils of N_1 and N_2 turns, respectively, and $V_B = V_2$. Note that this expression is really just another way of expressing Eq. (6.17), as specifically applied to the autotransformer.

The autotransformer may be used just as the previously discussed ordinary two-circuit transformers may be used: to transform power at a high voltage to a lower voltage, or vice versa, depending on whether V_A refers to the primary (input) or the secondary (output) voltage.

Actually, there is no requirement that we make a pronounced distinction between winding 1 and winding 2. In practice, one often has simply one continuous winding, separated only in the sense that somewhere between one end and the other a connection is made to the second circuit. With a number of possible connections to the second circuit, as shown in Fig. 6.14, various ratios of $(N_1 + N_2)/N_1$ are obtainable, and thus by Eq. (6.21) we see that a variable voltage supply is available. This latter modification of the autotransformer finds use in x-ray circuits.

At this point you may ask why an autotransformer is used when an ordinary two-circuit transformer could be used. The answer is that the

FIG. 6.14. Autotransformer with various taps to select the output voltage, V_B. This arrangement permits various values of V_B even though V_A remains constant. The connection shown yields the maximum output voltage and makes the autotransformer into a step-up transformer. Note that it is possible, by turning selector switch S into one of the lower positions, to make the transformer behave like a step-down transformer.

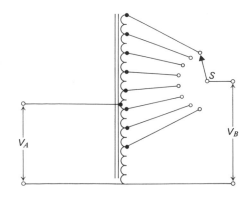

autotransformer has, in practice, a number of advantages such as smaller size, lower cost, greater efficiency, and smaller exciting current. For x-ray work the most significant advantage of the autotransformer is that it makes possible better voltage regulation than the ordinary two-circuit transformer does. Of course, along with these advantages is the quite significant disadvantage that the autotransformer produces high voltage, but with a conductive connection between the low-voltage and the high-voltage side. For this reason alone, an autotransformer would not be suitable as the high-voltage transformer required to develop the kV across the tube.

Transformers in X-ray Circuits

The largest transformer in the x-ray unit is the fixed-ratio high-voltage step-up transformer to which we just referred above. It supplies the kilovoltage across the tube. For example, such a transformer might be designed to step up from a mains (or supply) voltage of 240 volts to a maximum of 100 kV. The turns ratio required is about 1:400.

Although such a transformer usually has its secondary winding grounded at the center so that the actual potential difference between either end and grounded items like the transformer core, the transformer tank, etc., is only 50 kV, the insulation problem is still formidable. One can solve this problem by immersing the entire transformer in a tank of oil. This oil has excellent dielectric properties (see Table 3.1). Tackling the insulation problem by this means solves another problem, that of cooling the transformer. The oil's specific heat is sufficient to provide for effective heat removal from the core and windings. That is, the energy losses of the transformer—which, as we pointed out earlier, appear as heat—are absorbed by the oil, whose quantity and specific heat are such that they preclude any dangerously large temperature increase in the transformer.

Another requirement of a transformer in an x-ray unit is that it step down the supply voltage to the region of 5–10 volts, which is suitable for the heating of the filament in the x-ray tube and the valve tubes. Usually one such transformer is provided for each filament to be heated.

The chief remaining requirement of a transformer in an x-ray unit is that it be a device with which the primary input to the fixed-ratio high-voltage transformer may be changed in order to provide for a selection in kV across the tube. This requirement is met by an autotransformer of the type shown in Fig. 6.14. We shall discuss details of this transformer and its role in an x-ray machine in Chapter 8.

6.5 RECTIFICATION

Since the x-ray tube operates with a unidirectional current (that is, since the electrons always have to go in the same direction to strike the tube target), it behooves us to formally consider the matter of changing AC to DC; to summarize and expand on the relevant notions discussed and/or implied earlier.

The changing of an alternating current to a pulsating unidirectional, or direct current, is known as *rectification*. The circuit elements that achieve this rectification are termed *rectifiers*.

Rectifiers are essentially of two types: (a) vacuum or gas-filled tubes and (b) solid-state devices. Of these, still the most predominantly employed in x-ray machines are the vacuum tubes, sometimes called *diodes*, or thermionic diodes, because of the fact that two electrodes are sealed into the tube, one at each end, and one of the electrodes, the filament, is heated to give off electrons. In x-ray work, however, these tubes are most frequently called *valve tubes*. Since valve tubes have much in common with x-ray tubes, we shall discuss these rectifiers in Chapter 7 in conjunction with x-ray tubes.

Also to be considered further (in Chapter 8, which will deal with x-ray circuits) are the various types of rectification circuits employed in x-ray machines. For the moment, then, we shall consider only the basics of rectification and some elements of solid-state rectification.

Basic Rectification Circuits

We now confront the problem of how to convert AC to DC. The ideal rectifier to accomplish this task would be some device which would offer an infinite resistance when the voltage across it is applied in a given direction and zero resistance if the polarity of the applied voltage is reversed. We have now studied enough physics not to expect such a device. However, to be a rectifier a device has to meet this criterion in good measure at least. And for purposes of our waveform diagrams of input and output voltage and current comparisons, we shall assume the ideal rectifier. In truth, rectifiers, particularly the vacuum diode, are close enough to ideal to warrant such approximate analysis.

Readers who are not at all acquainted with the vacuum diode should turn ahead, right now, to Fig. 7.25 in the next chapter. This figure shows the essentials of a valve tube. For now it is enough if you are acquainted with the circuit symbolism and the fact that the tube will conduct current only when the plate (anode) is positive with respect to the filament (cathode). To say it another way: The tube will conduct only when the voltage across it is applied so that the anode is on the high-potential side of the circuit.

Let us now refer to Fig. 6.15 to establish the essential features of rectification. In part (a) of the figure we see the half cycle during which the anode of the valve tube is on the high-potential side of the circuit: The tube conducts and consequently there is a current, i, in the circuit. Since there is a current through the resistor R, there will be a voltage v_2 across the resistor which exactly follows the input voltage v_1. We may readily visualize the fact that this is the case by thinking of a DC case. If a dry cell is used as the input-voltage source in a circuit containing a resistor, then this voltage will appear across the resistor. If we now apply a greater EMF, or input voltage, by adding another dry cell in series, what happens? The current in the circuit is increased until again the voltage across the resistor, as determined by Ohm's law, equals the input voltage. And so on, if we add a

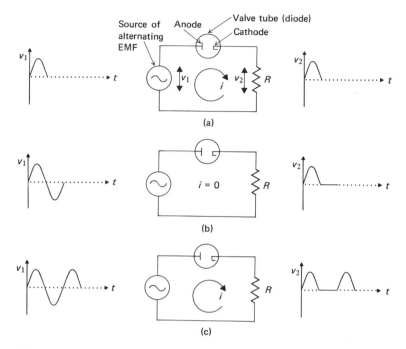

FIG. 6.15. Half-wave rectification employing a vacuum diode. (a) The first half-cycle, show-ing the input voltage v_1 supplied by the source and the output voltage v_2 across the resistor R. (b) The second half of the cycle, during which the tube does not conduct. (c) The first half of the next cycle.

third cell. Of course, if we go back to the lower input voltage of one cell, the voltage across the resistor drops again to its former corresponding value. Moreover, if we remove this dry cell, that is, make the input voltage zero, then the voltage across the resistor is zero. So v_2, the voltage across the resistor, follows (or behaves like) the input voltage v_1.

Next [see part (b) of Fig. 6.15] the input voltage makes its negative excursion which thus places the anode on the low-potential side of the circuit. The tube does not conduct. There is no current in the circuit. And hence there is no voltage across the resistor: v_2 is zero, even though v_1 is not.

In part (c) of Fig. 6.15 we have the same situation as in part (a). The tube conducts, there is a current, and there is consequently a voltage across R.

Now we see two things. First of all, when there is a current in the circuit, and consequently an output voltage across R, both the current and voltage, although pulsating as the input voltage, are always in the same direction. This unidirectional aspect is, of course, not a feature of the input voltage. So indeed AC has been changed to pulsating DC.

Second, we see that although the input voltage is only momentarily zero, the current and consequently the output voltage is zero for a whole

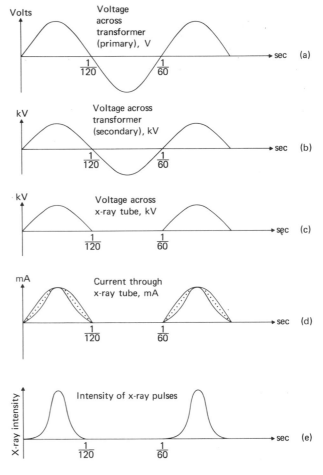

FIG. 6.16. Voltage, current, and x-ray intensity waveforms in a half-wave rectified unit.

half-cycle, in each cycle. We therefore call this particular rectification *half-wave rectification.*

A half-wave rectification circuit for an x-ray machine is shown in Fig. 7.24. We shall employ this circuit as a basis for reviewing the various waveforms and their meaning. We shall therefore refer to Fig. 6.16. In part (a) we see the input or primary voltage of the high-voltage transformer. This input is to all intents and purposes sinusoidal. From the calibration of the abscissa, the time axis, we see that 60-cycle AC is involved. The period, that is, the time for one complete cycle, one complete wave, is $\frac{1}{60}$ sec; and for half a wave, obviously $\frac{1}{120}$ sec.

In part (b) we see the stepped-up voltage across the secondary of the transformer. We present this waveform with a lower peak simply by chang-

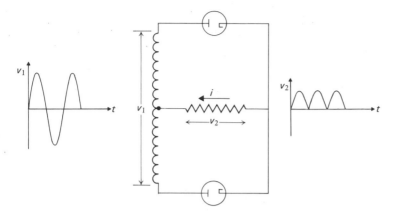

FIG. 6.17. Full-wave rectification, using two valve tubes.

ing the scale on the ordinate from the volts of (a) to kilovolts in (b). Note that there is no significant difference in wave shape, and certainly no difference in frequency.

Next, in part (c) of Fig. 6.16, we see the voltage that appears across the x-ray tube. We are making the simplifying assumption that when the secondary circuit is conducting, the voltage drop across the wires and the valve tube is negligible and therefore the peak of the voltage shown is the same as in (b). In actual practice this wave shape may show some distortion due to capacitive and inductive effects in the secondary circuit.

We turn from voltage to current in part (d). We see that the x-ray tube current is in one direction only and occurs in $\frac{1}{120}$-sec pulses, as is to be expected from the voltage across the tube as shown in (c). Note that three different wave shapes are presented for the current. These shapes are representative of any number of different wave shapes possible. The current is not strictly sinusoidal. How it varies depends considerably on the x-ray tube in question, particularly on the construction of the cathode.

Finally, in part (e), we see how the intensity of the x-ray pulses might vary. Note that significant x-ray production does not take place until well into the conducting half-cycle. The reason for this is that a high voltage is required for x-ray production. We should also note that, quite as to be expected with half-wave rectification, we get x-ray pulses during only half of each cycle.

Of course, for most purposes it would be desirable not to lose a half-cycle of the input voltage. This desirable end can be achieved: The process is known as *full-wave rectification*. One way of achieving full-wave rectification is shown in Fig. 6.17. The transformer which is the source of alternating EMF is tapped at the center as well as at each end. When the top end of the transformer is the high-potential end, then the upper tube conducts, with the current going through R from right to left. On the next half-cycle the lower end is at the high potential, the lower tube conducts, and the current again goes through R in the same direction as before.

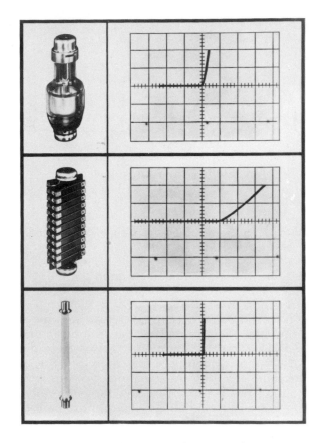

FIG. 6.18. Some rectifier types: comparison of rectifier size and current-voltage curves. Top: valve tube. Middle: selenium rectifier. Bottom: silicon rectifier. The current is plotted on the ordinate, graduated in units of 50 mA; the voltage is graduated in 0.4 kV units. (Courtesy *Medicamundi,* a journal on radiology, published by Philips, Eindhoven, in association with Müller, Hamburg, and Massiot Philips, Paris.)

Note, however, that in the case shown, the voltage across R is at best half the entire voltage across the transformer. Can we remedy this deficiency, if we want to? Yes. Such a circuit will be shown in Fig. 6.23, in connection with the mA meter.

Solid-State Rectifiers

The rectification described above can also be achieved by certain solid materials, which obviously must have non-ohmic characteristics. *Semiconductors* are such solids. In proper combination, with another semiconductor or with a conductor, semiconductors achieve a high resistance to current in one direction and a low resistance in the opposite, as shown in Fig. 3.12(b) and Fig. 6.18.

Because solid-state rectifiers have now been developed to the point of practicality in high-voltage x-ray circuitry, they are being more often used in x-ray circuits, although at the time of writing the valve tube appears still to be the rectifying element most commonly encountered in x-ray machines. The advantages of the solid-state rectifier over the thermionic valve tube are significant. The solid-state device is more rugged, lasts longer with proper usage, requires no heating current, does not produce x-rays as may a valve tube under certain conditions, and finally, the solid-state rectifier takes up much less room. Present silicon rectifiers about the size of a thick pencil can take the place of valve tubes usually somewhat larger than a large water glass (see Fig. 6.18).

Actually, there are three major different types of solid-state rectifiers, all of which depend in some measure on semiconductors: the metal-semiconductor combination, the p-n junction, and the conductivity modulation type. Examples of these types are the copper oxide rectifier, made of copper and Cu_2O, the germanium rectifier, and the silicon rectifier, respectively. Although the explanation of the behavior of these three types is different for each type, we can get some idea of the kind of behavior involved by considering what is probably the simplest type to explain: the p-n junction rectifier. Moreover, the p-n junction plays a key role in the conductivity-modulation type, like the silicon rectifier employed in the x-ray high-voltage circuit.

In order to understand this explanation, we need to know some elements of conduction processes in semiconductors. We shall have to come to grips with such nebulous electric charge carriers as holes!

In the first place, we need to realize that the conductivity of semiconductors is pronouncedly affected by slight amounts of impurities. Learning how to control the amount and distribution of these impurities is fundamental to semiconductor technology. Suppose now that a few arsenic atoms are added to a silicon crystal. What happens? Since arsenic atoms have five electrons in their outermost shell, while silicon atoms have only four, there appears a surplus electron, one not required for interatomic binding, that is, for the covalent bonds which bind silicon atoms to each other.

We do not wish to make an excursion into the various types of binding which may hold atoms together. Suffice it to say that all these types of binding involve the electrical characteristics of matter as pointed out in Chapter 1, and that covalent binding is one of the possible types. In covalent binding, adjacent atoms are held together in a unit by the mutual sharing of one or more electrons.

Now this apparently surplus electron requires very little energy to be detached from its arsenic parent: this electron is relatively free to roam around in the crystal. From the standpoint of the energy-level diagrams of Fig. 3.4, the effect of the added arsenic is to supply energy levels just below the conduction band. Therefore, only a little applied energy is required to boost electrons from these new levels into the conduction band.

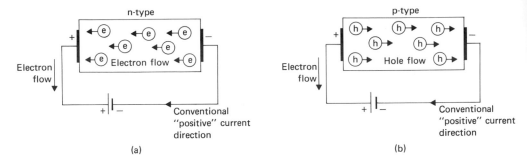

FIG. 6.19. Charge transfer in the two types of semiconductor materials. (a) The n-type with negative carriers, that is, electrons. (b) The p-type with positive holes as carriers.

These new energy levels just below the conduction band are called *donor levels,* and silicon doped with arsenic is called a *donor material,* or more frequently, an n-*type material.* Note that "n" is in the center of "donor"—a useful mnemonic device. In other words, a semiconductor owing its improved conductivity to a predominance of mobile electrons is called an n-*type semiconductor.* Another way to remember this designation is to realize that n means negative charge carriers.

If the silicon is doped with a small amount of gallium, which has only three outer electrons, then there occur in the silicon crystal places where an electron should be, but isn't. These vacancies are called *holes.* Since the absence of an electron is in some ways equivalent to the presence of a positive charge, a semiconductor of this type is referred to as p-*type;* or, since the hole can accept an electron, an *acceptor-type material.*

Now it doesn't seem surprising that if a hole exists and an electric field is applied, some electron will move toward the hole. This electron which has now filled the hole has, of course, itself left a newly created hole behind. Thus we have a progression of holes in a direction opposite to the direction of the migration of the electrons. Since in a p-type semiconductor the holes are in excess, and not the electrons as in an n-type material, we may conveniently consider the holes as the mechanism of charge transfer. We consider the holes as electric charges; positive charges to be sure.

If the semiconductor is an n-type one, that is, if it owes its conductivity behavior to a preponderance of electrons, the charge transfer through a complete circuit is readily imaginable. It is, in fact, just like the mechanism we are used to in metallic conductors. Figure 6.19(a) shows this behavior.

On the other hand, the situation with p-type material warrants a little closer look. In the metallic part of the circuit, of course, all is as we already know it to be. In this case, the electrons drift counterclockwise. But within the semiconductor the current is carried by positive holes moving clockwise from the positive to the negative terminal of the semiconductor. Consider the case of one electronic charge making the complete circuit in Fig. 6.19(b). At the left end of the semiconductor an electron is removed

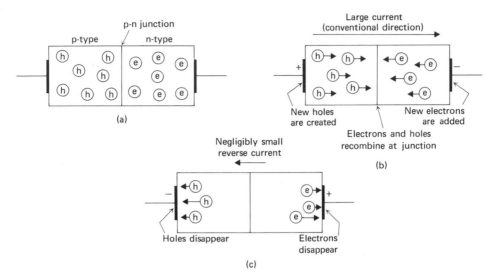

FIG. 6.20. A p-n junction solid-state diode. (a) No voltage applied. (b) Forward bias. Direction of applied voltage promotes a large current. This is the conducting direction. (c) Reverse bias. No appreciable conduction when voltage is applied in this direction.

from the semiconductor, leaving behind a positive hole. The electron drifts through the connecting wire to the battery, and once inside the battery, is forced to the negative terminal of the battery. Then, again under the influence of the electric field set up by the battery in the external part of the circuit, the electron continues its counterclockwise drift through the other connecting wire and ultimately into the right end of the semiconductor. In the meantime the hole has drifted from left to right in the semiconductor, so that at the right end the hole and electron again recombine. Mind you, the same original hole does not necessarily combine with the self-same electron. But on a statistical basis—that is, on the whole—holes created on the left are fulfilled on the right. In other words current, of equal magnitude, flows through the complete circuits. And the current through the semiconductor is one of positive charges, of holes, which are the surplus quantities in p-type material.

From the viewpoint of electric circuitry, of course, the n-type conduction and the p-type conduction of Fig. 6.19 are the same. One cannot distinguish one from the other. However, the fact that this distinction between n-type and p-type conduction does exist can be shown by the Hall effect, mentioned in Section 3.1. And it is upon this difference that the p-n junction rectifier depends. We shall now show that ordinarily current can flow through a p-n junction essentially in only *one* direction.

Refer to Fig. 6.20. In part (a) we see a p-n junction. In (b) the same junction is shown with a voltage applied so that the p-end of the junction device is positive and the n-end negative. This applied voltage results

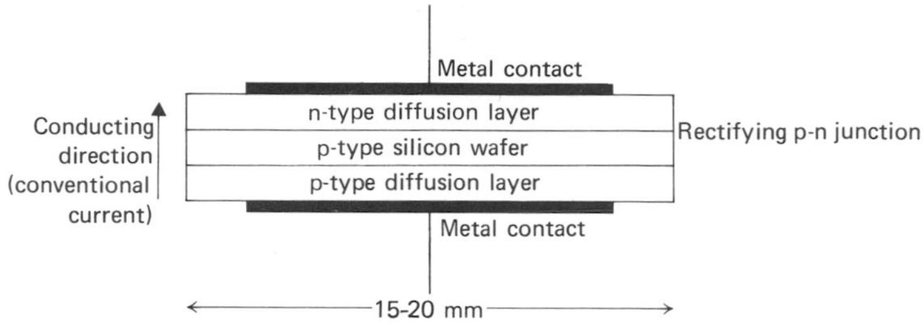

FIG. 6.21. Construction of a silicon rectifier such as is used in x-ray machine rectification circuits. More precisely, this device is known as a large-area silicon conductivity-modulation power rectifier. This type of rectifier can withstand higher peak inverse voltages than other solid-state rectifiers. A number of such rectifier units joined together in series can withstand the kilovolt inverse peak voltages experienced in x-ray circuits.

in a continual removal of electrons at the p-end and the consequent continual creation of holes at that end. In the meantime, electrons are being continually supplied to the n-end of the crystal. Two things we must note: First, the electrons and holes meet at the p-n junction and recombine there and again form part of the regular crystal structure, no longer acting as current carriers. Second, and most important, in spite of point one above, there is a continuous charge movement throughout the circuit. A current exists through a semiconductor in the direction of p-to-n.

Now let us reverse the applied voltage, as in part (c) of Fig. 6.20. The p-end is now negative, while the n-end is positive. The holes in the p-type material drift to the left and the electrons in the n-type material drift to the right. Soon there are hardly any holes in the p-type nor conduction electrons in the n-type. The current to all intents and purposes ceases. A significant current through a semiconductor in the direction of n to p does not exist. Consequently, a p-n junction has the property of a rectifier.

As we said earlier, the silicon rectifier is a little more complicated, but involves these same principles. Figure 6.21 shows the structure of a silicon rectifier unit. The pencil-like silicon rectifier of Fig. 6.18 is composed of a stack of such units.

The silicon rectifier has an exceedingly high conductivity in the "forward" direction, leaks only a very small current in the reverse direction, and can withstand large peak reverse voltages without a breakdown in its dielectric property in this direction. For these reasons, this type of solid-state rectifier is more useful in the high-voltage x-ray circuit than other semiconductor rectifiers, such as the copper oxide or selenium rectifiers.

Before we leave the solid-state rectifier let us now, in Fig. 6.22, redraw the circuit of Fig. 6.15, replacing the valve tube, or vacuum diode, with a solid-state diode. Note that the arrowhead in the symbol for a solid-state diode points in the (conventional) current direction the diode conducts.

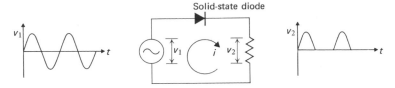

FIG. 6.22. Half-wave rectification employing a solid-state diode.

6.6 AC METERS

The problem of measuring currents and voltages in the case of AC introduces a new complication not encountered in DC. Let us look back at the moving-coil galvanometer of Fig. 4.25. If the current through this instrument changes in direction, the deflection of the pointer would have to change direction. If the current reversals are relatively frequent, the best one could obtain from this meter would be a wobbling about the zero mark. This is so because the coil and pointer have inertia. They oppose a change in motion. Thus, before they have moved far in one direction due to the torque exerted when the current is in a given direction, the current has changed direction and the torque now tends to produce rotation in the opposite direction. This means that DC instruments as we have considered them in Section 4.4 cannot be employed in AC, at least not directly.

What are the alternatives? Basically there are three possibilities. First, we could insert a DC instrument in an AC circuit, providing the moving-coil instrument had a rectifying circuit preceding it. This is done in the case of the mA meter, which we shall consider shortly.

Another alternative is to use a dynamometer (see Section 4.4). In this case, as you may recall, the magnetic field is produced by windings also connected to the circuit in question. Consequently when the current through the coil changes, so does the magnetic polarity of the field. As a rule, such meters are not found in x-ray machines, and hence we shall not refer to them further.

The third possibility lies in some system which is sensitive to AC but does not depend on the principle of the moving-coil galvanometer. For example, various magnetic and thermal effects offer possibilities. We shall restrict our discussion to the magnetic effect employed in a particular type of so-called moving iron meter, since this type is employed as the kV meter.

The mA Meter

The mA meter is an ammeter used to measure the current in the high-voltage part of the x-ray circuit. With proper compensation for extraneous effects which we shall not consider in this book, the mA meter measures the current through the x-ray tube. In most, if not all, x-ray units of today, the mA meter is a moving-coil meter similar in principle to the ammeter shown in Fig. 4.26.

In the case of half-wave rectification, this meter may be inserted directly into the circuit. For example, if in Fig. 6.15 the resistance R were to represent an x-ray tube, then the mA meter could be inserted anywhere in the circuit between R and the alternating source of EMF. The meter will "see" a pulsating half-wave current of wave shape similar to that of the output voltage v_2 in part (c) of the figure.

Analysis of the behavior of moving-coil meters shows that the meter deflection depends on the average value of the current over a cycle. For this reason the mA meter is calibrated in average values.

Now you might say: Why not calibrate this meter in RMS or peak values, since for sinusoidal current there is a definite relationship between these various quantities, as indicated in Fig. 6.5? One might well do this, except for the fact that the tube current measured by the mA meter, although almost sinusoidal, is slightly different, as indicated in Fig. 6.16(d). The wave shape may even change slightly with changes in kV and focal-spot selection, and may change if the original x-ray tube is replaced by a new tube. Hence, since the mA meter is exceedingly sensitive, these differences in wave shape are reflected in the meter reading. However, regardless of wave shape, within certain limits, the meter responds to the average value of the tube current, and there is thus merit in leaving the meter calibration in average values.

If a full-wave rectified unit is considered (and most if not all permanently installed units complete with x-ray table are full wave), then, as we shall show in Chapter 8, there is current through the secondary coil of the high-voltage transformer, each half of the cycle. This means that if we want to use a moving-coil meter to measure the current, we need to precede the meter by its own rectification circuit. Solid-state rectifiers, possibly of copper oxide, or of selenium, are employed for this purpose.

The appropriate circuitry is shown in Fig. 6.23. Let us see what happens. Following this behavior carefully now will pay dividends later, because the meter rectifying circuit is in principle the same as the full-wave Graetz-bridge circuit for supplying DC to the x-ray tube, to be discussed in Chapter 8. If you understand the present circuit your labors will be much reduced in Chapter 8.

Points X and Y are the connections by which the mA meter rectifier bridge is connected in series with the secondary coil of the high-voltage transformer. If you like, current flows in and out at points X and Y. Or, more precisely, electrons drift in and out at these points. Let us consider the time during which the side of the circuit to which point X is connected is at a higher potential than the side to which Y is connected. Rectifiers 1 and 3 conduct. The conventional current direction is as shown by the solid arrows.

During the next half cycle Y will be at the high-potential side. Rectifiers 2 and 4 will conduct, and the current direction will be as indicated by the dashed arrows. Note that in both cases the current through the meter marked mA is in the same direction.

In other words, although the current through the rectifying bridge is AC, the current through the mA meter itself is pulsating DC.

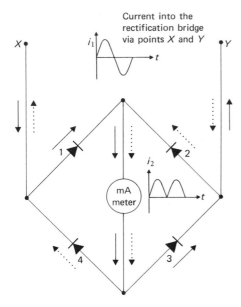

FIG. 6.23. Full-wave rectification bridge for mA meter, employing solid-state diodes. The input current to the rectification through points X and Y is i_1, while the current through the mA meter is i_2. Solid-line arrows show current direction during one half-cycle, and dotted-line arrows show the direction during the next half-cycle.

Now you might ask why all this concern about rectification. Why not use some other type of meter which works directly with AC? The answer is that such meters are on the whole insufficiently precise. The moving-coil, permanent-magnet DC ammeter employed is more sensitive and more accurate over a wide range of values than other meters working directly on AC. For example, the moving-coil meter, unlike the moving-iron meter employed for kV measurements, is not significantly subject to hysteresis effects and stray magnetic fields which lead to inaccuracies in the measurements indicated.

But no meter is perfect. For x-ray work the mA meter has a fault. In spite of the delicate construction, the carefully balanced movement, a moving coil cannot respond instantaneously to an applied force. As we have had occasion to state earlier, there is a certain amount of inertia: It takes time for the pointer to be set into motion and move to its final indicating position. For this reason, it is impractical to employ an mA meter for exposures less than, for example, $\frac{1}{4}$ sec. Therefore modern x-ray machines have a switching circuit which automatically switches from the mA meter to the mAs meter for short exposures. For fluoroscopy, of course, the mA meter is the one always employed.

The mAs Meter

The mAs meter, as its name implies, indicates the product of current and time: It measures the total electric charge flowing through the high-voltage circuit during the exposure. This meter could consequently be calibrated in coulombs. But in practice the meter is calibrated in milliampere-seconds, which is really another name for millicoulombs. (In terms of the calculus, the mAs meter is an integrating meter, integrating the current over the exposure time interval.)

The essential difference between the mA meter and the mAs meter is that in the case of the latter there is no hairspring or other device to produce a restoring torque which opposes the torque on the coil due to the electromagnetic forces. In other words, the mAs meter can continue to turn freely, except for minor opposition such as friction in the suspension mechanism, as long as any current is going through the coil. We can therefore see that it is plausible that, as careful analysis reveals, the total displacement of the coil from its original position depends not only on the force applied, which depends on the current, but also on the length of time during which the force is applied. Hence the meter measures current × time, that is, mAs (commonly written mAs; rigorously denoted mA-s).

The kV Meter

The kV meter is a voltmeter which is connected across the primary of the high-voltage transformer. It is calibrated to read the voltage across the secondary of this transformer, or more precisely, with certain automatically achieved corrections the actual voltage across the x-ray tube.

That a voltmeter connected to the primary side of a transformer can be calibrated to read the voltage across the secondary is, of course, no surprise. All we need to know is the turns ratio of the transformer, and then applying Eq. (6.17) enables us to make the appropriate adjustments, which can be incorporated right on the scale of the meter. This means, in effect, that while the meter is measuring volts across the primary of the transformer, the scale is actually showing the kilovolts across the x-ray tube. The advantage of this type of arrangement is obvious. It is much easier and safer to make measurements with low-voltage than with high-voltage equipment.

The kV meter is often referred to as a *pre-reading* kV meter. This terminology derives from the fact that the meter is so compensated that before the exposure it actually reads the voltage across the x-ray tube as it will be during the exposure. This is so because due allowance is automatically made for the various voltage drops which occur in the secondary, or high-voltage circuit, when current (mA) flows through it.

The kV meter does not need a rectifying circuit. It works directly on AC, and is of the moving-iron variety. Probably the most commonly employed type is the so-called *attraction moving-iron meter*. Sometimes, as we shall come to understand shortly, this type of meter is also referred to as a *solenoid meter* or a *sucking-coil meter*. Such a meter is shown in Fig. 6.24.

When current passes through the air-core solenoid of Fig. 6.24, a magnetic field is set up. This field in turn induces a magnetic field of opposite polarity in the movable iron vane. This behavior is just like that of a permanent magnet which temporarily so magnetizes a nail that the nail is attracted to the magnet. The larger the magnetizing current in the coil, the larger the magnetic field, and the larger the induced magnetic effect of the vane; consequently the greater the attraction, the farther into

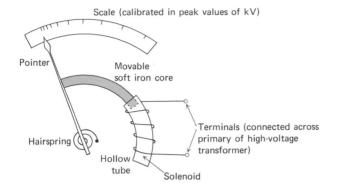

Scale (calibrated in peak values of kV)

Pointer

Movable
soft iron core

Hairspring

Hollow
tube

Solenoid

Terminals (connected across
primary of high-voltage
transformer)

FIG. 6.24. Mechanism of a
kV meter: attraction moving-
iron or sucking-coil type.

the coil the vane moves. Note that increasing the current is reflected not
only in an increase in the magnetic field of the coil but also in that of the
vane. From this fact it seems plausible that, as proper mathematical
analysis shows, the deflection of the vane, and hence of the pointer attached
to it, depends on the average value of the square of the current. For this
reason, as well as some other complications, the scale of the meter is
nonlinear. It has a larger space between successive numbers as the voltage
being measured, and hence the current through the meter, gets higher. To
repeat: The pointer deflection on the scale depends on the average of the
square of the current through the meter. And the current is presumed to
vary in the circuit as the voltage does, more or less at least, in accord with
Ohm's law, so that the pointer deflection depends on the average value
of the voltage being measured. That being the case, we can also say that
there is a definite relationship between the deflection of the pointer and
the square root of the average of the voltage squared. But this latter
quantity is the RMS voltage, V. So we could calibrate the scale in RMS
values.

Now, for the purposes of the measurements involved, there are no
significant differences between the voltage waveforms of the secondary
circuit and those of the primary, which we assume to be sinusoidal. On
this basis, we can employ Eq. (6.4) to determine the peak voltage value for
each corresponding RMS value. In other words, we can calibrate the
meter scale directly in peak values, peak values of the kV across the secondary circuit.

Although this type of meter is considerably sturdier than the moving-
coil type and does not need any associated rectification circuitry, it is not as
sensitive as the moving-coil meter and is far more subject to extraneous
magnetic effects.

6.7 MULTIPHASE AC

Up to this point our AC discussion has been based on the tacit assumption
that we were concerned only with single-phase AC. This does not make
our preceding discussions any the less valid, only less complicated than

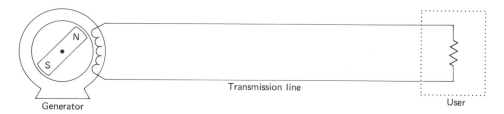

FIG. 6.25. Single-phase AC generator, showing the connection between generator winding (or windings) and the equipment of the user of the electrical energy supplied by the generator. The transmission, of two wires, may have several step-up and/or step-down transformers interposed between the generator and the user.

if, at each point, we had dealt with both single and multiphase. Moreover, it is probably safe to say that, as of the present, the vast majority of x-ray units, in North America at least, operate on single-phase AC, even though electrical power is generally distributed in three-phase systems.

We have, of course, already met the distinction between single and multiphase EMF's in Section 5.2. But a further look at this matter is warranted, since multiphase x-ray equipment is gradually becoming more widespread.

Single-Phase AC

First let us briefly review the essentials of single-phase AC. *Single-phase* means that the current (and voltage) rises from zero to a maximum, falls to zero, then rises to a maximum in the opposite direction, usually in a sinusoidal fashion. From the generating point of view this means, as discussed in Section 5.2, that the generator windings are connected in series, and that consequently there are only two terminals to lead off the current from the generator. Two wires are therefore required for the transmission of a single phase at a single voltage, as shown in Fig. 6.25.

If two single-phase voltages of the same phase but of different magnitudes are delivered to a consumer, then three wires are required. As an example, consider the situation common in North American homes. Three wires come into the house, thus providing both 120 volts or 240, as shown in Fig. 6.26.

From the standpoint of x-ray equipment, probably the major advantage of single-phase over three-phase is the relative simplicity of the switching circuitry controlling the exposure times: Only one circuit needs to be opened and closed, as opposed to three in the case of three-phase.

Three-Phase AC

Three-phase electric motors are less complicated and often less expensive, and hence, where three-phase supply is available, are sometimes used for tilting x-ray tables, for tomographic equipment, and for rapid film changers. But the most important aspect of three-phase AC in x-ray work is that it makes possible a more nearly constant voltage across the x-ray tube.

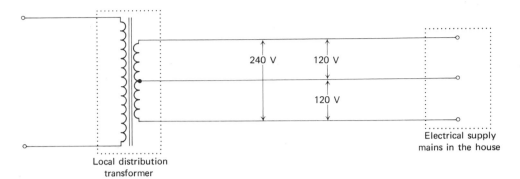

FIG. 6.26. Single-phase AC, with house mains supplying a choice of 120 volts or 240 volts. The 240 volts supplied in this way could be used in a hospital for single-phase x-ray machines.

We now draw upon our discussion of the generation of three-phase AC of Section 5.2. In particular, we refer the reader to Fig. 5.14(b). Note again that a sinusoidal voltage is produced by each of the three armatures of the three-phase generator, and that the three voltages are out of phase by 120°, or one-third of a cycle. This generator supplies three-phase AC. That is, by a three-phase voltage supply we mean three voltages of equal frequency, waveform, and magnitude, but each one differing in phase, each one lagging the preceding voltage by one-third of a cycle.

Note what happens if a three-phase voltage is rectified. Figure 6.27 shows this. The voltage does not go to zero as does the single-phase

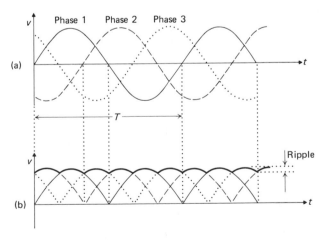

FIG. 6.27. Three-phase voltage. (a) As generated. (b) As full wave rectified. The solid line shows the voltage as it might appear across the x-ray tube. In actual practice this waveform is somewhat distorted. The ripple may be of the order of 15–20% of the peak voltage.

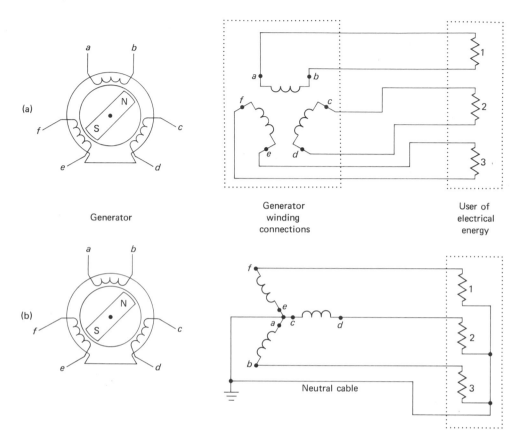

FIG. 6.28. Three-phase generation and transmission. (a) Six-wire system. (b) The more practical four-wire system, which gives the same service to loads 1, 2, and 3 as does the six-wire system of (a). The winding connection of (b) is called a star connection.

rectified voltage of Fig. 6.17. Therein lies the main interest in three-phase AC for the x-ray technician: the possibility of a more nearly constant voltage across the x-ray tube.

Let us now see how connection might be achieved between the three-phase generator and the user of the energy. The most obvious way would be to connect each of the three separate phase windings of the generator to the user with two wires as is done in single-phase. This arrangement would require six wires to give the user three different single-phase supplies. Figure 6.28 shows this arrangement as well as the alternative which is employed in practice because it uses less wire and is therefore considerably cheaper. One can see that it is possible, using only four wires, to make the three-phase distribution provide three separate single-phase supplies as well as the three-phase supply. As a matter of fact, it can be shown that if the user's loads are equal on each phase, then there

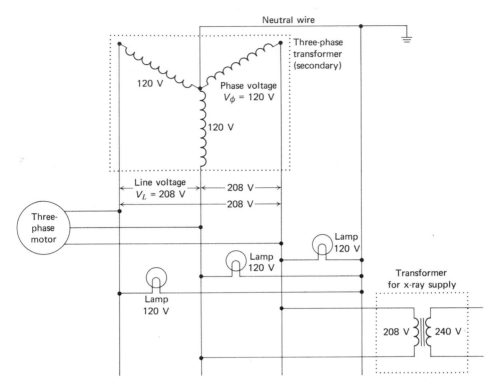

FIG. 6.29. Four-wire three-phase system, showing the connection of a three-phase motor and a lamp on each single phase. A possible connection, across the line voltage, for the transformer providing the mains voltage supply to a single-phase x-ray machine is also shown. In practice it is more likely that this transformer would be connected on the primary side of the three-phase transformer.

will be no current in the neutral cable and the distribution can be carried out with only three wires.

Let us now look at the voltages available with a four-wire, three-phase system (Fig. 6.29). In North America a common voltage across one phase, that is, across one secondary winding of a three-phase distribution transformer, is 120 volts. This voltage is called the *phase voltage*, V_ϕ.

Analysis, such as that found in the book by Lurch listed at the end of this chapter, leads to the result that, because of the 120° phase difference between the voltages, the voltage across any two of the windings, known as the *line voltage*, V_L, is given by

$$V_L = \sqrt{3}\, V_\phi.$$

Thus with a phase voltage of 120 volts we get a line voltage of 208 volts. In other words, a four-wire three-phase system can provide three separate single-phase 120-volt supplies, as well as single-phase supplies of 208 volts and a three-phase supply. (Note that V_L refers to line voltage here; not voltage across inductor.)

The corresponding common supply voltages in England are a phase voltage of 240 volts and a line voltage of 415 volts, while in continental Europe a phase voltage of 220 volts with a line voltage of 380 volts is common.

In North America, if the hospital has a three-phase supply (as is most likely) but, as is usual, has single-phase x-ray equipment, the heavy-duty x-ray machines are likely to have their own transformer. This transformer usually comes off one of the three phases of the three-phase supply transformer in order to provide 240 volts single-phase, since x-ray machines are generally designed to operate with a mains voltage of 190–260 volts. In the case of a single-phase supply to the hospital, then generally a 240-volt line is employed. In either case, some mobile units may work on 120-volt outlets.

Before leaving actual voltage values, let us point out that in the case of a three-phase voltage supply the relationship between peak values and RMS values (Eq. 6.4) applies only to the single-phase voltages across each individual winding. For the other cases the RMS value turns out, as we might expect, to be a higher fraction of the peak value.

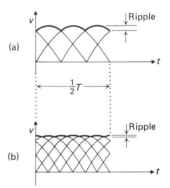

FIG. 6.30.   Multiphase AC rectified.   (a) Three-phase.
(b) Six-phase. Note the reduced ripple.

We now refer back to Fig. 6.27. If three-phase AC is better than single-phase for x-ray production, then six-phase would be better still; it would come closer to providing a constant potential, as shown in Fig. 6.30. And 12-phase would be better still. Although electrical energy is not generally available in these phases, it is possible to convert three-phase into higher-phase AC by appropriate circuitry. This is done with some x-ray equipment.

Another adjunct to provide a voltage across the x-ray tube that is more nearly constant is to introduce what is called a *filter* into the circuit. Referring to Figs. 6.27 and 6.30, we note that although the voltage across the tube does not go to zero during an exposure, there is a variation between a minimum and a maximum voltage. This variation is called *ripple*.

Circuitry comprising inductors and capacitors can be devised to reduce this ripple. Such circuitry is referred to as a filter, because it filters out the ripple.

We conclude by summarizing the advantages of three-phase AC over single-phase in general, and as specifically related to the x-ray department.

From the viewpoint of transmission, three-phase AC is cheaper: It saves copper. The comparison with three single-phase lines makes this obvious. Three-phase AC provides what three single-phase supplies do, and more, using only four wires where the three single-phase supplies need six.

On the whole, three-phase motors are less complicated. Both the motor itself and its control are cheaper.

From the standpoint of x-ray production, the principal advantage of three-phase AC lies in the more nearly constant voltage available across the x-ray tube. The resulting x-rays are consequently more homogeneous (more nearly of the same energy) and the intensity is increased, thus making shorter exposure times possible.

QUESTIONS

1. Sketch the voltage-time graph for 60-cycle sinusoidal AC for two full cycles. Mark in the various times (in seconds) at which $v = 0$, assuming $v = 0$ at $t = 0$.

2. a) What is the period of 15-cycle AC?
   b) What disadvantage would the above frequency have for illuminating purposes?

3. Would an AC current of 15 amp maximum (peak) result in the same temperature of a given heating element as a DC current of 15 amp applied for the same time? Explain.

4. Define the terms: root means square (RMS), peak, and average or mean, as applied to alternating voltages or currents.

5. It is usual to state the input or mains voltage to an x-ray unit in RMS values. However, the voltage across the x-ray tube is indicated in peak values, and the current through the x-ray tube in average values. Explain.

6. Define and/or explain the following: farad, impedance, inductance, frequency of AC, phase difference.

7. Refer to Fig. 6.31.
   a) Indicate to which type of circuit element each of the two graphs refers. Give the reason for your answer.
   b) Explain what is meant by applied voltage, current, and back EMF, as shown in part (b).
   c) Clarify the reasons for the phase relationships of the three quantities shown.

8. a) Explain why a coil of thick wire wrapped around an iron core is capable of limiting the flow of an alternating current, although the same coil will allow a direct current to pass easily.

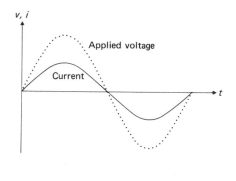

Current and voltage in phase

(a)

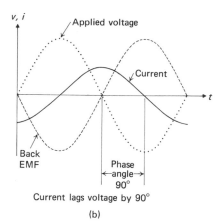

Current lags voltage by 90°

(b)

FIG. 6.31. Voltage-current relationships.

   b) Further explain why, when used to limit the flow of AC, such a coil does not become hot, whereas if a resistor were used to limit the flow it would become very hot.

9. What would happen to the inductance of an inductor with a diamagnetic core as opposed to one with no core at all?

10. If the x-ray tube filament were heated with DC, could one control the filament temperature with a variable inductor? Explain.

11. a) If a resistor, inductor, and capacitor connected in series have a resistance of 4Ω, an inductive reactance of 12Ω, and a capacitive reactance of 15Ω, respectively, what is their combined impedance?
     b) What value of the capacitive reactance would make the impedance a minimum?

12. What happens to the light when the iron bar is thrust into the coil, as shown in Fig. 6.32?

13. Consider AC power.
     a) State the general expression for AC power.
     b) What is the unit of power?
     c) Give the power expression in the form in which it would be applicable to both AC and DC.

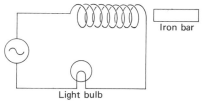

Iron bar

Light bulb

FIG. 6.32. Controlling current by means of a variable inductance.

14. If in an AC circuit a current of 20 amp at a voltage of 110 volts yields a power consumption of 2.2 kilowatts, what can be said about the current and voltage, and their values, and the nature of the circuit impedance?

15. Suppose that in an AC series circuit such as that shown in Fig. 6.6(a) the voltage across the resistor is 100 volts, across the inductor 40 volts, and across the capacitor 80 volts, while the current is 15 amp.

a) What current and voltage values (instantaneous, average, RMS) are presumably meant?

b) What is the individual power consumption of the capacitor, resistor, and inductor, respectively?

c) What is the power consumption of the entire circuit?

d) Is the input voltage V larger, smaller, or the same as the voltage across the resistor?

16. a) Should a transformer core be highly resistive or not? Comment.

b) A transformer core is generally built of thin sheets or laminations of iron. Explain.

17. A step-up transformer has a turns ratio of 500 to 1, and 100 volts are applied to the primary side of this transformer.

a) What is the output in kV?

b) If the secondary current is 100 mA, what is the primary current in amperes?

c) What is the power output of the transformer in watts?

d) What assumptions were made in your solutions to parts (a), (b), and (c) above?

18. a) Using a sketch, show the difference between a step-up transformer and a step-down transformer.

b) Explain how an autotransformer might be used to control the voltage in an x-ray unit.

19. What is the number of current pulses per second passing through the x-ray tube in a half-wave rectified x-ray machine operating on 60-cycle AC? Draw the appropriate current-time graph for the x-ray tube.

20. In the case of full-wave rectification, if one rectifying tube were burnt out, what would be the result on the voltage output across the x-ray tube?

21. a) What is meant by a solid-state rectifier?

b) What material is frequently used for solid-state rectifiers in x-ray circuits?

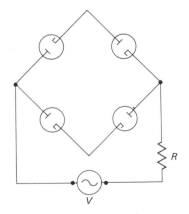

FIG. 6.33. A rectification circuit.

22. Refer to Fig. 6.33.

a) Is this full-wave or half-wave rectification?

b) Sketch the voltage-time curves for the sinusoidal AC voltage input V, and for the voltage across the resistor R.

c) What is the minimum number of rectifying tubes with which the same rectification could be achieved?

d) Draw a circuit using the minimum number of solid-state rectifiers which would achieve the same rectification.

23. a) What is the essential difference between the mA meter and the mAs meter?

b) Which of these two meters measures the total amount of charge which has drifted past a given point in the high-voltage circuit during the exposure?

24. a) Would the kV meter described in this chapter also work with DC? Would the calibration have to be changed? Comment.

b) Explain the nonlinearity of the kV meter scale; that is, tell why successive voltages are different distances apart on the scale.

25. Regarding three-phase AC circuits, state (a) an advantage, and (b) a disadvantage.

SUGGESTED READING

BEISER, ARTHUR, *Modern Technical Physics.* Reading, Mass.: Addison-Wesley, 1966. Chapter 29 provides a succinct quantitative treatment of AC circuits employing no mathematics beyond simple algebra and trigonometry.

JAUNDRELL-THOMPSON, F., and W. J. ASHWORTH, *X-ray Physics and Equipment.* Oxford: Blackwell Scientific Publications, 1965. Excellent reference for details, not likely to be found elsewhere in one and the same volume, on transformers, meters, and multiphase AC as specifically related to medical x-ray equipment.

LURCH, E. NORMAN, *Electric Circuits.* New York: John Wiley, 1963. A reference for those readers wishing to further analyze electric circuits, including polyphase systems.

SHIVE, JOHN N., *The Properties, Physics and Design of Semiconductor Devices.* Princeton, N.J.: D. Van Nostrand, 1959. An authoritative text by a member of the technical staff of the Bell Telephone Laboratories, where many semiconductor devices first saw the light of day. Beginning with descriptions of the various semiconductor devices, the book continues with a discussion of the whys and wherefores of their use and behavior. Some of the material is presented descriptively and hence is within the reach of any reader with a background knowledge of elementary general physics. Chapters 1 and 2, which deal with the scope and basic nature of semiconductors, along with Chapter 5 on large-area rectifiers, are particularly relevant.

STOUT, MELVILLE B., *Basic Electrical Measurements.* Englewood Cliffs, N.J.: Prentice-Hall, 1960 (second edition). Reference on AC meters. See comments at end of Chapter 4.

CHAPTER 7

X-Ray and Other Tubes

Now that we have investigated the basic electrical elements of the power supply of the x-ray tube, let us go on to a discussion of the x-ray tube itself. In Chapter 8, these two main x-ray machine components, the tube and its power supply, will be brought together to form, with other circuit elements, a complete example of a typical x-ray installation.

All radiography that uses x-rays is based on the discovery made by Röntgen (1845–1923) in 1895, and in this chapter you will learn something about the circumstances surrounding the discovery. As a student x-ray technician you may well come across many accounts of this period of history, and Röntgen's particular part in it, in books, magazines, and other literature. Most of these accounts will be brief and will vary a little, one from the other, depending on the intention of the author. From these accounts you will be able to gain some idea of the importance of the discovery as well as some of the relevant details. However, it must be made clear that such abbreviated accounts will never be able to provide the proper understanding and appreciation of the facts described, for these may be obtained only from reading the original papers published by Röntgen, or direct translations of them. These translations are readily available. Nothing can compare with reading them for yourself. In fact it usually comes as a surprise to find how clear and to the point the original papers are when compared with the so-called simplified accounts written by others after the event. This, of course, also includes the textbook you are now reading!

A book to be highly recommended is one written by Otto Glasser, called *Dr. W. C. Röntgen,* the second edition of which was published in 1958 by

Charles C. Thomas in Springfield, Illinois. (The book is also published in Canada by the Ryerson Press of Toronto.) This small volume of 169 pages is an account of the life of Röntgen, with six of its nine chapters devoted to the period of his discovery of x-rays and the publication of his three communications on the subject. Glasser has included translations of these papers.

Another historical highlight is the invention of the hot cathode tube by W. D. Coolidge in 1913. An interesting paper, presented by Coolidge in the *Physical Review* of December 1913 (Volume II, Number 6), entitled "A Powerful Röntgen Ray Tube with a Pure Electron Discharge," describes his invention, and we would recommend reading it. When you have read this paper you should realize, however, that modern x-ray tubes no longer resemble Coolidge's in outward appearance, even though they function on the same principles and may often be represented by diagrams similar to his. The shapes of some of the recent tubes are shown elsewhere in this book, and you may find opportunity to examine examples in your own department.

7.1 THE PRODUCTION OF X-RAYS

X-rays were discovered by Professor Wilhelm Conrad Röntgen on Friday, November 8, 1895, in Würzburg, Germany. But before we begin an account of this discovery, it will be of some value to briefly discuss some of the work by Röntgen and others which led up to his discovery.

Scientists had, for some time, been investigating what took place within a partially evacuated glass tube when an electric current was passed through it. The current, which was always a small one, in the order of microamperes, was produced by a high voltage applied between wire electrodes sealed in the ends of the tube (see Fig. 7.1). We know that this high voltage promoted ionization of the small quantity of residual gas and produced a flow of electrons and positive ions through the tube. (A low voltage would have been insufficient to give the same results.) Once started, the flow was replenished by electrons from the cathode. Depending on the amount of residual gas (in this case, air) and the voltage used (in the order of kilovolts), different effects were produced.

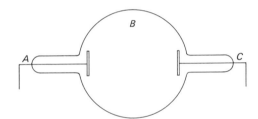

FIG. 7.1. A discharge tube: *A* and *C* are the metal, sealed-in electrodes; *B* is the glass tube or sphere in which only a little air or gas remains. Note the simplicity of the apparatus.

You may perhaps wonder why it was that this particular device should have excited so much curiosity. In Chapter 1 we talked about the fact that men have always been curious about the nature of things. They have, for example, wanted to find out about the ultimate particles of which matter is composed. They realized that the glass tube described here might give them some clues. For, in the tube, they now had to hand a few of the elements, in gaseous form, and moreover not very much of them, since the tube was pumped out to a considerable degree of vacuum. Anything which took place in the tube with the passage of electricity could only involve the gas itself and the electricity. No other significant factors intruded. It therefore seemed very likely that the behavior of the gas in these isolated circumstances would indicate something more about its innermost fundamental composition, or nature. And, as you know, this nature was gradually revealed.

One of the tubes put to frequent use in these investigations was devised by Sir William Crookes (1832–1919). It was with a tube of the Crookes type that Röntgen was working at the time of his discovery of x-rays (see Fig. 7.2).

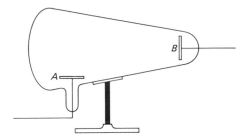

FIG. 7.2. Crookes-type tube, like the one used by Röntgen at the time of his discovery. *A* is the anode, and *B* the (possibly concave) cathode.

What happens in such a tube? As current is passed through it, the gas glows with a color depending on the kind of gas. (Neon glows with a red color, for example.) The glow shows light or dark rings or areas that change with the voltage and the degree of vacuum. At a pressure of 8 millimeters of mercury (atmospheric pressure, which is about 14.7 lb/in², will support a column of 760 millimeters of mercury at sea level), a crackling band of light appears through the tube between the electrodes. At 1 millimeter of mercury the tube is filled with light. As the pressure is further reduced various dark spaces appear in different parts of the tube until at 0.001 millimeter of mercury it becomes entirely dark inside, but its walls appear to light up.

During the passage of current through the tube, one can detect a stream of particles arising from the cathode. For instance, they can be made to cast a shadow of a metal object interposed between the cathode and the end of the tube (see Fig. 7.3). Or, if the walls of the tube are sufficiently thin, the particles may be detected beyond the end of the tube by means of suitable phosphors. (One of these, used by Röntgen for this purpose, is barium platinocyanide. This material fluoresces when struck by the cathode particles. We shall be discussing this more fully in Section 10.7.) In the Crookes tube the particles also could be focused by using a concave cathode so as to produce a bright spot of light on the glass wall. These particles were known as cathode rays. We now know them to be electrons.

During the month of October in 1895, Röntgen had been experimenting with cathode rays and on Friday, November 8, in the evening, was

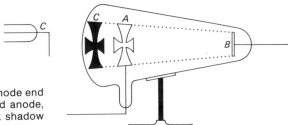

FIG. 7.3. A shadow cast on the anode end of the tube: *A* is the cross-shaped anode, *B* the cathode, and *C* is the dark shadow on the glass wall.

continuing his studies. He had covered the tube with a cardboard shield to shut in any light arising from the fluorescence of its glass walls. The room was dark and he was pleased to note that, when he passed a current through the tube, no light leaks appeared through the cover. He was about to turn off the current when he noticed a small glow coming from a nearby sheet of paper painted with a layer of barium platinocyanide. Something coming from the tube was causing the barium platinocyanide to fluoresce.

Despite his excitement at this discovery, he said nothing for several weeks but pursued his investigations more fully in this new direction. He published his findings in a paper at the end of December, calling the emanations from the tube "x-rays"; "x" for unknown. He found that the rays came primarily from the area of impact of the cathode rays on the glass.

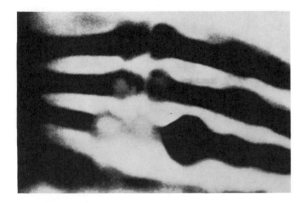

FIG. 7.4. A radiograph of the hand of Röntgen's wife, taken on Dec. 22, 1895. (Courtesy of Deutsches Röntgen-Museum, Remscheid-Lennep, West Germany)

In his first paper entitled "On a New Kind of Rays, a Preliminary Communication" and published in a journal of the Würzburg Physical Medical Society in December of 1895, Röntgen established that the degree to which x-rays penetrated materials depended on the thickness and density of any obstacle put in their path. He found that they could penetrate many substances to a considerable degree. He also noted the x-rays' properties of producing fluorescence and affecting photographic plates, and the absence of any measurable reflection from surfaces or deflection by magnetic fields. His paper was accompanied by radiographs of many objects, including one of a hand. This was probably the first radiograph of a part of the human body. Figure 7.4 is a print of the radiograph Dr. Röntgen took of his wife's hand on December 22, 1895.

A second paper was presented in March 1896 with a report of the use of platinum as a target for the cathode rays, a concave cathode, a target tilted at 45° to the cathode rays, and the use of the x-rays to discharge an electroscope in air.

Röntgen's third and last paper on the subject of x-rays was submitted to the Prussian Academy of Sciences in Berlin on March 10, 1897. In it he described the scattering of x-rays by air, the uniformity of emission of x-rays from the tube in different directions, the different penetrating abilities of the rays from tubes with different degrees of vacuum, and the gradual increase in vacuum which occurred in a tube with prolonged use.

You may see from the contents of these papers that nearly all the properties and uses of x-rays known today were to a considerable extent investigated and described between November 8, 1895 and March 1897. Indeed, much of the work was done in the first two months following the discovery.

While all this about Röntgen's work is well documented and certainly well known, what is not so well known is that around the same time that Röntgen achieved his success a young physics instructor in the United States also appears to have been producing x-rays. The man's name was Frank E. Austin, and the place was Dartmouth College in New Hampshire. Mr. Austin is reputed to have had spectators put metal objects in a cigar box and, without opening the box, would baffle his audience by telling them what was in it.

Unfortunately there seems to be no conclusive evidence to indicate whether Austin's work was actually done before, concurrently with, or after knowledge of Röntgen's discovery. Professor Austin himself left some doubt on this subject. Writing to a friend in 1958 he stated, "It may be a bit over-ambitious to presume to be the first in the world to have taken an x-ray picture, but I might well have been. I was certainly 'Johnny on the spot' because of the collection of tubes and the batteries to operate them." And "Johnny on the spot" he certainly appears to have been. Whether before or after Röntgen, his x-ray pictures may well have been the first in America.

Austin apparently tried to interest the medical profession in using his apparatus for diagnosing fractures of the bones. However, it appears that the medical people approached at the time were unimpressed, and nothing was done with Professor Austin's equipment until the publication of Röntgen's first paper became known in American medical circles. Then Dr. Gilman Frost of the medical staff of the Mary Hitchcock Memorial Hospital took the initiative to provide a subject, one Eddy McCarthy, who had fallen while skating on the Connecticut River. It is the picture of the taking of this x-ray which is found as the frontispiece of our book. Although Austin himself does not appear in this picture, there seems little doubt that his work with the tubes then available at Dartmouth College prepared the way for this momentous occasion. In fact, Austin claims to have earlier used the self-same equipment employed by Doctors G. D. and E. B. Frost to take an x-ray of his own hand. Unfortunately, Professor Austin died in 1964 without ever having received noticeable recognition for his pioneer x-ray investigations at Dartmouth College.

Back to Röntgen. He found that the new rays, which were able to penetrate matter to a far greater degree than any other sort of radiation, such as light, came from that part of the glass wall of the tube onto which the cathode rays fell. Something happened during the bombardment of the glass by the cathode rays to produce the new kind of ray. And whatever took place also occurred when a metal target was placed in the stream of cathode rays.

Somewhat simplified, the explanation is as follows. The cathode rays (electrons) produced in the tube undergo considerable acceleration under the influence of the electric field applied between the electrodes. This means that they gain energy. When they meet the atoms of the target material they are suddenly deflected by coming close to the nuclei of these atoms, which carry large positive charges (e.g., the number of protons in the platinum nucleus = 78). Sometimes, depending on the distance between a nucleus and an arriving high-speed electron, the deflection is small. The electron will then survive to meet with other deflections until it is finally stopped completely. Sometimes the electron is stopped at the first collision. Whatever occurs in the case of any particular electron, you can see that, as far as the total number arriving is concerned, the process gives rise to an infinite variety of degrees of deflection.

What is the outcome of this? Each electron, possessing considerable energy due to its acceleration through the tube, is deprived of much of this energy by being suddenly slowed down or deflected. The energy must go somewhere and a proportion of it appears from the site of collision as a parcel of energy in the form of a very penetrating electromagnetic wave. These waves are x-rays and the "parcels" of energy are the photons discussed in Chapter 1.

Now this description explains the appearance of radiation by talking about the fate of one electron. Any other electron may be slightly different in one important respect: that is, the relative energies involved. For example, any other electron arriving at the target may possess a different amount of energy. It may also have started out with more, or less, kinetic energy from its "home" in the residual gas, or the cathode. And, when it arrives, its particular collision event will almost certainly be slightly different from that of the first electron we considered. It may undergo a greater number of deflections before coming to rest. Or fewer. Or it may be deflected by different degrees at a similar number of collisions. The number of possibilities is certainly very large.

What does this now produce? Instead of each electron relinquishing the same amount of energy as all its neighbors in a neat and orderly uniformity of collision circumstances, many electrons give off energy in slightly different sized "parcels" or photons. The result is a heterogeneous beam of x-radiation emerging from the tube. There is a considerable variety in energy among the photons of which the beam is composed. These energies will vary from very low (with those rays just able to penetrate the glass wall of the tube) to a maximum which will depend on the kilovoltage applied across the tube.

This process accounts for most of the radiation produced in the tube and it produces a continuous spectrum between the limits described. At the moment this information is sufficient for our purposes, but we shall deal with the subject more fully in Chapter 9 when we give an account of the remaining radiation, together with other considerations of x-ray production.

7.2 THERMIONIC EMISSION

Thermionic emission is the emission of electrons from the surface of a conductor through the agency of heat (*therm*, from heat, and *ionic*, to do with ions).

Electron Emission from the Filament

We have previously discussed the place of electrons within a conductor (see Chapter 3) and the fact that there are many that are relatively free to move. We have seen that it is these electrons that constitute an electric current when they drift preferentially in one direction along the wire under the influence of an applied voltage. In a copper wire at room temperature, with no current flowing in it, all the electrons are in motion, most of them within their atomic shells. But those from the outermost shells, since they are bound only loosely, are in random motion throughout the substance of the wire. Their energy is derived from the heat of their environment (the room) but this is insufficient to allow them to escape from the surface of the wire. When they try to do so they are withheld at the boundary by the attraction of the positive nuclei close by. However, with an increase in energy, a stage is reached when some will escape. If the temperature of the wire is increased sufficiently the most energetic electrons will be emitted from the metal, at the expense of the thermal energy supplied.

When this process occurs in a vacuum, these electrons form a cloud about the wire and are in constant agitated motion. They increase in number as the temperature is increased, and are called the *space charge*.

In modern x-ray tubes a tiny coil of wire is used as one of the electrodes, the cathode, and by means of heating it is made to supply electrons by the process described above. This coiled wire or filament which forms the cathode is heated by an electric current supplied from outside the tube. The filament is made of tungsten with which a suitably efficient electron emission for purposes of x-ray production takes place from 2300–2500°C. Let us examine in some detail the heating of the cathode filament.

The energy dissipated as heat from the filament will be given by the equation

$$W = I^2 Rt, \qquad (3.12)$$

where W is the energy in watt-seconds or joules, I is the current through the wire in amperes, R is the resistance of the wire in ohms, and t is the time under consideration in seconds. The value of current, I, is an RMS value in this equation because the filament is heated by an alternating current. If the value of W is raised by increasing either I or R, this will mean a greater rate of heat production in the wire and therefore an increase in temperature. But as R, the resistance, remains constant for all practical purposes (we shall ignore any small change in the value due to a temperature change), the only possibility is to change I, the current in the wire. And this is what is done. As the current is increased, the filament becomes hotter and glows brighter. When the current is made smaller the temperature of the filament drops.

Now refer again to the equation $W = I^2Rt$. It will be seen that, when R and t are kept constant, W will vary as the square of I. That is to say, a relatively small change in I, the filament current, will give rise to a large change in W and therefore a pronounced temperature change in the filament, and consequently a considerable increase in thermionic emission.

You may have realized by now that a filament of this sort could be used as a source of electrons in an x-ray tube. In fact most modern x-ray tubes utilize this principle, and a tube of this type is called a *Coolidge tube* or a *hot-cathode tube*. We shall have more to say on this subject in the next section. Meanwhile let us examine the function of this source of electrons when it is built into an evacuated glass tube. What we have to say will certainly apply to hot-cathode x-ray tubes but may also be extended to apply to other vacuum tubes in a more general way.

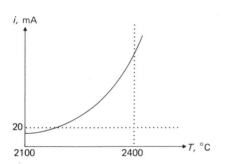

FIG. 7.5. Tube current as a function of filament temperature in the case of a tungsten filament.

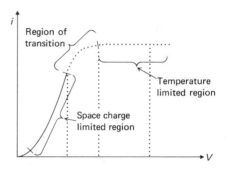

FIG. 7.6. Tube current as a function of tube voltage.

We have seen the plausibility of a small change in the filament current producing a pronounced change in filament temperature and a corresponding increase in electron emission. Figure 7.5 shows the nature of the relationship which exists between the temperature of the filament and the current through a tube when all the electrons emitted by the filament are drawn across to the anode. Of course, different tubes produce different curves, but they all have this characteristic shape. Note how equal increments of temperature produce larger and larger increases in tube current. This fact makes the filament temperature an extremely useful control factor in the selection of tube current, and consequently this is the method used for the control of x-ray tube currents.

The tube current not only depends on filament temperature in the manner shown, but it also depends on the tube voltage. An example is shown by the curve of Fig. 7.6, which represents the case of constant filament temperature. The rising part of the graph indicates that as the voltage is increased more and more electrons from the space charge are drawn toward the anode, and the tube current increases. This part of the graph is known as the *space-charge-limited region of operation*.

The horizontal part of the graph indicates that no increase of tube current is produced by increasing the tube voltage. Here all the emitted electrons are being drawn across to the anode as rapidly as the filament produces them; that is, there is no longer any significant space-charge cloud around the filament. A relatively constant current is the result. Only a change in filament temperature can appreciably alter the value of current in this region, so it is called the *temperature-limited region of operation.* The value at which the tube current no longer increases with tube voltage is known as the *saturation current.* Any increase in tube voltage beyond this point, although it will not increase the number of electrons crossing the tube, will, however, increase their acceleration. They will therefore strike the anode with greater energy, and in the x-ray tube will thus produce x-rays of greater energy.

Now let us see what the significance of all this is in the matter of radiography. If x-ray tubes were operated in the temperature-limited region, the tube current would be quite independent of the tube voltage. What are the advantages of this in the x-ray department?

First, without such independence, a change in one factor (e.g., tube voltage) would always produce a change in the other (e.g., tube current). The changes involved would not always bear the same constant simple relationship to each other. Exposure factors would therefore become much more difficult to formulate. Also the relationship between tube current and voltage would vary to some extent from machine to machine and make the interchangeability of exposure techniques impossible.

Unfortunately x-ray tubes do not operate in the temperature-limited region, although they do very nearly. It so happens that at the relatively large tube currents demanded in modern medical radiography (200 mA or more), the inherent characteristics of tube designs make it necessary to apply tube voltages in considerable excess of the usual diagnostic range, that is, 40 to 140 kV, in order to reach the region of temperature limitation. Figure 7.7 shows a family, or group, of curves relating tube current and tube voltage for an actual x-ray tube. Each curve has been produced by a different filament heating current I_f. Only the lowest curve demonstrates a near-horizontal region of temperature limitation. The other curves get progressively steeper as the filament current is increased. Note the values of tube current and tube voltage for the most "ideal" curve; about 50 mA and up to 150 kV.

Space-Charge Compensation

To overcome the disadvantages which would otherwise be brought about by operation of x-ray tubes in the space-charge-limited region, it is necessary to compensate in some way for the changes occurring in the tube current due to variations in tube voltage. This is accomplished by the *space-charge compensator,* which is composed of circuitry which automatically decreases the filament heating current appropriately as the kV is increased so that the tube current (mA) remains constant. We shall discuss the space-charge compensator further in Section 8.3.

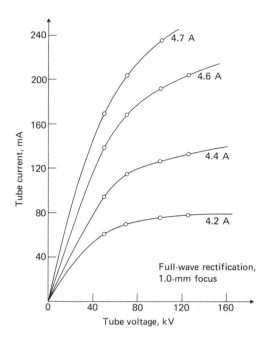

FIG. 7.7. Tube current as a function of tube voltage at four different filament currents.

7.3 COOLIDGE TUBES

In 1913, William Coolidge (1873–   ), reported the invention of the hot-cathode tube now named after him. This event marks a significant turning point in the history of the x-ray tube.

Prior to this time, gas tubes were used for radiography, but they suffered greatly from at least two disadvantages. The production of x-rays was by no means steady, as stated earlier; from minute to minute during the exposure there was often a considerable variation in the tube's radiation output. Also, as you will readily appreciate from what has already been said about the gas tube, the fact that it was impossible to control the current through the tube, and therefore, the intensity of radiation, independently of the kilovoltage applied across it, severely restricted the gas tube's technical flexibility. What was required was a source of electrons other than that provided by the residual low-pressure gas in the tube; a source that could be turned on or off and the output of which could be controlled. Then all the gas could be removed, and with these two factors the production of x-rays would become a matter of considerable precision.

Coolidge achieved these aims by making the cathode from a small spiral of tungsten wire, heated by an electric current, and completely evacuating the tube. (Tungsten has a high melting point, good mechanical strength, and does not vaporize readily. You can see the advantages of these properties in this type of x-ray tube.) He overcame the technical difficulties of making hard, brittle tungsten into a fine wire and then supported this filament within the tube. Now, when x-rays of greater pene-

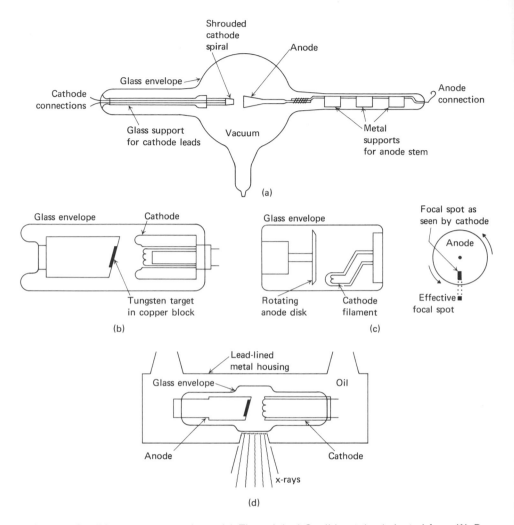

FIG. 7.8. Coolidge-type x-ray tubes. (a) The original Coolidge tube (adapted from W. D. Coolidge's paper in *Physical Review,* December 1913). (b) A stationary-anode tube. (c) A rotating-anode tube. (d) A stationary-anode tube inside its housing.

trating ability were required (for the radiography of thicker parts of the body for example), it was only necessary to increase the kilovoltage across the tube. This accelerated the electrons to a greater speed, and in their collisions with the target material they gave rise to radiation having a greater energy and consequent greater penetrating ability. At the same time there was no increase in the number of electrons, so that the tube current remained the same. Compare this with the behavior of the gas tube. See Fig. 7.8 for diagrams of Coolidge-type tubes.

Of course, if for some reason it became necessary to increase the intensity of radiation (that is, the number of rays emerging from the tube port), for example to compensate for an increase in the anode-to-film distance, this could be done by passing more current through the filament. This rise in filament current would then raise the temperature of the filament, thereby increasing the number of emitted electrons, thus in turn (by increasing the number of collisions at the target) increasing the intensity of radiation.

In the Coolidge tube we therefore have an x-ray tube in which it is possible to vary the tube current independently of the voltage across the tube. This means that we may vary the intensity of the x-ray beam for the purpose of making greater or smaller radiographic exposures simply by changing the filament current. We may also change the penetration ability of the beam by increasing or decreasing the kilovoltage across the tube, without affecting the tube current, with the reservation previously discussed; that is, that for tube currents much in excess of 50 mA, a space-charge compensator must be employed. There is thus a great deal of independence between the factors controlling these two important properties of the beam. In fact, from what has gone before you might suppose that with the advent of the space-charge compensator this independence is complete. But some other process intervenes to prevent this from being so.

You may recall from reading Section 7.1 that x-rays are given off during the interactions of high-speed electrons with the atoms of the target material. Any particular electron follows a path in the material which results from a number of deflections due to adjacent nuclei. At each deflection the electron loses energy, some of which is radiated as a photon of x-radiation. Clearly, the number of deflections and photons produced depends on how long a path the electron can follow, and this in turn depends on its energy to begin with. This amount of energy is determined by the voltage difference between the tube electrodes. Therefore it is evident that a rise in kilovoltage will not only produce more penetrating (that is, higher-energy) x-rays, but also more of those having less than the maximum energy. Kilovoltage changes, therefore, alter the intensity of the beam as well as its penetrability. Later, in our discussion of tube efficiency, we shall find that the intensity of the x-ray beam varies approximately as the square of the kilovoltage. That is, if the kilovoltage is changed from 30 to 60 kV, or multiplied by 2, the intensity of radiation will be increased by a factor of 4, even though the tube current remains constant.

Other refinements which Coolidge introduced besides this major change in the basic tube design included a filament shrouded by a cylindrical metal cup, which, since it was at the same potential as the cathode spiral and connected to it, focused the electrons onto a small spot on the anode, called the *focal spot*, or simply the *focus*. Instead of flying out widespread toward the anode, the electrons were now repelled from the metal sheath surrounding their points of origin and were thereby concentrated into a relatively small cone (see Fig. 7.9). The size of the truncated tip of this electron stream falling on the target could be arranged at manufacture by suitable positioning of the focusing-surround relative to the spiral filament within it. Thus the size of the focal spot could be

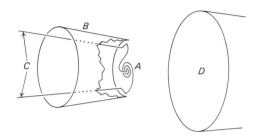

FIG. 7.9. Details of the Coolidge cathode: The filament spiral, *A*, is supported inside the focusing cup, *B*, and connected electrically by the wires at *C*; *D* is the circular face of the anode. (Adapted from Coolidge's paper in the *Physical Review*, December 1913)

predetermined. He also devised a target made of tungsten in the form of a small plaque inset in the face of a copper block. The high melting point of the tungsten (3370°C) raised the limits of operating voltage of the tube, while the copper block into which it was set conducted heat away from the target through a copper stem to the outside of the tube. Sometimes, in the early Coolidge-type tubes, this stem expanded outside the glass envelope into a number of fins to provide a greater surface area for the purpose of more rapid heat dissipation. Sometimes the copper anode stem was hollow and water circulated through it. This water either boiled in an open container at the outside extremity of the anode, or was cooled through a system of pipes (see Fig. 7.17).

7.4 X-RAY TUBE POWER OUTPUT AND RATINGS

Now that we have discussed x-ray tubes qualitatively in terms of their principles of operation, we may at this stage look a little more closely at some of the quantities involved. After all, it is with numbers that you will be dealing as an x-ray technician when you consider exposure factors, and especially how closely those factors approach whatever maximum exposure the tube will safely stand. If such a maximum limit exists (and it sounds reasonable to suppose that it does) you may ask how large it is, how to find it (in advance of an exposure!), and the reason for it.

Tube Efficiency

You may recall from Section 7.1 that in the account of energy transfer from a deflected electron within the target material to the photon of x-radiation which that electron produces, we stated that only a part of it appears from the site of collision as a photon of x-radiation. There is still some energy left to account for.

This energy is of considerable importance because it appears in the form of heat. As the bombardment of the target continues, the metal becomes hotter. So far, we have been primarily concerned with the x-ray production of the tube, but as x-ray technicians you will also have to

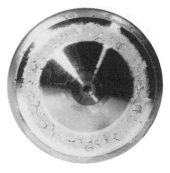

FIG. 7.10. Peeling of tungsten from an anode face. A rotating anode (see Section 7.5), showing the damage due to overheating.

consider the heat produced, because if the target becomes too hot it may easily be damaged or destroyed (see Fig. 7.10).

The quantity of heat produced at the anode as a proportion of the total energy supplied to the tube is exceedingly high. Within the range of kilovoltages used in conventional diagnostic radiography, that is, in the region of 40 kV to 140 kV, only 1% or less of the total energy supplied to the tube appears as x-radiation. The remainder, 99% or more, appears as heat.

The actual efficiency of the process of x-ray production is dependent on two factors: the material of the target and the tube voltage. The x-ray output will increase with a target material of higher atomic number, with a higher tube voltage, and with a larger tube current. These quantities have been found to be related to a close approximation by the simple formula:

$$P_x = kZIV^2, \qquad (7.1)$$

where P_x is the x-ray power output in watts, Z is the atomic number of the target material, I is the RMS value of the tube current in amps, V is the RMS value of the tube voltage, and k is a numerical coefficient, 1.4×10^{-9}/volt, which is experimentally determined. This constant is affected by the nature of the applied voltage (e.g., single phase, three phase) and is at best only an approximation.

Note that it is the RMS value of tube voltage which is employed in Eq. (7.1). In the x-ray machine it is the kV peak which governs the upper limit of x-ray photon energy (see Section 7.1) and therefore, the penetration ability of the most energetic rays in the x-ray beam. For this reason, kV meters in control panels are always arranged to read kV peak, and are often labeled in this manner. In this text you may regard "kV" as meaning the peak value unless we state otherwise, as was done in Eq. (7.1). Both kV and kVp are widely used synonymously in the literature of radiology.

To get the total energy output, of course, one would simply multiply the power by the time of operation. If one were to multiply watts by seconds one would get the energy in watt-seconds, or joules. As will be shown later in this section, the actual energy unit most commonly employed in medical radiography is a so-called "heat unit," which is slightly smaller than the watt-second, or joule.

When we study Eq. (7.1), several things are readily apparent: the obvious desirability of a target material which has a high atomic number; the simple effect of I, the tube current, on the x-ray power output; and finally the effect of V, the RMS value of tube voltage. Note that this factor in the right-hand side of the equation plays a more important part in helping to determine the total x-ray power output than do the other two factors discussed. As the voltage is increased the x-ray power output is increased as the square of the voltage. We shall return to this point when we consider the units in which heat is measured in medical radiography.

The percentage efficiency is given by:

$$\text{Efficiency} = \left[\frac{\text{x-ray power output}}{\text{cathode ray power}} \times \frac{100}{1}\right]\%,$$

where the cathode ray power (in watts) equals VI, the voltage and current being expressed in RMS volts and amps, respectively. (The power factor $= 1$; that is, only ohmic resistance is significant.) Substituting Eq. (7.1) in the numerator of the above expression for efficiency, we get

$$\text{Efficiency} = \left[\frac{kZIV^2}{IV} \times \frac{100}{1}\right]\%,$$

which may be simplified to

$$\text{Efficiency} = [kZV \times 100]\%,$$

or simply

$$\text{Efficiency} = [KZV]\%, \tag{7.2}$$

where $K = 100k = (100 \times 1.4 \times 10^{-9})\text{volt}^{-1} = 1.4 \times 10^{-7}\text{ volt}^{-1}$.

Example: What will be the percentage efficiency of a tungsten target in an x-ray tube operating at a setting of 100 kV?

First we must realize that the kV setting on the machine refers to peak values, and the voltage in Eq. (7.2) refers to the RMS value. Hence we must first determine V, the RMS value corresponding to V_p, the peak value of 100 kV:

$$V = 0.707\ V_p = 0.707 \times 10^5 \text{ volts} = 7.07 \times 10^4 \text{ volts}.$$

Next we employ Eq. (7.2):

$$\text{Efficiency} = (KZV)\% = [(1.4 \times 10^{-7}/\text{volt})(74)(7.07 \times 10^4 \text{ volts})]\%,$$

where 74 is the atomic number of tungsten, chemical symbol W, formerly known as wolfram. Note that the units "volt" cancel out, yielding

$$\text{Efficiency} = (1.4 \times 74 \times 7.07 \times 10^{-3})\% = (734 \times 10^{-3})\% = 0.734\%,$$

which, if we assume that the tube voltage is precise to only two significant figures, means that the efficiency is 0.73%, that is, less than 1%.

In the early days of x-ray tube manufacture, a platinum target was used. Platinum has an atomic number of 78 and could therefore be expected to produce a corresponding increase in efficiency over tungsten.

However, the trouble with platinum is that it has a lower melting point than tungsten (1770°C as opposed to 3370°C), and therefore has a lower operating limit.

This figure of 0.73% tube efficiency means, of course, that in this case over 99% of the input energy is converted to heat. This heat is measured in heat units in radiography and these units are included in a number of factors listed together by the tube manufacturer to indicate the maximum limits of tube operation. These factors, of which heat units are probably the most frequently considered on the part of the technician, are collectively called *tube ratings*.

Tube Ratings

X-ray tubes are rated by the manufacturers in terms of the maximum permissible limits within which the tube may be operated. In order to provide a safety factor, it is a common practice to set the rating at some figure lower than that required to damage the tube. But despite this leeway it is inadvisable to exceed the stated ratings. Even though no damage is apparent, the life of the tube will be shortened by abuse.

The factors quoted are usually the following:

1. The maximum permissible voltage, in kVp, which limit is set by insulation considerations. At voltages greater than this, there is danger that the insulation will break down between regions of different potential in the tube.
2. The maximum tube current, mA average, which is limited by the permissible filament temperature. (A typical current through the filament may be from 3 to 5 amps.)
3. The maximum energy dissipation, in heat units, that is, the amount of energy in the form of heat which the tube can safely produce in a given interval of time.

For the purpose of any consideration of heat units in tube ratings it is assumed that all the tube output is in the form of heat. After all, so little of the output is in the form of x-radiation and the small error involved in this assumption only increases the tube's margin of safety.

As we know from Chapter 3, units of heat may be defined in watt-seconds, where watts = amps × volts. In this term watt-second (or volt-ampere-second), we have three variables for which, at first glance, it would seem easy to substitute figures from the mA, kV, and time factors of the x-ray exposure. But in Chapter 6 we found that to legitimately substitute in this way we must consider RMS values of the voltage and current. You may recall that the relationships (assuming a sinusoidal AC waveform) are as follows:

The RMS value is 0.707 of the peak value of current or voltage, and the average value of these quantities is 0.636 of the peak value in full-wave rectification.

Perhaps you can anticipate what is before us. Each time you (the technician) wanted to compare an intended set of exposure factors with the maximum rating of the tube you were using, you would have to employ some simple but tedious and time-consuming arithmetic in order to do so; that is, if the tube rating chart used the unit of heat defined as the watt-second.

To avoid this unwelcome labor, it has become customary to use a hybrid unit known simply as a *heat unit,* in which

$$1 \text{ heat unit} = 1 \text{ kVp} \times 1 \text{ mA} \times 1 \text{ second.}$$

In this unit the value of mA given by the meter on the x-ray machine control panel is the average value. Yet another complication! But you already know the reason for this from your reading in Chapter 6.

The Conversion of Radiological Heat Units to Watt-Seconds

The following calculation will show us the precise relationship between our own units of convenience and the more scientific watt-second.

First we calculate the heat associated with a given set of exposure factors (kV, mA, and time) in terms of the radiological heat unit (HU) and then, for purposes of comparison, we shall repeat the calculation in terms of the watt-sec.

Heat (in HU) = [(kVp)(mA)(s)]HU, or, recalling that by kV is meant kV peak:

$$\text{Heat (in HU)} = [(kV)(mA)(s)] \text{ HU,}$$

where kV is the peak value of the tube voltage in kilovolts, mA is the average value of the tube current in milliamperes, and s is the exposure time in seconds. Hence

$$\text{Heat (in HU)} = [(V_p \times 10^3)(\bar{I} \times 10^{-3})(s)] \text{ HU,}$$

where V_p is peak voltage in volts, written V_p to emphasize peak value here, and $\bar{I}$ is average current in amperes. Finally

$$\text{Heat (in HU)} = [V_p \bar{I} \text{ s}] \text{ HU.}$$

Now repeating the calculation in terms of watt-seconds:

$$\text{Heat (in watt-sec)} = [V_{\text{RMS}} I_{\text{RMS}} \text{ s}] \text{ watt-sec}$$
$$= \left[(0.707 V_p) \left(\frac{0.707}{0.636} \bar{I} \right) (s) \right] \text{ watt-sec.}$$

These numerical substitutions, of course, follow from the relationships among peak, average, and RMS values for sinusoidal AC, full wave rectified, as discussed in Chapter 6. Thus we have:

$$\text{Heat (in watt-sec)} = [(0.785) V_p \bar{I} \text{ s}] \text{ watt-sec.}$$

So we see that the same amount of heat as expressed in $[V_p \bar{I} \, s]$ HU is expressed by $[0.785 V_p \bar{I} \, s]$ watt-sec. In other words,

$$1 \text{ HU} = 0.785 \text{ watt-sec.}$$

In conclusion we convert this radiological heat unit into the calorie, the commonly used heat unit of the world of science. Recall that a watt-sec is simply a joule. And 1 calorie = 4.186 joules. Thus

$$1 \text{ HU} = (0.785 \text{ joule}) \left(\frac{1}{4.186} \frac{\text{cal}}{\text{joule}} \right) = 0.188 \text{ cal.}$$

That is, 1 heat unit may be expressed as about 0.2 calorie.

The Use of High kV

Under the general heading of this chapter we may consider two advantages to be gained from the use of high kV techniques. (There are also other advantages which, however, we shall not discuss here.) First, from our consideration of radiological heat units, you can see how the three factors involved, kV, mA, and time, have similar effects on the total. That is to say, a doubling of any one of them, for example, will lead to the same result: a doubling of the total.

But this is not the case when photographic effect is concerned. True, doubling the mA or time will, in general, produce twice the photographic effect, but for kV and photographic effect there is no such simple relationship. For one thing, the x-ray output rises whenever the kV is increased. We have already discussed this earlier in this section. Also, more energetic photons may give rise to a latent image in other than the silver halide crystals they strike. Adjacent crystals may be affected by photoelectrons and recoil electrons arising from the initial interaction of the x-ray photon and the halide grain. This will lead to a greater photographic effect at higher kilovoltages.

The relationship which does exist between photographic effect and kV shows that a doubling of photographic effect results from an increase of about 8 kV. Even this is merely a rule of thumb which, moreover, is only valid in the 50-to-60-kV range. At lower kV's, less increase is required for the same effect, while at high kV's (up to 140 kV, for example), a somewhat greater increase is needed to produce double the photographic effect. It thus turns out that a greatly increased photographic effect will result with a relatively small proportional increase in kV, while at the same time the total heat units produced will not be very much greater.

The Use of Tube Rating Charts and Cooling Curves

Refer now to Fig. 7.11, a tube rating chart for the rotating-anode tube, Model HRT B 1–2. The chart shows a series of 6 curves. The x-axis of the graph represents maximum exposure times between $\frac{1}{120}$ second and 20 seconds. The y-axis represents kilovoltage peak (kVp), and varies from 50 kVp to 130 kVp. The manufacturer has provided 6 curves, each of a

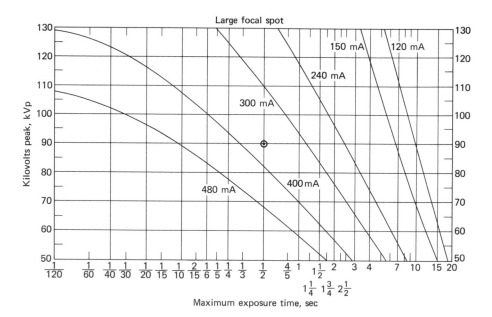

FIG. 7.11. Tube rating chart for rotating-anode x-ray tube, Model HRT B 1–2, when operated on full-wave-rectified equipment, single phase, 60 cycles. The point circled is discussed in the text as an example. (Courtesy of General Electric Co., X-Ray Department)

different mA value, which indicate the maximum values at which the tube should be operated in terms of kVp and time.

In order to use such a chart, all that is necessary is for us to take our proposed exposure, say 90 kVp, 400 mA, and ½ second, and refer it to the chart thus. When we find the point of intersection of 90 kVp and ½ second, we see that it lies above the 400 mA curve and is therefore outside the limits set by this curve. So it is unsafe for us to proceed with this exposure. Some other approach will have to be adopted; perhaps the procedure in which we are engaged will permit us to shorten the anode-film distance.

You may ask why the chart states "When operated on full wave rectified equipment, single phase, 60 cycles." The answer is that with some other sort of supply, say half-wave rectification, or 100 cycles per second, the heat produced at the target per unit time will be different and the rating chart in its present form will no longer hold true.

The question of rectification and tube rating is one which often arises in the x-ray department. It is not unusual for a technician to use a major x-ray unit, which may have full-wave rectification, and then perhaps use a mobile unit, or a dental x-ray machine, which are often half-wave rectified machines. In such a case it is as well to note that the operating limits of the mobile machine with half-wave rectification are lower. That is, the maximum exposure time permitted for any given combination of mA and kVp is shorter than for these same exposure factors on the major unit

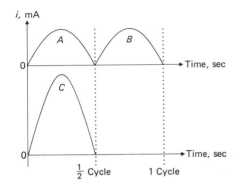

FIG. 7.12. Two graphs to show heat-production rates with two different types of rectification. The areas $A + B$ = area C.

whose tube is supplied with a full-wave rectified voltage. If we examine Fig. 7.12, the reason becomes evident.

Suppose that the total area $A + B$ below the first curve is equal to the area C below the second curve. These areas represent in each case the product of a rate (millicoulombs per second = milliamperes) and a time. This product will therefore give us a quantity, in this case millicoulombs. What we have done in effect, then, is to set each of our machines at the same mAs. We shall also presume that the kVp is the same in each case so that it will not interfere as a variable. But, when we look at the figure, we see that the quantity C millicoulombs is passed through the tube in $\frac{1}{2}$ cycle, whereas the quantity $A + B$ millicoulombs, equal in size to C, passes through the tube in one complete cycle. The difference in rate is due to the type of rectification. This will mean that heat is produced more rapidly at the anode of the tube which is half-wave rectified, and so, if similar tubes are used in each case the rating of the half-wave rectified tube must be set lower than the other. Separate rating charts will have to be used for each tube in these two circumstances, even though the tubes in the two machines may be identical.

Frequently an x-ray machine is designed so that it is impossible to make an exposure with the controls adjusted for a set of exposure factors that exceeds the tube rating. Although everything else appears to be in order apart from this exceeding of the tube limits, pressing the exposure button produces no result. In these cases, the design of the machine is such that an arrangement of mechanical and electrical interlocks operates to open the exposure switch circuit and no exposure is possible. Any combination of mA, kVp, and time which exceeds the tube rating will cause this safety lock to operate. We shall make further reference to this and other safety devices in Chapter 8.

You may think that such a device would absolve the technician from any responsibility as far as the tube ratings are concerned. But this is not the case. It is sometimes possible to "beat the system" and obtain exposures greater than the maximum permissible. If a person sets the controls just below the point at which the safety interlock begins to function and then uses this exposure two or three times in rapid succession, the total exposure is greatly increased. Although you may then be pleased to find that your radiograph is at last adequately exposed, you will have damaged the tube and perhaps ruined it altogether. Intelligent use of the machine and its tube rating chart is still a necessity.

Anode Cooling Curves

We have seen that the chief reason for the existence of tube loading limits has to do with the question of heat. An amount of heat (that is, really, an amount of energy), greater than a certain quantity will damage the tungsten target. Either the target will be pitted or it will begin to peel (and both these effects will change the geometry of the focal spot and so give rise to image distortions), or else, if it reaches a very high temperature, due to the heat energy absorbed, it may liberate electrons from its surface. If these electrons are then accelerated toward the cathode during the reverse half-cycle of voltage in a self-rectified tube, they will bombard the filament of the cathode and destroy it.

So far, we have chiefly considered single exposures. But what about a succession of exposures which are all within the tube rating limits? How long should one wait between these permissible exposures to avoid their summation becoming a total impermissible exposure? How long does it take the anode to cool down sufficiently to allow us to add more heat to it? The answers to these questions are indicated by the Anode Cooling Curve for the tube concerned.

Figure 7.13 shows one of these curves. This curve is for the same tube as the previous rating chart. The two types of graphs are often made available on a single sheet.

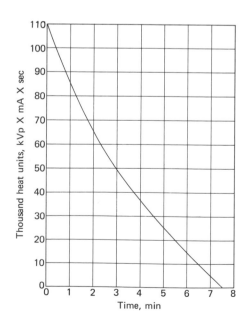

FIG. 7.13. Anode cooling curve, showing the rate at which heat leaves the anode of a rotating-anode x-ray tube, Model HRT B 1–2, when operated on full-wave-rectified equipment, single phase, 60 cycles. Anode heat characteristics: heat storage capacity, 110,000 heat units; maximum cooling rate, 30,000 heat units/minute. (Courtesy of General Electric Co., X-Ray Department)

The curve shows the rate at which heat leaves the anode. The rate is given in thousands of heat units per minute. Note that the rate of cooling is not quite constant. If it were, the curve would become a straight line.

Remember that heat units = kVp × mA × s. For this particular tube's anode, the maximum heat storage capacity is given as 110,000 heat units. With this amount of heat the anode would be a very bright red. If more heat than this is added to the anode, the temperature of the tungsten will be increased so as to bring it into the danger range we wish to avoid. Therefore this is the upper limit of safe function. A single exposure of 110,000 heat units, or a series of rapid exposures producing in total more than 110,000 heat units, must not be used. Moreover, for this maximum value of 110,000 heat units, the chart indicates that it will take 7.5 minutes for the anode to cool again to a value of zero heat units, that is, the heat of the target at room temperature.

If any smaller exposure is used, producing, for example, 50,000 heat units, the anode cooling curve shows that in order for the anode to give off this amount of heat and so reach zero again, it will follow the curve from this point at 3 minutes and 50,000 heat units down to 7.5 minutes and zero heat units. The elapsed time for this to occur will therefore be 4.5 minutes. By referring to the cooling curve then, you may quite easily see how many heat units it is safe to produce within a given time and how long you should wait before making another exposure.

7.5 X-RAY TUBE TARGETS

A typical target arrangement is shown in Fig. 7.14. In this case the anode is of the stationary type. The target material, usually tungsten, is a small plaque embedded in the anode, which is a larger piece of copper.

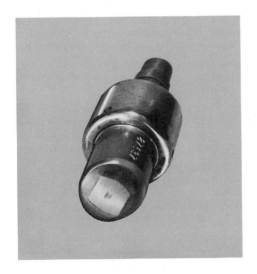

FIG. 7.14. The target face. This is a stationary anode. Note the relative sizes of the tungsten insert and the central spot or roughened area made by the electron bombardment.

The function of the x-ray tube target is to provide an obstacle in the path of electrons originating from the filament. To fulfill the purpose of the tube, the subsequent energy release should appear in the form of x-radiation. Any heat resulting from the collision is unwanted and will have to be dissipated by the target area as rapidly as possible, to avoid damage to the target material or the anode stem. We have already found, in Section 7.4, that the highest efficiency of x-ray production can be achieved by using a target metal of high atomic number and high melting point. We have also seen that this efficiency is still very low; less than 1% of the total energy input is available as x-rays when the tube is operated at voltages in the usual diagnostic range, say, 60–100 kV. The rest of the energy appears as heat.

The speed with which heat may be transferred from the target depends, in large measure, on the type of metal of which the anode is made, as well as its physical dimensions. In any case, there is always a practical upper limit of heat transfer and therefore of tube loading.

We may arrive at a simple approximation of the size of this upper limit by using the figure of 200 watts per square millimeter of target area for one second of exposure. The question of tube loadings is so complex that no single figure can be given to suit every case, but for a stationary anode this figure will serve the purposes of our discussion. Above this load limit we may assume that the temperature of the target will rise to a critical level.

From what has just been stated, you will see that any consideration of x-ray tube targets consists almost entirely of the consideration of methods by which the problems of heat production may be overcome, while still retaining those tube design features which are essential for radiographic purposes. We shall now talk about the more important of these methods.

Line Focus

Obviously, there is a simple way in which one could greatly increase the loading limit: One could increase the focal spot or target size. Such a procedure would mean that a greater mass of metal would be made available for heat energy absorption. That this procedure would result in a smaller increase in temperature of the anode is fairly obvious. Contemplate, for a moment, the fact that it requires a lot more heat energy to warm up a pailful of cold water than a thimbleful.

Examining an example of a target shows that the area of tungsten presented to face the filament of the tube is approximately 1 cm², while the focal spot size is only 1 mm². There is evidently a difference between these two areas. The reason for this is that the focal spot size refers in some way to the area onto which the electron beam is focused by the curved face of the cathode, whereas the first-mentioned area refers to the size of the piece of tungsten.

Why then, you may ask, is the electron beam confined to this tiny spot when so much more tungsten is available? In brief, the answer is that for the x-ray beam to project a sharp radiographic image onto a film or screen it is essential for the x-ray beam to originate from a point source, or a source which is as small as practicable. You can illustrate this by casting the shadow of your hand onto a wall; first use a lamp with a small filament, and second a large fluorescent tube light. When the larger light source is used, the shadow on the wall becomes so blurred and diffused as to be almost unidentifiable, but with the small source the shadow is sharp.

So if we want the focal spot to remain very small for radiographic purposes and yet as large as possible to increase the maximum permissible loading, perhaps we can "cheat" in some way in order to achieve both aims. Fortunately, this is in fact the case.

One setup commonly used in diagnostic tubes is the tungsten target arranged at an angle of about 20° to the central ray of the useful beam, and the filament made in the form of a coil (see Fig. 7.15). With this arrangement, the focal spot, when seen from the position of the film, appears to be square, and of a certain size, say 1 mm², while from the filament the focal spot appears rectangular and about three times larger. The electrons strike a relatively large area, but the utilized x-ray beam originates from what appears at the film to be a relatively small area. The requirement of increased loading, while maintaining an apparently small source of the x-ray beam, has been satisfied to some degree. This arrangement is known as a *line focus*.

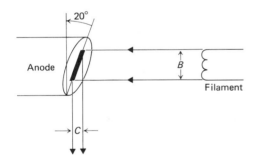

FIG. 7.15. The angulation of the x-ray tube target. Here the target is at an angle of 20° to the vertical. This means that the electron beam width, B, is three times the apparent focal spot width, C.

Double Focus

The single-line focus arrangement is somewhat restricting in practice because of the conflicting necessities of large-tube currents and fine focal spots. When the part to be x-rayed is apt to move it will surely be more important for us to use a high tube current and a corresponding short exposure time than to try to produce fine detail from a small focal spot and have movement blur spoil the result. From this point of view a larger focal spot is to be preferred. But such is not always the case. Some parts of the body are small, have fine structures, and may be easily immobilized. In these cases the high tube current is a secondary consideration. If one wants to achieve the sharpest possible detail, a fine focal spot is more desirable. These and other circumstances may be dealt with by having two foci in the tube (see Fig. 7.16). Two filaments are arranged side by side

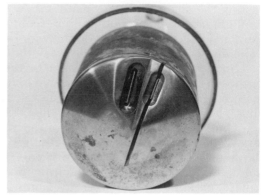

FIG. 7.16. Photograph of a twin-filament cathode. This is the aspect seen by the anode of the x-ray tube.

in the cathode, one larger than the other, and their electron beams bombard two separate areas of the target. One focal spot is the small one, commonly about 1 millimeter square, and the other the large one, perhaps about 2 mm square (that is, 4 mm²). The supply circuits for these two filaments are arranged so that only one can be used at a time. Two focal spot sizes in one tube are usually sufficient for most radiography, and they may be in a variety of sizes to suit various purposes. The technician then selects the focus he wants by means of a switch on the control panel. By this means he can choose between a higher tube loading or a smaller focal spot.

Anode Design

Another obvious way in which the loading limit may be raised is to try to take heat away from the target area as quickly as it is produced. There are several ways of doing this.

Probably the most universal approach to heat dissipation is to mount the tungsten target in the face of a block of copper. Copper is a much better conductor of heat than tungsten. Thus, by such an arrangement, heat is transferred quickly away from the target. This is the first step. Beyond this point there are several alternatives. The copper block or stem may not project beyond the tube envelope, but may provide a sufficiently large reservoir to absorb all the heat produced during the use for which the tube has been designed. In this case there is merely a metal connection of some other type passing through the glass to provide an electrical contact.

On the other hand, the copper stem may protrude and be connected to a series of fins, or a large copper block, which, by increasing the surface area, permits a more rapid heat loss from the anode. This loss of heat may take place to the air, or, if the tube is immersed in oil, to the surrounding oil. Direct transfer to the air is now mainly of historical interest because of the associated hazard of electric shock.

Another way of increasing the rate of heat transfer from the anode is to make it hollow and to pump a coolant such as water or oil through the cavity. The use of water, of course, raises a problem of electrical insulation because it is not a good electrical insulator and the anode is commonly

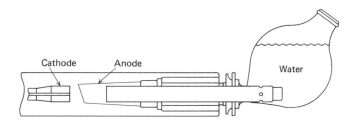

FIG. 7.17. A hollow anode (with water cooling).

at a high voltage relative to ground. The water therefore has to be conveyed to and from the anode in rubber hoses with high electrical insulating properties, free from leaks. The water also has to be disposed of with special care, unless the anode is designed to operate at ground potential, which may be done in some cases, especially when the x-radiation is to be applied therapeutically via a body opening. For these reasons, water is used as a coolant in a hollow anode of the type shown in Fig. 7.17. This anode stem terminates in a vessel in which the water boils while exposed to the open air. For obvious reasons of protection against electrical shock, this method also is now only of historical interest.

Oil as a coolant poses no such electrical hazards. Special insulating oil, which may be circulated through the hollow anode, is indeed a very efficient cooling agent, and hence such an arrangement is frequently used in larger therapy x-ray machines which are employed for long exposure times. The oil is pumped rapidly through the anode by an electric pump, and the removal of heat is accomplished so effectively that the oil, cool when it enters the anode, leaves it at a considerably higher temperature, and has to be cooled again before it is recirculated. The oil is cooled by passing it through a system of pipes around which cold tap water is constantly running. Figure 7.18 is a diagrammatic representation of this process. In such an installation, any breakdown of oil circulation during exposure would cause almost immediate overheating and damage to the tube. Therefore it is common practice to include in the electric pump circuit a switch which connects with the x-ray exposure circuit. If the pump stops the exposure is stopped too.

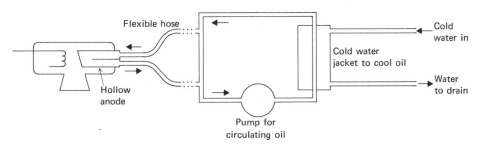

FIG. 7.18. Schematic of anode cooling system employing oil and water. The pump circulates oil through the hollow anode and the water jacket. Heat is transferred in the water jacket from the oil to the water.

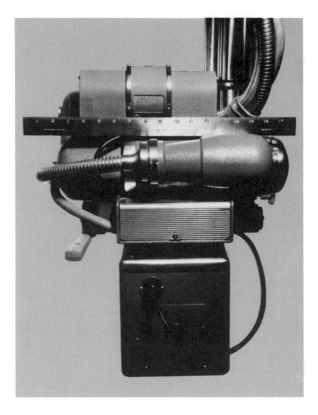

FIG. 7.19. The x-ray tube. The glass x-ray tube proper is inside the cylindrical metal casing immediately below the ruler. Above the ruler is the casing for the cooling fan. The large square box toward the bottom is the beam collimator. (Ruler is calibrated in inches.)

Oil Immersion

Most modern x-ray tubes used for radiography, rather than therapy, make use of oil as a cooling medium, but in a way that is slightly different from that described above. Most such tubes are now enclosed within metal casings in which all the space not occupied by the glass tube and necessary electrical connections is filled with oil. The outside of such a case is shown in Fig. 7.19. This is the very common appearance of the "x-ray tube" in the diagnostic x-ray department. The anode is cooled by the radiation of heat from itself, through the vacuum to the glass walls of the tube and to the surrounding oil. From the oil closest to the tube, heat is transferred by conduction and convection to the outer case, and from the case by radiation and convection to the air. To assist this final transfer a small electric fan is often built onto the outside of the case. Figure 7.19 shows this feature.

Among the advantages of this type of cooling are these: the oil, of a nonconducting type, acts as an electrical insulator, and the casing can provide radiation shielding. If the case is made of steel of sufficient

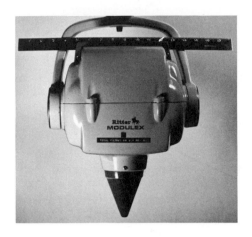

FIG. 7.20. A dental tube head. The x-ray tube is inside this case at about the level of the manufacturer's name.   Above this are the filament and high voltage transformers.   Compare the size and contents of this case with the one shown in Fig. 7.19. (Ruler is calibrated in inches.)

thickness or if it is lined with lead, and with joints which are designed to overlap, no significant amount of unwanted radiation escapes from the tube case or housing and radiation hazards connected with the x-ray machine are greatly reduced. Only a relatively small area in the bottom of the casing is left so that the x-ray beam can emerge, and at this part of the casing the cones or collimators necessary for further beam limitation are attached. This "open" area in the casing may be glass, or aluminum, or some other relatively radioparent material.

We have just mentioned oil as an electrical insulator but, of course, the risk of electric shock is not confined to the tube itself; the high-tension cables connected to it also have to be considered as a possible hazard. You may know that this problem is dealt with in the design of the cables. They are sheathed with thick rubber, which acts as an insulator and even makes it possible to handle them during an exposure (although naturally this is not recommended).

But in certain circumstances the use of an oil-filled casing for the x-ray tube has made it feasible to do without the high-tension cables as well. We refer now to low-power x-ray units, such as dental or mobile machines, as shown in Fig. 7.20. Here there are no visible, external, high-tension cables, and their apparent absence has made the tube-head unit much neater and easier to support and use. Note, however, that this unit is somewhat larger than that shown in Fig. 7.19. The reason is that the casing contains not only the x-ray tube but the high-tension transformer and the filament transformer as well. The high-tension cables are still present, but they are inside, much shorter, and do not have to be rubber-covered, since the oil effectively insulates them from their surroundings. Cable wear is also obviated. Figure 7.21 is a sectional drawing of such an arrangement.

Another feature of this and the previously mentioned tube housings is the provision which must be made for the oil to expand as it gets hot. This is done by including somewhere inside the case a small metal or

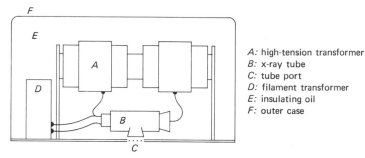

A: high-tension transformer
B: x-ray tube
C: tube port
D: filament transformer
E: insulating oil
F: outer case

FIG. 7.21. X-ray generator and tube head, of the type commonly used in dental and mobile x-ray machines.

rubber bellows filled with air. As the oil expands the bellows are crushed and the air inside is compressed. Without this air, which is readily compressible to the small extent required, the expanding oil would either leak from the casing or smash the x-ray tube. Sometimes a switch is incorporated in connection with the bellows, so that any undue collapse of them activates the switch, thus opening the x-ray exposure circuit. This arrangement makes it impossible to use the tube if its temperature and that of the oil have risen too high. Thus this constitutes a useful safety device.

Rotating Anodes

Rotating anodes, introduced in 1936, represent yet another method of overcoming as far as possible the loading restrictions imposed on the use of the x-ray tube by its great heat output. The principle is a simple one. It is based on a removal of the target from the electron beam before it reaches too high a temperature, and the rapid replacement of it by another, cooler target. In practice this change is carried out continuously many times during the course of an exposure; the targets are joined together, as it were, and form the face of a rotating disk, or the end of a rotating cylinder. As you can see by looking at Fig. 7.22, the tube filament is offset to one side

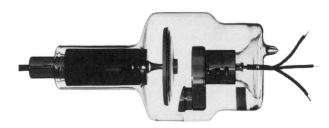

FIG. 7.22. Rotating anode with offset filament. In this photograph the filament is hidden by its focusing shroud. (Photograph courtesy Siemens A. G., Wernerwerk fuer Medizinische Technik, Erlangen, Germany)

so that the electron beam is focused onto a portion of the rotating anode close to its circumference. Note that the target face is angled in the same way as that of the stationary anode we discussed earlier. The anode is either faced with tungsten or is a solid tungsten disk. Immediately before the exposure begins, the anode is made to rotate at a high speed, so that, during the exposure, no single area of the anode face is bombarded for more than a moment, and before this same area comes round for bombardment again it has radiated much of its heat away. The rotation takes place at about 3000–3600 revolutions per minute, depending on the design of the tube and the frequency of the AC supply. With high-frequency anode supplies, such as 180 cps, the anode may rotate at up to 10,000 rpm.

One of the problems associated with the rotating anode concerns the lubrication of its bearings. Since the anode is in a vacuum it is impossible to use oil for lubrication purposes. Therefore the surfaces of the ball bearings of the spinning shaft are operated dry, but are coated with a thin layer of lead, which acts as a lubricant. A nonsolid lubricant would spread throughout the tube and destroy the high vacuum. This is the reason you can hear a typical dry, rasping sound from the rotating anode tube once the anode has been set spinning. This noise continues after the exposure has been terminated, and you can hear the anode turning with less and less speed until it finally stops. This time may be 10 minutes or more in some cases. If, while the anode is running down, you turn the tube on its mountings from, say, a horizontal to a vertical position, you will hear the note of the sound change as the bearings on the shaft meet the slightly different distribution of weight.

The anode is rotated by means of an induction motor, all of whose wires are outside the x-ray tube. Figure 7.23 shows a typical arrangement of this. Only the metal rotating shaft of the anode is inside the tube and no electrical connections to it are required for motor operation. (Recall that the operation of this induction motor was described in Section 5.3.)

If you were able to look at a rotating anode after a series of heavy exposures, you would see it glowing red hot. Of course you would have to remove any metal filters from the tube port so that you could see in through the glass, and also you would have to make certain that the x-ray machine

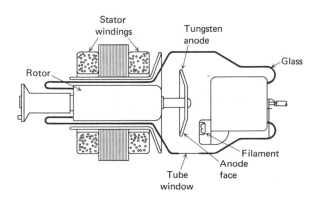

FIG. 7.23. Induction motor and rotating anode.

was properly switched off! The reason that the tube is designed in such a way as to permit such a high temperature is to allow radiation of heat from the anode. The rate of heat radiation increases rapidly with higher temperatures, the rate varying as T^4—that is, the fourth power of the absolute temperature—and radiation is the primary method of transferring heat from a rotating anode. If there were much transfer of heat by conduction through the anode stem, this would bring heat to the vicinity of the induction motor, with the consequent risk of damage to the stator windings.

You will probably note that, when an exposure is made with a rotating-anode tube, it is impossible to press the rotor switch and the exposure switch and obtain the exposure all at the same time. A delay of 1 second after starting the rotor is usually necessary before the exposure begins. The purpose of this delay is to allow the rotor to reach its working speed before exposure and so avoid damage from overheating.

In these two sections (7.4 and 7.5), we have examined various aspects of the function and design of x-ray tubes. We have seen that the production of x-rays by this method is inherently inefficient, but that constant research and the continuing development of tube design make the inefficiency a little less as time goes by. We can expect this trend to continue, but unless there is some significant difference in the principles employed, the gains will always be small. However, in the meantime, a sort of leapfrog process occurs. As various features of the tube (the filament, the anode, the efficiency of vacuum production, etc.) are developed, there is always at least one factor which limits tube life. This year's tubes have their lives terminated perhaps by failure of one component, which is then improved, so that next year's tubes will fail for some other reason. Meanwhile the average life span of x-ray tubes in general is being slowly increased. At present, as a very approximate rule of thumb, one can expect something like 50,000 exposures from an average tube. Naturally this figure depends greatly on the size of the exposures and other factors of tube use, but it will give you some idea of the life to be expected.

7.6 VALVE TUBES

The valve tube is basically similar to an x-ray tube; that is to say, it is a *diode*. But although the x-ray tube is of course used for x-ray production, this is not the object of the valve tube. As its name implies, this is a device which permits the passage of electricity in one direction, but prevents a current through it in the opposite direction. It is therefore said to act as a rectifier, and can convert an alternating current to a unidirectional current. The essential difference between the valve tube and the x-ray tube is that, although the x-ray tube operates in (or as close as possible to) the temperature-limited region of thermionic emission, the valve tube operates in the space-charge-limited region (see Section 7.2).

The diode as a rectifier is used in the x-ray machine and inserted in the circuit between the high-tension transformer and the x-ray tube. The high-tension transformer converts mains voltage (120 or 240 volts) to the various voltages required for operating the x-ray tube (about 30,000 to 140,000 volts). The valve tube immediately precedes the x-ray tube in the chain of electrical events represented by different components in the x-ray circuit, and is connected to the x-ray tube by the high-tension cables you can see on many x-ray machines. The valve tube comes as an interruption of the high-tension pathway and is installed in the large oil-filled transformer tank from which the cables to the x-ray tube may be seen to originate. There is usually at least one valve tube connected in the pathway of each high-tension cable, connected so that current will flow only through it to maintain the positive polarity of the anode of the x-ray tube and the negative polarity of the cathode. This is shown in Fig. 7.24. Current cannot flow in the reverse direction, as there is no source of electrons at the anodes of the valve tubes to produce it. Therefore an alternating supply from the transformer is converted in this instance to a unidirectional supply to the x-ray tube. Note that the valve tubes are connected with one of them one way round and one the other. (We shall give more details on this subject of rectification circuitry in the next chapter.)

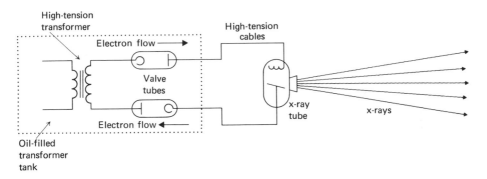

FIG. 7.24. Diagram of valve tubes in the x-ray circuit. Two valve tubes are shown; usually there are four, but the principle is more clearly shown by two.

The characteristics required of the diodes used in these circumstances are: (a) a low internal resistance to permit large current flows and (b) a small voltage drop across them, 3000 volts or less (that is, all or nearly all the voltage supplied by the transformer should appear at the x-ray tube).

The low internal resistance is obtained by having a large tungsten cathode filament in close proximity to the anode, perhaps surrounded by the anode, so that the electron flow is short in length and large in cross section. Figure 7.25 demonstrates examples of this sort of structure. The *kenotron* is a type of valve tube with one end of metal, forming the anode, as shown.

When a valve tube is not conducting, the inverse voltage across it is very high. This has to be taken into account when the tube is being designed.

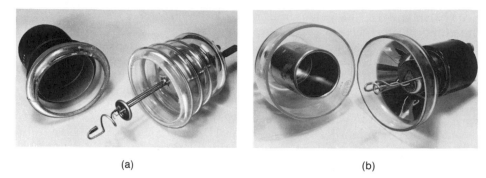

(a)   (b)

FIG. 7.25. Valve tubes. The left-hand photograph shows a kenotron, a valve tube with one end made of metal and forming the anode. The right-hand photograph shows a glass envelope. Both diodes have been cut in half and in both cases the anode normally surrounds the cathode spiral.

There are usually four valve tubes in the transformer tank of a typical x-ray machine. When the machine is switched on ("switching on" does not require making an exposure), the filaments are heated and light up inside the tank. You may be able to see this happen in your department, for very often there is a window in the top of the tank. The oil in which the valve tubes are immersed as insulation against high-tension short circuits is very clear, and as it fills the tank completely you may not at first realize it is there at all. In some cases a suitable nonconducting gas, such as freon, is used instead of oil. Gas has the advantage of being lighter. Generally, in most situations other than x-ray high-voltage circuits, the valve tube has been replaced by solid-state components, referred to in Chapter 6. As previously mentioned, such components are now becoming available for x-ray equipment.

As time goes by, the characteristics of the valve tube filaments may change so that their electron output is diminished. If this happens, the internal resistance of the valve tube will be increased, and for a given current the voltage difference across the tube will rise. This will cause a greater acceleration of electrons and their subsequent collision with the anode may produce x-radiation. Since the valve tube is immersed in an oil-filled steel tank it is unlikely that this radiation will constitute a hazard; but, of course, the x-ray tube output will diminish in some way. The output of the high-tension transformer will be taken up increasingly by the valve tubes and so the kV set at the control will not all appear across the x-ray tube. The penetrability of the beam will therefore decrease and you, the technician, may be unaware of it. You may only notice that gradually, as time goes by, all your exposures have to be increased.

If a valve tube ceases to function (because the filament breaks or for some other reason), it will not permit current to flow through it in either direction. We shall talk about the exact consequences of this in the section dealing with rectification. At present it is enough to point out that the result is an x-ray tube current of about half the expected value. This deficiency will show up on the mA or mAs meter and is thus a very good clue for locating the possible explanation of why, for some unknown reason, a film is underexposed. Confirmation can be made by visual inspection of the valve tube in the transformer tank. Of course, the malfunctioning tube will not light up like the others. The faulty component should be replaced by a qualified x-ray equipment serviceman.

7.7 THE TRIODE

A *triode* is a thermionic tube that has three electrodes. The provision of one electrode more than the diode has resulted in certain additional and important characteristics. As we shall see, some of these characteristics of the triode are of use in medical radiography.

The additional electrode in the triode is called a *grid*, and it is usually schematically represented as in Fig. 7.26(a). Part (b) of the same figure shows one form of actual construction. As you can see, the grid consists of an arrangement of parallel wires between the anode, or plate, and the cathode.

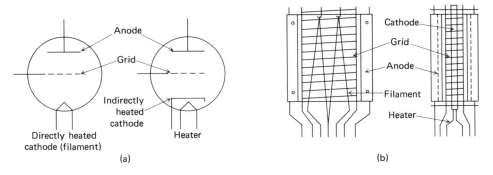

FIG. 7.26. The triode. (a) Diagrammatic representation. (b) Construction details.

If the triode is used in a circuit with only the cathode and anode connected, it will function more or less as a diode. Electrons will flow in one direction only: from cathode to anode. But if the grid is made sufficiently negative with respect to the cathode, there will be no electron flow through the tube. The negatively charged grid will repel the electrons emitted at the cathode. These electrons will therefore be unable to reach the anode, even though the anode is positive with respect to the cathode. This situation is shown in Fig. 7.27.

The voltage by which the grid is made negative is known as a *negative grid bias*. Because of the proximity of the grid to the cathode, the amount of negative bias required to hold the tube current at zero is relatively small.

In order to permit electrons to flow through the tube, we may reduce the negative grid bias. As the value of the grid voltage approaches

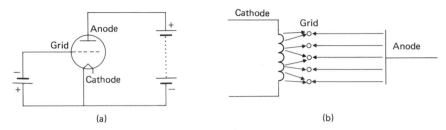

FIG. 7.27. Negative grid bias. (a) The circuit diagram containing the triode. (b) The electric field (approximate) in the tube. The arrows show the direction of the field during negative grid biasing.   Recall that, conventionally, the field direction is shown with reference to positive charges.

zero, the effect of the distant but relatively large positive potential of the anode will predominate. Because electrons are emitted from the cathode with a range of energies, some electrons will pass through the grid, which is now less negative than before. With a grid bias of zero, electron flow will be virtually unimpeded.

FIG. 7.28. The dependence of tube current on grid voltage in a triode. Small changes in grid voltage produce large changes in tube current. (The tube, or plate, voltage has been kept constant.)

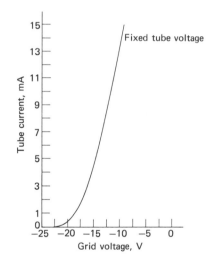

The significant relationship in the triode is that between the tube current and the cathode to the grid voltage, or grid bias. For a fixed tube or plate voltage (that is, voltage between cathode and anode), the tube current will vary greatly with small changes of grid voltage, as shown in Fig. 7.28. Therefore the application of a small varying voltage between the grid and the cathode, that is, a small variation in the grid bias, results in large changes of tube current. If the tube current is passed through a suitable resistor, the voltage across the resistor will then, quite in accordance with Ohm's law, also vary greatly. Such an arrangement, shown in

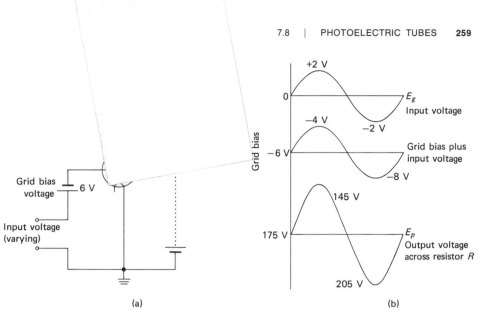

FIG. 7.29. The triode voltage amplifier. (a) The circuit. (b) Input and output voltages. The numerical values shown could be those of an actual circuit.

Fig. 7.29(a), is called a *voltage amplifier.* Part (b) of the same figure shows graphically the relationships between the three voltages, input voltage superimposed on grid bias voltage, resulting grid voltage, and output voltage.

The voltage amplifier not only has widespread application in radio and television equipment, but it is also used to amplify small signals in electro-cardiography and electroencephalography, for example. The vacuum-tube form of the triode, as described here, is at present rapidly being replaced by solid-state amplifiers, which, however, operate by means of somewhat similar principles.

In the x-ray machine, the triode is used as a switch in control circuits (see Section 8.5). We shall also refer to the triode in its role as an amplifier in Section 11.4.

The x-ray tube itself may be made in the form of a triode. The grid electrode is then used as a switch to start or stop the exposure by con-trolling the tube current. We shall have more to say about the triode x-ray tube in Section 12.3.

7.8 PHOTOELECTRIC TUBES

The Photoelectric Effect

As you know, electrons are bound to the atoms of any particular substance by electrical forces that hold them to the nucleus. If energy is transferred from an outside source to these electrons in sufficient quantities, they may overcome this binding force and be detached from the atom. The nature of the energy given to the electrons may differ from case to case. We have already seen that this energy may be in the form of heat in the case of thermionic emission. It may also be in the form of light energy. There are certain metals—for example, selenium, cesium, and lithium—which are composed of atoms having some electrons in such energy levels that, when light is permitted to fall on the surface of the metal, electrons may be emitted from it. Under suitable conditions it may therefore be possible to measure the quantity of electrons emitted from a particular metal when light falls on it, and by this means to determine the quantity of incident light, providing the relationship of the two is known. This is the case because (although whether or not any electrons are emitted depends on the wavelength, or color of the light), if electrons are emitted, then the quantity of emitted electrons depends on the light intensity and not on the wavelength. It was primarily on account of his theoretical explanation of this phenomenon—that is, the photoelectric effect—that Einstein was awarded the Nobel prize in 1921, although the actual paper on this photoelectric effect was published in 1905. Inherent in his explanation is the fact that electrons can accept light energy only in discrete bundles, the quanta or photons of Chapter 1.

By somehow collecting the electrons after emission from a photoemissive material, one might be able to devise an instrument which could perhaps turn off the light or perform some other task after a predetermined number of electrons had been emitted.

The Phototube

These circumstances and possibilities are employed in the x-ray department in automatic phototimers. These timers operate to terminate an x-ray exposure when the film has received enough radiation to produce a density suitable for the purpose involved. At the heart of this apparatus is the photoelectric tube, or *phototube*.

FIG. 7.30. A photoelectric tube. *A* is the anode and *C* is the photocathode, which emits electrons when illuminated. Both are enclosed in the evacuated glass tube represented by the outer circle.

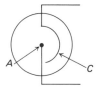

It may consist of a glass envelope from which the air has been pumped. Again, it is somewhat similar to an x-ray tube, but usually much smaller (see Fig. 7.30). Inside the tube is a small curved piece of metal coated with a photo-emissive material, selenium, for example. This piece of metal is the cathode of the tube; adjacent to it is the anode. In use, the two electrodes are connected to an external source of EMF, but when they are in darkness no current passes through the tube. When light falls on the tube and reaches the cathode through the glass, electrons are detached from the surface and tend to form a cloud adjacent to the metal. Under the

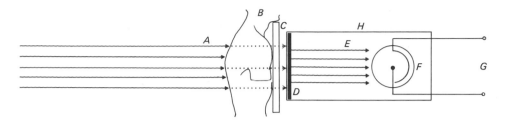

FIG. 7.31. A phototimer unit. *A* is the x-ray beam; *B*, the patient; *C*, the cassette; *D*, a fluorescent screen with active layer facing *F*, the photo-electric tube which is inside the light-tight box, *H*. *E* is the light coming from the fluorescent screen, and *G* represents the connections to an external circuit. The different elements are not to scale; an actual photo-timer is quite small compared with the cassette.

influence of the applied voltage these electrons are accelerated to the anode, thereby constituting an electric current through the tube. This current flows through the external part of the phototube circuit, where it may be utilized in several ways.

As suggested before, the most common application of this photo-electric circuitry in the x-ray department is as a phototimer, whose construction is shown diagrammatically in Fig. 7.31. Shown at *D* in the figure is a small piece of fluorescent screen with its light-emitting surface directed to the right into a light-tight box or enclosure. Inside the box is a photo-electric tube. As shown, this device is positioned underneath or behind the x-ray cassette, so that x-radiation passes through the patient into the cassette, where it will produce a radiographic image. Some of the beam will continue through the back of the cassette and so reach the small fluorescent screen. When this happens, the screen will fluoresce and the light from it will be received by the photo-electric tube. (X-rays are not used directly for stimulating photo-emission, since the efficiency of the process is much lower than for visible light.) As the light reaches the metal plate inside the tube, electrons are emitted from its surface and under the influence of the voltage difference between the electrodes they pass from the cathode to the anode and so into the external circuit. At this point, the current can be made to flow into a capacitor (see Section 2.6) of variable capacity. The values of the capacitor and other components of the circuit can be so arranged that the current produced by an exposure which gives a satisfactory radiographic result will be sufficient to fully charge the capacitor. The voltage across the fully charged capacitor can be used to trigger another circuit, which in turn terminates the x-ray exposure. You can see from this that the x-ray controls may be set at one value for a series of patients, and that the length of exposure in each case will be controlled by the phototimer. All that the technician has to do is to set suitable values of mA and kV, arrange a timer setting longer than any time interval anticipated during the series of films, and then let the phototimer take over. The general density of the radiographs is chosen by adjusting the

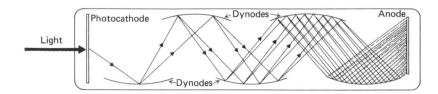

FIG. 7.32. A photomultiplier tube. Note how many electrons arrive at the anode and how many leave the photocathode. (The number of electrons shown is not to be taken literally.)

capacitance of the variable capacitor, or the resistance of a resistor in series with the capacitor, thereby varying the time constant (see Section 2.6) in the phototimer circuit so that it will terminate the x-ray exposure following a greater or smaller dose. Obviously for thicker patients it will take a longer time for a given dose to be received at the fluorescent screen, while for a thin patient this dose will be received in a shorter time. In either case, the phototimer will produce a film of a consistent density.

The Photomultiplier Tube

Since the light intensities in the phototimer are quite low, the simple photoelectric tube has been superseded in today's x-ray equipment by the *photomultiplier* tube, which is shown diagrammatically in Fig. 7.32. Between the anode and the cathode are several intermediate electrodes called *dynodes*. Each of these is maintained at a voltage higher than the one preceding and each is coated with a material which emits secondary electrons when bombarded with electrons from the dynode before. Although the primary electrons are emitted as a result of light energy, the secondary electrons are emitted as the result of the energy imparted to them by the primary electrons, a phenomenon known as *secondary emission*. Let us follow these events through the photomultiplier tube.

When light falls on the cathode, electrons are emitted. They are then accelerated to the first dynode, where they produce secondary electrons. These electrons are accelerated to the second dynode, where each produces more than one new secondary electron. As this process is repeated through the photomultiplier tube, the final electron flow is many times—perhaps 10^8 times—greater than the original. This flow is hence large enough to be easily utilized directly to operate an x-ray exposure circuit, whereas using only the simple phototube would make it necessary to have additional amplifying circuits.

Limitations of the Phototimer

The phototimer has some limitations, of course. For example, for very large patients, the phototimer may end the exposure even though insufficient dose has reached it to produce a satisfactory radiograph. In this case a safety factor may be involved. Usually the phototimer has an upper limit, set at the time of installation, designed to avoid overloading the x-ray tube.

Occasionally, on the other hand, when the patient is very thin, a radiograph is produced which is overexposed, even though nothing is wrong with the phototimer. This happens because a lower limit of operation is often made necessary by the minimum time required for mechanical contacts to operate in other parts of the x-ray circuit. Even though the phototimer could perhaps function efficiently for shorter times, shortcomings in the rest of the machine lead to inconsistent results.

QUESTIONS

1. Why can an x-ray tube be destroyed by operating under conditions of inverse emission?

2. For comparable current ratings, why would a tube operated on a self-rectified circuit require a larger focal spot than a tube operated on full-wave rectification? (Assume the same kV.)

3. Discuss the phenomenon of thermionic emission. Illustrate your answer with graphs which show how the current flowing through the valve depends on (a) the filament temperature, and (b) the tube voltage.

4. What information do you get from a tube rating chart? Explain how you would use such a chart.

5. Describe the principle of line focus.

6. Discuss the use of oil in the x-ray machine.

7. Show by calculation the relationship between joules and radiological heat units.

8. What is the photoelectric effect?

9. By means of a diagram and a brief description, explain the function of a photomultiplier tube.

10. Calculate the percentage efficiency of an x-ray tube operating at 90 kV and using a tungsten target. Assume K to be as given in the text.

11. Discuss rotating anodes in x-ray tubes.

12. Compare the valve tube with the x-ray tube.

13. Describe the production of x-rays in a diagnostic-type x-ray tube and include an explanation as to why the resulting x-ray beam is heterogeneous.

14. The production of x-rays may be compared with the noise produced when a steel plate is bombarded by bullets from a machine gun. What quantities in x-ray production are analogous to the sound and the bullets?

SUGGESTED READING

GLASSER, OTTO, *Dr. W. C. Röntgen.* Springfield, Ill.: Charles C. Thomas (second edition) 1958. This is a short and interesting account of the life of Röntgen. We referred to this book in the historical preamble to this chapter.

COOLIDGE, W. D., "A Powerful Röntgen Ray Tube with a Pure Electron Discharge," *The Physical Review*, December 1913, Volume II, Number 6. This paper reporting the invention of the Coolidge tube in one of the leading physics journals of the world is surprisingly readable. Students will be pleased to find that the limited mathematics involved is very manageable.

JAUNDRELL-THOMPSON, F., and W. J. ASHWORTH, *X-Ray Physics and Equipment.* Oxford, England: Blackwell Scientific Publications, 1965. Chapter 12, "X-ray Tubes," gives a discussion of the subject that is much more comprehensive than we have provided.

CHAPTER 8

X-Ray Circuits

Now that we have finished our discussion of the x-ray tube (Chapter 7) and have the relevant physics groundwork presented in the previous chapters, we are in a position to bring together all the principal components of the complete x-ray machine. None of the material in the present chapter involves new physics, and we shall touch on only a few new ways of applying previously discussed physical principles. What will be new is the assembling of various familiar units into new patterns. These patterns are called *circuit diagrams.* And we have seen a number of circuit diagrams on various previous occasions.

At the risk of redundancy, let us now emphasize that in essence a circuit diagram is a schematic representation intended to show how a certain electrical apparatus works, how its parts are connected electrically. Such a diagram does not show what the apparatus looks like. It does not even show the relative relationship of its parts, that is, whether one part is, for example, above or below, or beside, another. The circuit diagram is arranged in the simplest possible way to convey to the reader which EMF's produce currents where, what voltages appear across what circuit components, and how a change in current and/or voltage in one part of the circuit affects the other circuit components. Consequently, a single basic circuit diagram may explain the principles of operation which underlie numerous x-ray machines that appear to be quite different. In this ability to reduce apparently complex matters to relative simplicity lies the great value of the circuit diagram for the medical radiographer. Of course the circuits to be discussed do not necessarily show how a particular x-ray machine is made to function. But from a study of the circuits the student should be able to gain an understanding of how x-ray machines in general function.

Now a word of warning about circuit diagrams: Do not skip over the simplest diagrams, nor be nonplussed by the more complicated ones. We recommend that in each case the student draw the diagram for himself. What we said regarding diagrams at the beginning of this text may be repeated here, in somewhat amended form. One good circuit diagram is better than a hundred words: Spend your time on the diagrams accordingly.

We would like to direct your attention to Fig. 8.2. This figure represents the basic x-ray machine and, as such, is a culmination of much of the material in this chapter. An understanding of the components of this circuit could well be all, or nearly all, that the student is required to have. For the more ambitious, we suggest going on to Fig. 8.29 and its constituent parts. Wherever you stop will depend in some measure, of course, on the particular training program you are following.

We further recommend the reader to discover for himself the parts which go to make up the x-ray machines around him. Of course, he should get assistance where necessary and, most important, before he looks inside any machine he should *TURN IT OFF AT THE MAINS* and not merely at the control panel.

Historically, the components of the x-ray circuit which have undergone the most significant changes in design are those dealing with transformation of voltages and with rectification. Of these components, the Snooks Interrupterless Transformer of 1907 was probably the most outstanding. Previous to this date it was necessary to interrupt the primary current to an induction coil by mechanical means. These mechanical interrupters were noisy, erratic in operation, and required frequent cleaning.

In 1918 Coolidge introduced a tube which acted as its own rectifier. Later, in the early 1930's, half-wave and full-wave valve tube rectification began to be used. At about the same time, in the later 1920's, better insulating materials made it possible to enclose generators, high-tension wires, and x-ray tubes in shockproof covers.

We can see from these few facts, then, that x-ray equipment has been in essentially its present form for about 40 years.

Finally, we would note that, as we have done in the past, we shall use the terms "high voltage" and "high tension" as meaning the same thing. In the medical x-ray world, in fact, the use of H.T. for high tension is quite common in most English-speaking countries.

8.1 BASIC COMPONENTS

Before we use our first circuit diagram, let us state clearly, with the help of a block diagram in Fig. 8.1, which components we have to consider and how they are linked functionally. For purposes of clarity, we have here omitted some of the components, which we shall get to later in the chapter. The omitted components are refinements of the simple circuit, which make the circuit more effective for practical radiography. It will not be difficult to include these additional components as we go along.

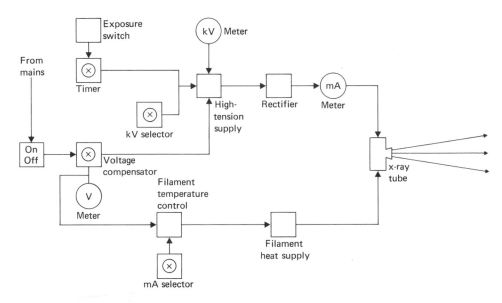

FIG. 8.1. Block diagram of basic x-ray machine components, shown in order from the mains supply on the left to the x-ray tube on the right. Circles denote meters on the control panel. Crossed circles denote control knobs on the control panel.

When we study Fig. 8.1, we see two main lines of electrical supply to the x-ray tube. One, the upper line of components in the figure, functions to produce a high voltage which is then applied across the tube's anode and cathode. The H.T. (high-tension) or high-voltage supply is the heart of this system. Then, because the H.T. supply is an AC one, that is, a high-voltage step-up transformer, rectification follows. By means of rectification, a pulsating DC high voltage is applied to the tube. The current through the tube follows the H.T. pathway and is measured by the mA meter.

The kilovoltage produced by the H.T. supply must be known in advance of an exposure; the kV meter gives this information. It must also be possible to change the kV between exposures: a kV selector is included.

The duration of application of kV will determine the length of the exposure (assuming that the filament of the x-ray tube is heated). The timer and exposure switch control the H.T. supply, and thereby the time of the exposure.

The mains voltage to the H.T. supply may vary. But if the voltage to the H.T. supply changes so will the output, that is, the particular kV we wish to use. For this reason, something is done to compensate for changes of mains voltage: the voltage compensator, along with its own voltmeter, is included.

The on-off switch explains itself; it is to be found on the control panel.

The second line of electrical supply concerns the heating of the x-ray tube filament. This filament must have its own supply and a control. As we already know from Section 7.3, it is the filament temperature which controls the tube current or mA. Therefore the filament temperature control has an attached mA selector, as shown in Fig. 8.1.

The filament supply line is taken from the mains voltage-compensated autotransformer because the filament, too, requires a stable voltage. In fact, so important is this last requirement that most of the extra items missing from Fig. 8.1 belong in the filament supply circuit. Their refinements are necessary to meet the demands for filament voltage and current stabilization.

This Fig. 8.1, then, gives the basic outline of a typical major x-ray machine. We recommend that you study this figure thoroughly if you wish to understand the remainder of this chapter.

8.2 THE PRIMARY SIDE AND MAIN CONTROL CIRCUITRY

Now let us translate Fig. 8.1 into a circuit diagram, as shown in Fig. 8.2.

Note how the three transformers are connected. The autotransformer (Section 6.4) is energized from the mains and is in turn connected directly to the primary of the step-up transformer (Section 6.4). The high-voltage output of the H.T. transformer supplies a high AC voltage across the x-ray tube. Of course, normally no current can flow through the x-ray tube when the anode is negative with respect to the cathode. For this reason, the tube current is a pulsating DC. However, a rectifier unit may be included (dashed lines in Fig. 8.2) to supply a DC voltage to the tube. This aspect will be discussed at greater length in Section 8.4.

A circuit somewhat similar to the H.T. circuit is used to heat the x-ray tube filament. A suitable voltage supply is tapped off the autotransformer and used to energize the primary of the step-down filament transformer (Section 6.4). The output current of the filament transformer goes through the tube filament, thereby heating it.

Control Circuits

How is our x-ray machine controlled? We shall talk about the timer in Section 8.5, but for now we should note that it is connected in some way to the exposure switch. When this switch is closed the H.T. circuit is completed, the heated filament of the x-ray tube supplies electrons, and x-rays are produced. At the end of the exposure the timer opens the exposure

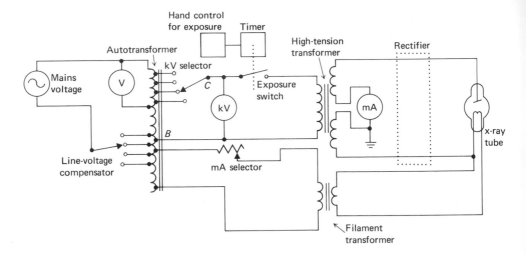

FIG. 8.2. Basic x-ray machine components. This circuit diagram shows a simplified but complete x-ray machine.

switch and, although the tube filament is still hot, no more x-rays are produced. The timer's action is started by the technician pressing the exposure button. Both these controls, exposure switch and timing selector, are at the control panel.

Tube current, or mA, selection is also shown in Fig. 8.2. The size of the current in the primary of the filament transformer is controlled by the size of the variable resistor (see Section 8.3) in that circuit. If the resistance is larger, the voltage across the primary of the filament transformer is smaller; so will the voltage and the current in the secondary be smaller. But this latter current is heating the tube filament. Therefore adjustment of the variable resistor changes the temperature of the filament and thus the size of the tube current. As you may know, the operator sets the temperature of the filament and consequently the mA before the exposure. The mA selector is installed in the control panel and may be in the form of a knob or a series of push buttons.

The tube voltage, or kV, also set before an exposure, is selected by means of another knob or a series of buttons on the control panel. The place of this selector in the circuit is shown in Fig. 8.2. By changing the output tapping from the autotransformer to include more or fewer turns, we can make the input voltage to the H.T. transformer greater or smaller. Since the output voltage at the transformer is related to the input voltage by a fixed turns ratio, we can, in this manner, by adjusting the output tapping from the autotransformer, adjust the output voltage of the high-voltage transformer and hence control the kV across the tube.

Sometimes two kV selector knobs are found on the control panel, one major and one minor. Changing the kV major selector from one position to the next may change the kV by 5 or perhaps 10 kV; changing the minor selector by one step will change the kV by only 1 or 2 kV. The major selector is connected to the autotransformer with many turns between taps, while the minor selector has only a few turns between taps. Figure 8.3 shows these arrangements. Although only five positions for each selector are shown, in practice ten or more positions may be provided. By means of the two selectors, one can vary the kV from about 40 kV to about 140 kV (depending on the machine) in steps of, perhaps, 2 kV.

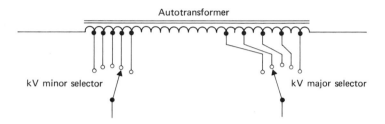

FIG. 8.3. The kV major and minor selectors. The major selector may have 10 or 20 turns between taps, while the minor may have, in that case, only perhaps 2 turns between taps.

The student should note, in Fig. 8.2 and elsewhere throughout this chapter, that as far as possible controls, meters, and switches are included in the primary low-voltage side of x-ray circuits. This means that although in general currents may be larger, voltages are much smaller. By arranging these circuit elements to operate in low-voltage conditions, one can avoid much expense for insulation and ensure safer operation for the operator who has to touch the various controls.

Meters

If we measure the output voltage from the autotransformer and multiply this reading by the H.T. transformer ratio, we have the kV which will appear as H.T. output, even before it occurs. This is the role of the pre-reading kV meter shown in Fig. 8.2. This prereading kV meter is a moving iron meter described in Section 6.6. The meter measures volts but is calibrated in kilovolts. In fact, it reads kV peak values, although this fact may not always be clearly indicated; the meter may be labeled kV or kVp. Since the kV meter is read before an exposure, it is logical that it be placed on the control panel.

The tube current is the current in the secondary circuit. Therefore the mA meter must be placed somewhere in the secondary circuit. Since it is advantageous from the insulation viewpoint to ground the secondary winding of the H.T. transformer in the center, as shown in Fig. 8.2, it becomes imperative, from the viewpoint of safety, to connect the mA meter at this point. After all, the mA meter will have to be on the control panel which the technician touches. So an interruption is made at this grounded central point and the mA meter is inserted there. Now neither terminal of the mA meter will be at a voltage much different from ground, but all the tube current will pass through the meter, which can be mounted in the control panel by using long wires from the H.T. transformer. Sometimes, however, the secondary winding of the H.T. transformer is not center-grounded, but grounded at one end. In this case the mA meter is inserted at the grounded point, not in the center of the winding.

We can read the mA meter, of course, only during an exposure. During the exposure this meter responds to the average value of the current. As we said in Section 6.6, this meter is a moving-coil ammeter preceded by its own rectification circuit, as shown in Fig. 6.23. Further, as we also pointed out in Section 6.6, because the mA meter operates only while tube current is on (that is, while the exposure is in progress), the needle may not have time to register properly for a high tube current and a very short exposure. So, for short exposures an mAs meter is used. This meter measures the product of mA and time, as we described in Section 6.6.

Since the mAs meter has no hairspring mechanism, the mAs meter needle has to be returned to zero by a small reverse current. This reverse current may be supplied either automatically at the "prepare" stage of the next exposure, or sometimes by pushing a special button close to the meter.

Switching from the mA meter to the mAs meter is now usually accomplished automatically, on the basis of the exposure technique selected. In some cases, however, the selection may be made manually, by moving a switch. In the latter case, one should take care not to exceed the full-scale deflection of the mAs meter by inadvertently using the mAs meter for a technique which demands the mA meter.

Voltage Compensators

Figure 8.2 shows a line (otherwise called "mains") voltage compensator with an associated voltmeter above it. Let us have a closer look at this part of the circuit now.

We have previously stated that, in order to get a desired x-ray output from the x-ray machine, it is necessary for a constant value of AC voltage to be supplied from the mains. And yet we know that the line voltage may change from time to time during the day. For example, demands by other users of electricity in the vicinity may produce voltage fluctuations. These changes are compensated for by the line voltage compensator, even though the device cannot stop the changes from occurring.

You may recall from Section 6.4 that the output voltage between two fixed tappings of an autotransformer depends on the ratio of volts per turn. Thus, if there is an induced EMF of $\frac{1}{2}$ volt for every turn, output tappings which include 400 turns will produce 200 volts. The important requirement for a constant voltage output is a constant volts-per-turn ratio.

Let us suppose that originally the input voltage was 230 volts and that it was applied across 460 turns. This would induce $\frac{1}{2}$ volt per turn throughout the transformer. Now, suppose that the line voltage were to drop to 220 volts. We cannot raise it again, but by applying 220 volts to only 440 turns we reestablish our ratio of $\frac{1}{2}$ volt per turn. By changing the input tapping we maintain the output voltage. The change is brought about by the line voltage compensator, the function of which is shown in the figure. On the control panel the compensator tapping is changed by turning a knob.

The voltmeter associated with the compensator indicates the voltage across a fixed number of turns. The actual value indicated is of no great importance to the technician. All that matters is that it should always be the same before an exposure is made. For this reason, the voltmeter may have only a red mark on its dial. The needle is adjusted to this mark by the line voltage compensator. In other words, both the meter and the compensator are concerned with the volts-per-turn ratio.

The other compensator with which the technician has some concern is the kV meter compensator. From Section 6.4 we see that the problem is this: The technician uses the kV meter shown in Fig. 8.2 to determine what the kV will be across the tube at the time of the exposure, but he reads the meter before the exposure is made. Let us assume, for example, that he has set the kV selector so that the meter reads 80 kV. Then he makes the exposure, but in accordance with Ohm's law and our discussions in Sections 3.5 and 6.4, the voltage output of the autotransformer (which is what the kV meter responds to) drops to a lower value. This voltage drop across a source depends on the current drawn from the source, so that the voltage drop in this case will ultimately depend on the tube current or mA. For a larger mA the voltage drop will be greater. In our example, during the exposure the kV meter may read 72 kV. This, of course, is a true indication of the kV at the time of the exposure.

We can clearly see the practical difficulties of this. The technician does not know by simple means what the kV will be during the exposure before he makes it, while during the exposure the knowledge comes too late, even if he were able to make the reading. What we need then is some voltage compensation of the meter before the exposure. Then in our example the meter would read 72 kV before the exposure.

This is accomplished by the kV meter compensator, as shown in Fig. 8.4. Instead of the kV meter reading between points B and C, as in Fig. 8.2, one lead from the meter is taken to A. The connection through A is made to a short section of the autotransformer which is wound in the reverse direction to the main section. This means that between A and B there will be a small voltage opposite in polarity to that between B and C. The kV meter will therefore operate on the voltage $BC–AB$, where AB is designed to be of such a size as to just compensate for the voltage drop which will occur during the exposure.

We have already said that the voltage drop varies with the mA used, and this is why the tapping at A is variable. It must be set at a different value for different mA settings of the machine. This is what is meant in the figure by "ganged to the mA selector": A kV meter compensator is connected mechanically to the mA selector, so that for larger mA selections a slightly larger voltage AB is applied to compensate the kV meter.

Although the technician may never see the kV meter compensator and certainly will not adjust it independently of any other control, neverthe-

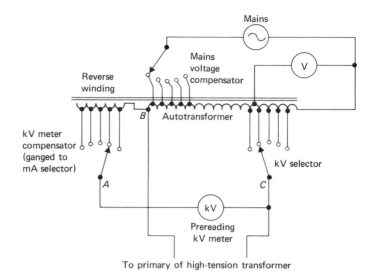

FIG. 8.4. A diagram of kV meter compensation. (There is very little difference between the connections of the kV meter in this figure and in Fig. 8.2, but the difference is important.) Note that only one kV selector is shown.

less he must, to some extent, bear in mind what is going on here, because the compensation is carried out when the mA is selected. This means that the technician must select the mA to be used before he reads the kV meter. If the kV is set first, then the meter reading will change if the mA is changed thereafter. A further point to note is that the kV reading will still drop during the exposure, but the relationship between its reading during the exposure and the actual tube kV is now of no consequence.

8.3   X-RAY TUBE FILAMENT SUPPLY

A very important part of x-ray output control is concerned with the heating of the filament of the x-ray tube. We have already seen (in Section 7.3) that a relatively small change in filament temperature will produce a large change in current through the tube. This, in turn, produces a large change in the intensity of the radiation produced. The present section is therefore concerned with methods of filament temperature control and stabilization.

Filament Heating

As we have already seen, the heating current for the x-ray tube filament is supplied from the filament transformer. Typical values of voltage and current in the tube filament are, for example, 6 to 12 volts and 3 to 5 amp. The primary of the filament transformer is supplied from the autotransformer. The voltage across the primary of the filament transformer is typically something close to mains voltage. The value of current in the

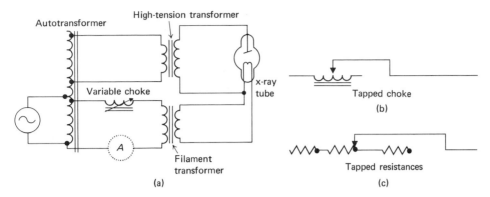

FIG. 8.5. A diagram of mA selection. The x-ray tube filament heating may be controlled by any one of these three methods. (a) The complete simplified circuit. Alternative (b) or (c) would replace the variable choke in the circuit diagram (a).

primary of the filament transformer may be something like 0.5 amp, a value which follows from the transformer equations (6.17) and (6.18). In some older machines one may still find an ammeter connected in the circuit as shown by the dashed meter in Fig. 8.5(a). In more modern machines this meter is unnecessary and is not included.

Looking again at Fig. 8.5(a), we see one method of controlling the filament current. In the primary side of the circuit there is a variable choke (see Section 6.2). The variable choke constitutes a greater or smaller reactance to alternating current in this circuit, and thereby controls the size of the total current flowing to the filament transformer.

An alternative to the variable choke is the tapped choke shown in part (b) of Fig. 8.5. Here the core remains fixed within the inductor. One connection to the device is made to the end of the coil, as shown in the figure, while the other is made variable, to some other part of the coil. Depending on whether more or less of the coil is included in the circuit, the value of inductive reactance is made greater or smaller. This method of mA control can be made continuous or stepwise.

The third method of mA control, shown in part (c) of Fig. 8.5, is that most commonly found in modern x-ray machines. It consists of a type of rheostat discussed in Section 3.6, a number of resistors in series, with a variable tapped connection. The variable connection is so arranged that it makes contact with one resistor or another, but is variable only with respect to separate resistors. The variable contact is always made to the same point on each resistor. This produces the stepwise control of mA required by modern exposure techniques.

Note once again that the controls for the mA circuit are arranged in the primary side of the filament supply circuit. This is because the secondary side of the circuit is at a large voltage with respect to ground, as we shall see shortly.

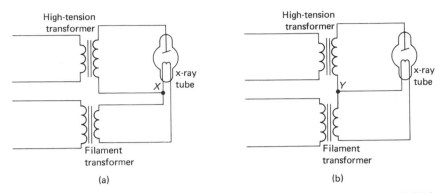

FIG. 8.6.   The connections between the H.T. circuit and the filament heating circuit; (a) is equivalent to (b).

A Digression on Connecting Two Circuits

In the x-ray tube two circuits come together. One is concerned with the high-tension supply between anode and cathode and is produced by the secondary winding of the H.T. transformer. We might imagine the H.T. connection to the cathode to be made anywhere on the filament. For practical reasons it is easiest to make this connection at one of the filament terminals just outside the tube. This is shown in Fig. 8.6(a).

But then we have to heat the filament. For this purpose we require a separate circuit, one from the filament transformer. Connections to the filament are made via its two terminals. This second circuit is shown added to the first in Fig. 8.6(a). Point X shows where the two circuits are joined.

Part (b) of Fig. 8.6 shows an entirely equivalent circuit, but now the connection between the two circuits is made at point Y. In this case only two wires are required along the distance from the region of Y to the x-ray tube. This will be of practical significance when we discuss high-tension cables in Section 8.6.

When we look at the circuit loop from the filament transformer to the x-ray tube filament in Fig. 8.6(b), we note that at the point Y, which may be as much as 50,000 volts with respect to ground, a high-tension connection has been made with the filament heating circuit. We can therefore regard the filament heating circuit as being more or less completely at 50,000 volts with respect to ground. The complete circuit will therefore have to be well insulated from its surroundings (such as the technician and the primary side of the filament transformer).

Let us look for a moment at what results from the connection of these two circuits. Figure 8.7(a) shows them joined together in yet another configuration, but one which is again equivalent to both the circuits of Fig. 8.6. We have deliberately drawn the filament transformer quite separate from the H.T. transformer. The values of voltage and current shown have been chosen merely as examples, but they are all fairly

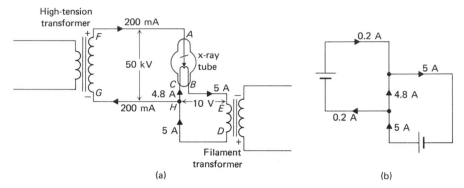

FIG. 8.7. Some values of voltage and current in the x-ray tube circuits.

reasonable figures with regard to practice. We shall assume RMS values throughout, although you know, of course, that the kilovoltage figures given are invariably expressed as peak values in an actual x-ray machine, and the tube current figures are average values. We have further assumed the instantaneous polarities shown at the two transformer secondary terminals, but the digression could as well be conducted with opposite polarities.

We already know that the current through the tube, shown by the dashed arrow from anode to cathode in the figure, may be 200 mA, for example. (Remember that electrons pass through the tube in the opposite direction.) This current flows through the conductor from C to G, through the transformer secondary winding to F, and around again to A; this is shown in the figure.

A typical current in the filament circuit might be, for example, 5 amp. This will flow completely around the circuit $EDHCB$, as shown.

What happens between H and C? Here the two currents are in opposition, but one is much larger than the other. The resulting current will therefore be:

$$5 \text{ amp} - 200 \text{ mA} = (5 - 0.2) \text{ amp} = 4.8 \text{ amp}.$$

An ammeter in the circuit between C and H would therefore register 4.8 amp.

If we investigate the situation in any other part of the circuit where the two currents may be involved, we still find a reasonable result. For instance, 5 amp leaves the filament at point B but only 4.8 amp is seen to enter it at point C. But we know that 200 mA arrives at the filament after the current crosses the tube from the anode. An equivalent circuit is shown in Fig. 8.7(b). These results are perhaps intuitively plausible, in that one expects that there will be no more current leaving a point in a circuit than entering it. This fact—that the algebraic sum of currents at any branch point in a circuit is zero—is actually an important law in electricity: *Kirchhoff's first law.*

Let us now look at the various voltages concerned, viewing the respective transformer secondaries simply as generators of EMF. Let us say that *GF* produces 50,000 volts and *ED* 10 volts. Now note that *H*, being a common point on both circuits, might thus provide us with a good reference point. But assuming the connecting wires to have negligible resistance, the potential of point *C* is the same as that of point *H*. So we shall use point *C* as our reference point, common to both the high-voltage tube circuit and the low-voltage filament-heating circuit.

Again assuming no potential drops across the connecting wires, we can say that the voltage from *C* to *A* is 50,000 volts. The voltage across the filament, on the other hand (that is, from *C* to *B*), is −10 volts, *B* being at a lower potential than *C*. Thus the voltage from *A* to *B* turns out to be (50,000 + 10) volts = 50,010 volts.

What does all this mean? It means that the interconnection of two circuits with separate voltage supplies will still produce results which follow basic laws of electrical circuits. In the case of the x-ray tube it leads us to see that the potential difference between one end of the filament and the target (anode) is not the same as that between the other end of the filament and the target. The voltage between *A* and *C* is as given by the kV meter, but that between *A* and *B* is 10 volts greater. But 10 volts compared with 50,000 volts is such a small fraction that we may ignore it.

We suggest that the interested student may gain a further insight into the analysis of the two circuits involved in the x-ray tube supply by drawing other variants of the circuit of Fig. 8.7 and using his own voltages, currents, and polarities.

Stabilization of Filament Heating

In Section 7.3, and in Fig. 7.5 in particular, we saw that small changes in the x-ray tube filament-heating current produce relatively large changes in the x-ray tube current, that is, the mA. For example, a variation in the filament supply voltage of 5% may cause sufficient change in the filament-heating current to result in a tube current (mA) change of about 30%, a percentage which can pronouncedly affect film exposure. Therefore it behooves us to make every effort to maintain a constant predetermined value of current in the filament-heating circuit. To look at it another way, we may say that it is imperative to supply the primary winding of the filament transformer with a constant AC voltage. Moreover, it will also be necessary to automatically modify this AC voltage to achieve space charge compensation.

Before we embark on a more detailed discussion of the various circuit components, we refer the reader to Fig. 8.8, which, in block form, indicates the positions of the main circuit components ultimately leading to the x-ray tube filament.

We see that naturally the voltage supply for the filament heating emanates from the mains voltage. Thus the filament transformer voltage will be subject to whatever fluctuations occur at the mains. But slowly occurring changes in the mains voltage pose no serious problem. They are

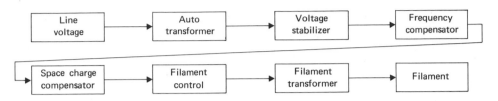

FIG. 8.8. The positions of the voltage stabilizer, frequency compensator, and space-charge compensator in the filament supply circuit.

compensated by the mains voltage compensator (Section 8.2). Since this mains voltage compensator provides the autotransformer with the properly adjusted voltage per turn, the filament transformer, which is supplied from the autotransformer, will thus also be protected against slow changes in mains voltage.

However, for rapid changes in the mains voltage which occur during the actual x-ray exposure, the mains voltage compensator is useless. What is required is some device which will stabilize the voltage to the filament transformer more or less instantaneously. Such a device is called a *voltage stabilizer*. Its position in the scheme of things is apparent in Fig. 8.8.

In addition to this stabilizing device, there is also a frequency compensator, referred to in Section 6.4, to compensate for voltage changes across the primary of the filament transformer due to frequency-dependent impedance changes in the primary circuit. This component is also shown in Fig. 8.8.

At this point one might suggest that the most important issue for the radiographer is probably the knowledge of the existence of these stabilizers and/or compensators and the reasons for their existence. We have now covered these points. We present the following paragraphs for those wishing some insight into the workings of these stabilizing circuit components.

The Voltage Stabilizer

Voltage stabilizers may take many forms, but we shall describe only one here, to indicate some principles which could be employed. In actual practice, although the working of these stabilizing units involves similar physical principles, these units tend to be considerably more complex than our simplified description indicates.

Figure 8.9 is a diagram of a *static voltage stabilizer*, that is, a stabilizer having no moving parts. It consists essentially of a transformer with the primary and secondary coils wound on the core piece as shown. The core has two noteworthy features: the limb on which the secondary winding is wound is of a much smaller cross section than the other two; and the center limb, which has no winding, has an air gap at one end.

The input winding is supplied from the autotransformer, and the current in the input winding sets up a magnetic field throughout the core. As the peak value of the input voltage, and thus the current in the primary

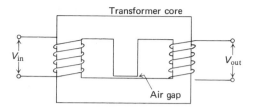

FIG. 8.9.   A static voltage stabilizer.   By means of the saturated choke (secondary coil), V_{out} remains fairly constant for rises in V_{in}.

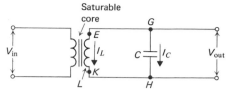

FIG. 8.10.   A static voltage stabilizer with capacitor added. The addition of C to the transformer of Fig. 8.9 produces further stabilization of voltage output.

winding, increases, the magnetic field (the B of Chapter 4) within the core grows until a point is reached at which the output limb is magnetically saturated.   Further increase in the input voltage V_{in} therefore cannot significantly increase the magnetic flux Φ through the output limb.

This means that as long as the frequency remains constant there can be no further increase in $\Delta\Phi/\Delta t$ on the secondary side. To all intents and purposes, therefore, further increases in V_{in} will thus produce no significant increases in V_{out}. To that extent the filament voltage has been stabilized.

At this point let us draw attention to the above restriction regarding constancy of the frequency of the input voltage.   In other words, this stabilizer is frequency dependent, and thus requires the frequency compensator which we referred to earlier (Section 6.4), and which we shall discuss further shortly.

Incidentally, you might ask what is going on with the magnetic flux during the variations in the peak values of the input voltage. Increasing V_{in} increases the value of the magnetic field B in the primary, since the primary is operating below saturation, and hence increases the flux Φ through the core.   But we said that when the secondary limb is saturated Φ does not increase there. What of the excess flux through the primary? This magnetic flux now passes through the center limb with the air gap. Since the average permeability of this center limb, including the air gap, is lower than the permeability of the metal of the core, this center limb very nicely helps to keep as much flux as possible in the more permeable path of the secondary limb: It helps to keep the secondary limb near saturation and takes care of the excess flux when saturation is reached.

From all these considerations we can see that this stabilizer results in stabilization only with respect to input voltages in excess of normal, because only then is the secondary limb more or less saturated. But what if V_{in} drops below normal values? Then V_{out} will also drop, unless some modification to this static stabilizer is employed.

A suitable modification is shown in Fig. 8.10, in which we see that a capacitor has been added in parallel with the transformer secondary. We shall not discuss the details of the effect of this capacitor here. Suffice it to say that decreasing V_{in} below normal takes the secondary limb out of the region of saturation: V_{out} also drops. This drop in V_{out} results in a change in the currents I_L and I_C in the loop $EGHK$ such that the voltage drop across the secondary winding will be reduced, and hence V_{out} raised to its former value. All this, of course, happens more or less instantaneously.

Thus, by means of the static voltage stabilizer, rapidly occurring variations from the mains and the autotransformer, which take place during an exposure, are stabilized before they reach the filament transformer. For example, when there is an input voltage variation of ±10% the output voltage may change only ±0.5%.

The Frequency Compensator

As we mentioned, a voltage stabilizer of the type we discussed above will operate as intended only while the supply frequency remains constant. But if this frequency changes, the output voltage of the stabilizer will also change, because although the stabilizer bucks (or opposes) increases in $\Delta\Phi$, we see that if Δt is reduced, $\Delta\Phi/\Delta t$ is increased; that is, if the frequency is increased, the output voltage of the secondary is increased. For example, if the frequency increases, say, 1 cycle per second, the voltage output of the stabilizer may rise by 3 or 4 volts. A frequency compensator is required, as indicated in Fig. 8.8.

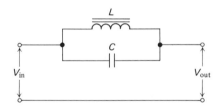

FIG. 8.11. A frequency compensator. The V_{out} from this component forms the input of the x-ray tube filament transformer; V_{in} comes from the voltage stabilizer.

This compensator may take the form shown in Fig. 8.11, in which we see that it consists of an inductor and a capacitor connected in parallel. This parallel group is then connected in series with the supply to the filament transformer. The voltage drop across the parallel group will depend on X, the total reactance (assuming ideal components), but we already know from Section 6.2 that $X_L = 2\pi fL$ and $X_C = 1/2\pi fC$. Because X_L and X_C are frequency dependent, it is possible, by means of suitable choices of values for L and C—which values depend on the line frequency—to arrange that the impedance of such a parallel group will rise as the frequency rises, at least until a certain maximum value is reached; and fall as the frequency falls.

Now suppose that the supply frequency rises; the impedance of this parallel group will rise and a larger voltage drop will occur across the group. Therefore V_{out} will drop relative to V_{in}. This fall in V_{out} from the frequency compensator can be designed so that it exactly offsets the frequency-dependent voltage increase from the voltage stabilizer.

The inverse effects take place when there is a fall in the supply frequency.

The Space-Charge Compensator

As we saw in Section 7.3, space charge around the x-ray tube filament results in an increase in mA as the kV is increased. This undesirable feature, which prevents independent variation of mA and kV, is circumvented by a *space-charge compensator*. It is the function of the space-charge compensator to apply a small opposing voltage to the supply voltage of the filament transformer. This small reverse voltage is increased as the kV is increased, so that the resulting decrease of emitted electrons from the filament, now at a lower temperature, just balances the increase in the number of electrons crossing the tube from the space charge.

The principles of a space-charge compensator are shown in Fig. 8.12. A small transformer called a space-charge transformer is supplied from the autotransformer. The output voltage of the space-charge transformer is variable and the winding direction is such as to provide voltage in opposition to the filament transformer supply voltage. The variable control of the space-charge compensator is ganged to the kV selector of the x-ray machine: As the kV is raised, so is the voltage from the space-charge transformer.

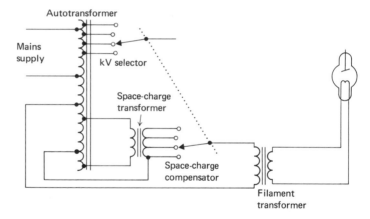

FIG. 8.12. A space-charge compensator. The compensator is ganged to the kV selector by a mechanical linkage, represented by the dotted line.

8.4   THE SECONDARY SIDE: RECTIFICATION CIRCUITRY

Self Rectification

As we have already noted, it is possible to use an x-ray tube in conjunction with an alternating high-tension supply voltage and obtain a pulsating DC current through the tube. A simple circuit of this type, and the associated voltage and current variation, are shown in Fig. 8.13. Although the filament remains heated and the anode is maintained at a temperature too low to emit electrons, current flows only during those half cycles of voltage in which the filament, which provides thermionically emitted electrons,

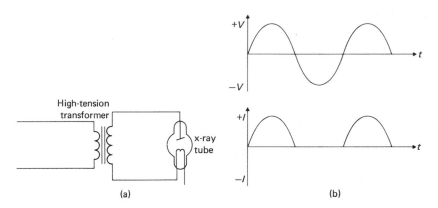

FIG. 8.13. Self rectification. (a) The circuit diagram. (b) The voltage and current waveforms at the x-ray tube.

is negative with respect to the anode, that is, the target. No current flows in the reverse direction unless either the target emits a significant number of electrons as the result of overheating or an excessively large inverse voltage is somehow applied, or both.

Self rectification, as we can see, is a form of half-wave rectification, and is commonly employed in small mobile and dental units. This type of equipment is generally limited to a maximum output of about 100 kV and 100 mA. Many machines of this type have maximum tube currents of only 15 or 20 mA. The common practice in such machines is to install the high-tension transformer, the filament transformer, and the x-ray tube in one casing, known as the *tube head.* This casing is oil-filled; the oil acts as an insulator for the high-tension components. (See Fig. 7.21.)

Peak Inverse Voltage

When self rectification is used and current flows during one half cycle only, there is an IR drop across the high-tension secondary during that half cycle. During the nonconducting half cycle, because of the absence of current in the secondary circuit, the full voltage output of the transformer appears across the x-ray tube. This effect is shown in Fig. 8.14,

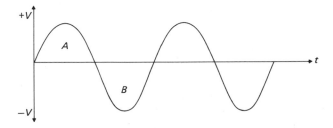

FIG. 8.14. Inverse voltage: *A* is the conducting half cycle, *B* the nonconducting half cycle.

where A is the voltage waveform during the conducting half cycle, and B is the voltage waveform during the inverse or nonconducting half cycle. Note that the inverse half cycle reaches a higher maximum value.

Because of these considerations, the design of the high-tension circuit components has to take into account kilovoltages higher than those nominally obtainable, i.e., as indicated on the control panel. An example of the difference between the voltage during the forward and inverse half cycles is 10 kV, when the tube is operated at 15 mA and 65 kV. For these reasons, insulation problems are more severe, and the x-ray tube must be constructed to withstand a higher voltage than would be the case if the two voltages concerned were of the same magnitude. All told, these factors require an undesirable increase in the size and complexity of the various x-ray machine components, making the unit more expensive and more cumbersome. Consequently, in order to minimize these problems, an inverse voltage suppressor is included in the x-ray machine.

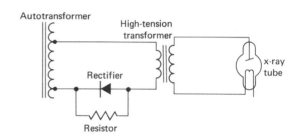

FIG. 8.15. An inverse voltage suppressor. Only the essentials of the primary and secondary x-ray circuits are shown.

Figure 8.15 presents the essential features of such an inverse voltage suppressor. In the primary circuit of the high-tension transformer, there is a rectifier in parallel with a resistor, both components being in series with the autotransformer. Let us consider first what happens when the lower end of the autotransformer is at the low potential, that is, is negative with respect to the upper end. According to our discussion of Section 6.5, the rectifying diode conducts in this situation, presenting a negligible resistance. Since the resistor is in parallel with the diode, the total resistance of the parallel combination is even less than the resistance of the conducting diode. Hence there is a reasonably large current in the primary, and a voltage across the secondary in such a direction that it causes the x-ray tube to operate.

During the next half cycle, when the upper end of the autotransformer is at the low potential, what happens? Now the diode will not conduct, but there will be current just the same, since the resistor provides an alternate route. But the resistor is chosen large enough to result in a significant voltage drop across it. This voltage drop means a lower input voltage to the high-tension transformer. Consequently during the inverse half cycle there is a correspondingly lower output voltage at the high-tension transformer. If the resistance of the resistor is properly chosen, it is possible to have the inverse peak voltage be the same size as the forward peak voltage, that is, the peak voltage during which the x-ray tube conducts. In other words, the larger inverse peak voltage has been suppressed.

Half-Wave Rectification

Half-wave rectification means that an AC voltage is rectified to produce a current which is a DC pulsating one. This topic was amply discussed in Section 6.5; and the reader is also directed to Fig. 7.24, which shows a typical half-wave-rectified x-ray circuit. Perhaps you are wondering: Why this arrangement, as opposed to self rectification?

One of the dangers in an x-ray machine that utilizes self rectification is that, because of overloading, the tube target may reach a temperature sufficiently high that it emits an appreciable number of electrons. If this happens, electrons will be accelerated to the filament during the inverse half cycle of voltage and the filament will be damaged or destroyed. For this reason, two valve tubes may be included in the high-tension conductors, as shown in Fig. 7.24. Of course each valve tube has to have a filament transformer and supply circuits; these components can, of course, be omitted if solid-state rectifiers are employed in place of the valve tubes.

This half-wave rectification circuit is not very widely used in diagnostic x-ray machines because the addition of the valve tubes and associated circuits increases the weight and the cost of the machine, which still, however, produces x-rays only on every alternate half cycle. For another slight increase in weight and cost, it is possible to obtain x-ray production on every high-tension supply half cycle. In other words, full-wave rectification is possible.

Full-Wave Rectification

Full-wave rectification in the x-ray machine means a DC pulsating current through the x-ray tube during every half cycle of AC voltage from the high-tension transformer. This may be accomplished as shown in Fig. 6.17, using two valve tubes, but the standard method adopted in the x-ray machine employs four valve tubes. The relevant circuit diagram is shown in Fig. 8.16.

At this point we would warn the student against trying to memorize this circuit diagram, or indeed any others, because such labor is usually misplaced. It is much easier and, in the long run, more satisfactory to study this arrangement until you understand what it is the circuit is intended for. This particular figure is one variant among many which are used to show the four-valve full-wave-rectification circuit.

Students who have already mastered the full-wave rectification circuit given in Fig. 6.23, in connection with the discussion of the mA meter, may now take full advantage of this knowledge. Others may be interested in the following advice: An easy method of reproducing a circuit for this purpose is to first draw in the high-tension transformer and then the x-ray tube and decide in which direction through the x-ray tube the current should flow. The student is, of course, free to choose conventional current or electron flow for this purpose. The next step is to

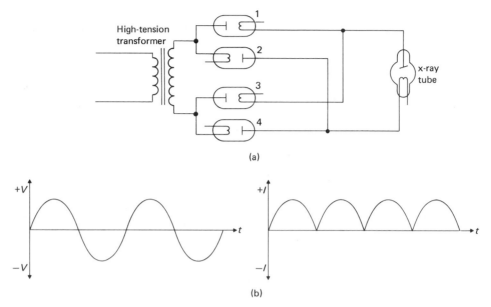

FIG. 8.16.   Four-valve, full-wave rectification. The valve tubes are numbered 1 through 4.
In part (b) *V* refers to the H.T. transformer output voltage and *I* refers to the x-ray tube current. This circuit is sometimes called a Graetz bridge.

draw in the four valve tubes. The pattern they make is of no great moment,
but neatness in the diagram is an obvious advantage. Then, arbitrarily
deciding on a polarity for the transformer output terminals, make one
negative and one positive. Next connect the negative end through one
valve tube to the filament of the x-ray tube and connect the positive end,
through another valve tube, to the anode of the x-ray tube. Make sure that
the electrodes inside those two valve tubes are then included correctly.
Now reverse the polarities of the high-tension output terminals and repeat
the connections to the x-ray tube, using the other two valve tubes. After
you make a few practice tries on rough paper, you will find this procedure
to be simple indeed.

Now then, for your own satisfaction, trace the current pathways
through the valve tubes in Fig. 8.16 with the polarities of the H. T. output
first one way round and then the other. Note that, although sometimes
there seems to be an alternative pathway for the current being considered,
nevertheless one alternative leads to an H.T. terminal which is of the same
polarity as the starting point for the current. This fact will obviously rule
out that alternative.

Figure 8.16 also includes the AC voltage waveform produced at the
H.T. transformer output terminals, and the current waveform through the
x-ray tube. We can see clearly that every half cycle is utilized for x-ray
production, which makes for a much more efficient machine than would be
the case if there were half-wave rectification.

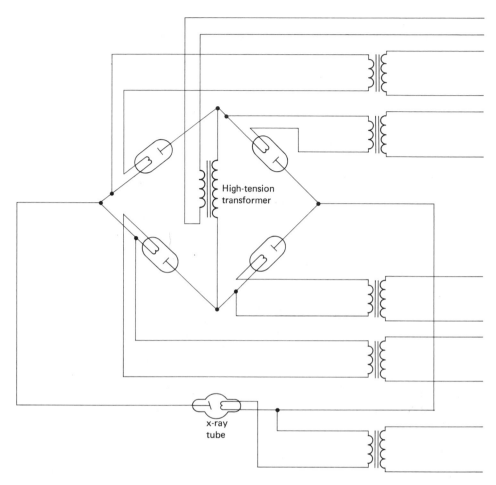

FIG. 8.17. Another Graetz-bridge circuit, which includes five filament transformers. All the leads on the right of the figure are connected, via suitable controls, to the autotransformer.

The arrangement to provide full-wave rectification with four rectifiers, as discussed and featured in Fig. 8.16, is sometimes known as a *Graetz bridge*. And often the Graetz bridge circuit is drawn as shown in Fig. 8.17. The reader should convince himself that this arrangement is entirely equivalent to that of Fig. 8.16.

Figure 8.17 is different from Fig. 8.16 only in that it includes all the filament supplies for the valve tubes and the x-ray tube, so that you may learn two things: that the total circuit diagram begins to look formidable, but also that, after you have already dealt with the component parts separately, the drawing of such a diagram is really quite simple. Try it for yourself.

Finally we should note, as mentioned earlier in Chapter 6, that in the case of high-tension rectification in the x-ray machine the rectifiers used may be valve tubes, as indicated in Fig. 8.17, or solid-state rectifiers, which are finding increased use in modern machines.

8.5 TIMING DEVICES

Timing and Testing

If the length of the exposure is to be controlled, the x-ray machine must have in it some sort of timer. Unless, of course, one were content to use the primitive equipment shown in our frontispiece, in which one can see Professor E. B. Frost doing the timing by looking at a pocket watch!

Timers vary widely in their methods of operation. Before we discuss some of the more common ones, let us look first at the position and role of the timer in the x-ray circuit.

In Fig. 8.18 we see the timer in a circuit in series with the exposure button or switch. This circuit also contains a solenoid and a source of EMF, that is, a part of the autotransformer output.

First let us assume that the x-ray machine is switched on and that the x-ray tube filament is at working temperature. When the exposure switch is closed two things happen. First, current flows through the solenoid and closes the x-ray contactor, which in turn permits current to flow through the primary of the high-tension transformer. Consequently a kV is applied across the tube and x-rays result. Second, depressing the exposure button energizes the mechanism, whatever it may be, of the timer. At the end of the selected time interval, this timer mechanism in turn opens a switch, in series with the hand switch. This switch (not shown in the figure), inside

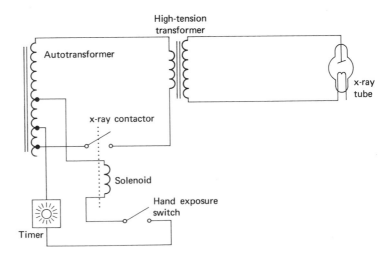

FIG. 8.18. The timer in the x-ray circuit. Note that in this case the exposure switching is carried out in the primary circuit.

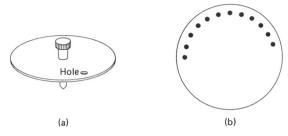

FIG. 8.19. The spinning-top timing test. (a) The top (in practice this may be supported in a stand). (b) The nature of the radiographic appearance at $\frac{1}{10}$ sec and full-wave rectification with 60-cycle AC.

the timer, interrupts the current flowing through the solenoid. The x-ray contactor is pulled open again by a spring: The x-ray exposure is terminated.

Incidentally, this simple circuit also makes sense when you recall that if you take your finger off the dead-man-type exposure button before the timer has had a chance to terminate the exposure, the exposure will end anyway. This is obviously the case because the two switches—hand switch and timer switch—are in series. Either will interrupt the current.

There is a simple test that one can use to test timer accuracy. A spinning top or disk of metal with a single hole punched near the periphery, as shown in Fig. 8.19, can be used. A radiograph is taken of the top while it is spinning. Depending on the type of apparatus, a number of images of the hole will result (see Fig. 8.19b). For instance, at $\frac{1}{10}$ sec with a full-wave-rectifying x-ray unit, twelve half cycles should normally occur at the tube if 60-cycle AC is employed. Twelve pulses of x-radiation will occur, one after the other, so that between each pulse the hole has had time to move round in its rotation. Any other number of images will indicate timer inaccuracy. (Of course, this is true only if the exposure is started and stopped when the tube current is zero.)

For half-wave-rectified equipment there would obviously be half as many (i.e., six) hole images shown in the same time interval.

There is some risk that if the top or disk is spun too rapidly the images of the hole may overlap in a little more than one complete circle. If the top spins too slowly, the images may merge into each other. However, with a little practice, the technician performing this task will usually not encounter any great difficulty.

It is of interest to note here, with reference to Section 7.6, that if there should be a failure of one of the valve tubes in a four-valve-rectified unit, then only half as many pulses of x-rays as normal will be produced in a given time. This, of course, will result in half the expected number of images of the hole in the top. Since, with properly operating valve tubes, such an observation would lead to the conclusion that the timer is twice as fast as it should be, the observation would suggest that probably the rectification circuit is at fault.

Exposure Switching

Exposure switching is a large subject in its own right, and one into which we shall not go very deeply in this text. Nevertheless we must describe briefly some of the methods used, as well as some of the further implications.

As we saw in Fig. 8.18, the x-ray switching device known as the x-ray *contactor* is frequently included in the primary circuit of the H.T. transformer. The contactor is a heavy mechanical device constructed as a unit, including its solenoid. The parts that make actual contact when the switch is closed have to be of fairly large surface area, perhaps the size of a dime, and should make even contact over the entire surface. In the operation of an x-ray machine you may have noticed a distinct thump as the exposure commences: This noise comes from the x-ray contactor. It is normal. But when the contacts are "made" at the beginning of the exposure, they must not bounce unduly. Also, some provision has to be made for the "breaking" of contacts at a time when the AC voltage is at or near zero, unless some other method can be devised to diminish arcing (see Section 5.5).

Because of the mechanical nature of this type of contactor, there is an inevitable delay during the movement of its parts. Although this delay can be tolerated for exposures of say $\frac{1}{60}$ sec or longer, for exposures much shorter than this the contactor is inadequate.

Other methods of x-ray switching include the use of the triode in either the primary or the secondary circuit. In the secondary circuit, a gridded x-ray tube (see Section 7.7) or a separate gas-filled triode may perform the switching function. If the switching is to be accomplished in the primary circuit, the x-ray tube itself obviously cannot be employed. Here a special gas-filled tube, capable of conducting a fairly large current, must be employed. Gas triodes for use in the primary circuit may be required to conduct as much as 100 amp or more, whereas in the secondary circuit only small currents, up to perhaps 1000 mA, need be conducted.

One gas-filled tube that is commonly employed is the *thyratron* shown in the circuits of Fig. 8.20. Once conduction through the thyratron is estab-

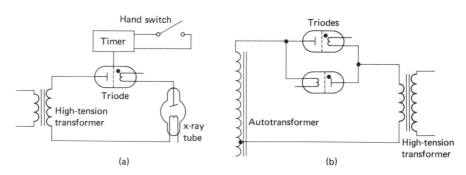

FIG. 8.20.   Triode-controlled x-ray switching.   (a) The switch in the high-tension circuit. (b) Triode switching in the primary circuit.

lished, that is, once ionization of the gas occurs, a large tube current is possible, and the grid loses control of the current. Hence making the grid of the triode less negative starts the exposure, while decreasing the plate voltage until the discharge through the gas tube stops terminates the exposure. At this time the grid regains control and is thus ready to initiate a new exposure. All this is accomplished by circuitry which produces the necessary potentials, and controls the time interval between the beginning and the end of the exposure. These relatively complicated details are omitted in Fig. 8.20, although the place of the timer is indicated. The hand switch, of course, initiates the whole series of events.

An alternative use of the triode for x-ray switching is shown in Fig. 8.20(b), in which triodes are included in the primary side of the high-tension transformer. In one particular line from the autotransformer to the high-tension transformer, two oppositely connected triodes are necessary, so that both forward and inverse half cycles of the AC supply can reach the high-tension transformer. Switching by means of the grids has to be accomplished in both triodes. Of course, these triodes require their own power supplies and associated controls.

Solid-state devices, called *silicon-controlled rectifiers* (SCR), are increasingly being used as switches in the primary circuits of high-output x-ray machines. This growing application is due to their very rapid response; they change from on to off, or vice versa, in 1 to 4 μsec.

Essentially, the SCR is a four-layer PNPN semiconductor device which can be made conductive on the application of a small-signal current to one of its three electrodes.

Unlike the mechanical contacts discussed earlier, both the triode and the solid-state switches operate silently. Because of this silent operation, it has been found useful to add a discreet buzzer to the x-ray circuit. When he hears the buzzer, the x-ray technician can tell that an exposure has been made, even though he may be watching the patient.

Whatever type of radiographic contactor or exposure switch is used, the time it remains "closed" is determined by some sort of timer mechanism. We shall next consider various timers.

The Spring-Driven Timer (Hand Timer)

The basic mechanism of the *spring-driven hand timer* is shown in Fig. 8.21. The solenoid that operates the x-ray contactor is energized when the hand switch is depressed and when the clockwork-driven timer arm—which, as the figure shows, rotates counterclockwise—is in any position other than that shown by the solid lines. When it is at rest, at zero, the arm of the clockwork motor pushes the timer contacts apart so that no exposure is possible.

Before he makes the exposure, the technician winds the clockwork motor in a clockwise direction against a scale marked in seconds, to the required time. When the exposure button is pressed in the side of the timer, the clockwork mechanism is released and the contactor solenoid is energized. The timer unwinds at a constant speed until it reaches zero again; then the timer contacts are opened and the exposure is terminated.

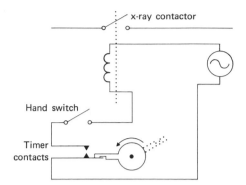

FIG. 8.21. The spring-driven timer. The rotating arm opens the timer contacts at the end of its travel. The dotted out-line of the arm denotes the setting before the exposure.

This is the simplest of timers. Its use is now confined to some older mobile and dental machines with outputs of 10 to 15 mA. The range of the timer usually varies from 0 to 8 or 12 sec, the dial usually being calibrated in increments of $\frac{1}{4}$ sec. For exposure times shorter than $\frac{1}{4}$ sec, this type of timer becomes increasingly unreliable.

The Synchronous Timer

The *synchronous timer* is quite similar to the spring-driven timer described above, except that its movement is caused by a synchronous motor. This type of motor is an AC motor which runs at a constant speed that depends on the frequency of the voltage supply. When the x-ray machine is turned on, the synchronous motor runs constantly. When the exposure button is pressed an extension of the motor shaft grips a mechanism similar to that shown in Fig. 8.21 and rotates until, at the end of its travel, timer contacts are opened and the exposure is terminated. The distance of travel of the rotating mechanism is set on the timer face in the control panel. The face, or dial, of the timer is calibrated in seconds. Exposure times as short as $\frac{1}{20}$ sec are possible with the synchronous timer.

The Impulse Timer

The *impulse timer* is somewhat like the synchronous timer, in that it is driven by a synchronous electric motor. However, the impulse timer's moving parts are driven faster than those of the synchronous timer. This makes it possible to time shorter intervals, giving the impulse timer a timing range commonly from $\frac{1}{120}$ sec to $\frac{1}{5}$ sec.

The important feature of the impulse timer is that its mechanism is synchronized with the mains supply frequency, so that the x-ray contactor is always opened and closed when the x-ray tube current is at, or almost at, zero.

The Electronic Timer

Another type of timer, the *electronic timer,* is shown in Fig. 8.22. As we can see, the figure consists of three circuits drawn one below the other. The upper circuit is the circuit between the autotransformer and the high-tension transformer. Only a small part of this upper circuit is shown:

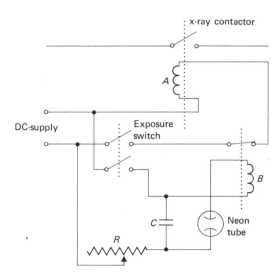

FIG. 8.22. An electronic timer. The exposure switch, which energizes the x-ray contactor solenoid, is ganged to a switch which permits the charging of the capacitor C.

the part that contains the x-ray contactor. The second circuit, in the center of the figure, contains the exposure switch and the solenoid, A, which closes the x-ray contactor. This circuit initiates the x-ray exposure. This and the lower circuit are connected to the power supply. When the exposure switch is depressed, the lower circuit energizes the solenoid, which opens a switch in the exposure switch circuit, thereby terminating the exposure. However, this termination does not occur immediately. The amount of time that elapses between the lower circuit being closed and its solenoid operating depends on how long it takes the capacitor C to reach a certain critical voltage, sufficiently high to cause the neon tube to conduct and thereby permit current through the solenoid B. The time C takes to reach this voltage depends on the value of R, the variable resistor. If R is smaller, C will charge more quickly. Therefore the dial of the electronic timer is calibrated in seconds, but adjusts the value of R. (You may recall our discussion of the time constant and related matters in Section 2.6.)

[An aside on the neon tube: This tube is a neon-filled diode. At a certain voltage across it, ionization occurs; the tube conducts and has a low resistance. Below the "firing" voltage, no current will flow. The tube then acts as an open switch.]

A variant of this timing circuit is one which includes a triode instead of a neon tube. In this case the critical voltage is the voltage on the grid of the triode.

The Photoelectric Timer

We discussed the phototube and its place in the photoelectric timer to some extent in Section 7.8. Now we see how the phototube forms part of a timer circuit. The circuit diagram is given in Fig. 8.23.

The x-ray contactor is closed by a solenoid (not shown in the figure) and the exposure starts. At the same time, light from a small fluorescent

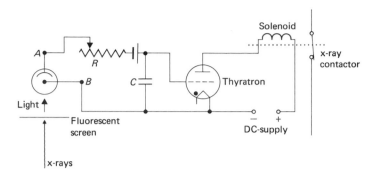

FIG. 8.23. A phototimer. By means of the capacitor C, charged via the phototube, the grid of the thyratron becomes positive and the solenoid is energized.

screen (about 4 × 4 in.), made to fluoresce by the x-ray beam, reaches the phototube in the figure. This permits current to flow through the variable resistor R, thus charging the capacitor C. When the voltage across this capacitor reaches a certain critical value, the triode, a thyratron, fires, or conducts, and thereby energizes the solenoid which opens the x-ray contactor.

The time taken to charge capacitor C, and therefore the resulting density of the film, may be adjusted by changing the value of R. This is usually done at the control panel of the phototimer.

Both the phototube and the ionization chamber, which we shall discuss shortly, have somewhat similar limitations, as mentioned in Section 7.8. The most practical comment we might make about these two types of timers is that the technician must position the patient very accurately. If the position of the patient is such that some anatomical structure other than that intended covers the phototube or ionization chamber area, then the film will be exposed to produce a standard density for that region rather than the region of interest.

The Ionization Timer

We shall discuss ionization chambers at greater length in Section 11.4. At present, let us just say that an ionization chamber is somewhat like a capacitor, but has its two electrodes inside an enclosed chamber. This chamber contains a small quantity of gas, often air.

In operation, the two electrodes have between them a difference of potential and the chamber is exposed to x-radiation. This radiation produces ionization in the chamber, dependent on the intensity of the radiation. The resulting ions will produce a current in the circuit, external to the chamber, which is supplying the potential difference between the electrodes.

In the case of ionization-type timing circuits, a large 14 in. × 17 in., very thin-walled ionization chamber, about $\frac{1}{4}$ in. thick, is placed between the patient and the cassette. Within this area of 14 in. × 17 in., it is usual to include two or three smaller regions of functional chamber, any one of

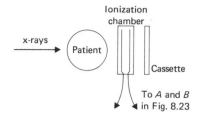

FIG. 8.24. An ionization timer. Unlike the photo-tube, the ionization chamber is placed in front of the x-ray film.

which regions may be selected, depending on the anatomy of the part being examined.

The exposure is started by means we are already familiar with. Ionization occurs in the chamber, a current flows in the external circuit, and may be used to trigger a thyratron, which will terminate the exposure after the film has received a predetermined amount of radiation.

The details of the ionization-chamber part of the circuit are shown in Fig. 8.24. The chamber may then be substituted for the phototube in the circuit of Fig. 8.23, between points A and B.

8.6   SAFETY DEVICES

Many parts of the x-ray machine present electrical hazards to the x-ray technician, or could possibly be operated in a manner which could cause damage to the machine itself. In this section we shall talk about some of the *safety devices* incorporated in x-ray equipment to overcome some of these hazards, particularly with regard to the position of these devices in the x-ray circuit.

Switches

The three switches which concern the x-ray technician most are the *mains switch,* the *on-off switch,* and the *exposure switch.*

The mains switch for a fixed x-ray machine is usually found on a wall adjacent to the control panel. By operating this switch, one can isolate the whole of the x-ray machine completely from the electrical supply. Before any maintenance or service is carried out on the machine, this switch should always be turned off.

Figure 8.25 shows the electrical symbol for the mains type of switch. Note that both supply wires to the apparatus are opened when the switch

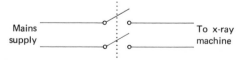

FIG. 8.25. The mains switch. The double blades are ganged together, as indicated by the dotted line, so that, when the switch is open, the x-ray machine is completely isolated from the electricity supply.

is in the off position, and that really this switch is a double switch. The two parts of it are connected mechanically, although not, of course, electrically. For this reason the switch is known as a *single-throw, double-blade*, or *double-pole* switch. Another point to note is that the blades of the switch are spring-loaded; that is, one can't operate the switch slowly. When the technician moves the lever of the switch, he may move it just so far, as slowly as he likes. But then the spring mechanism inside will operate the blades so that they make or break contact very rapidly. This rapid movement minimizes burning of the contacts if the switch should be opened or closed while a current is flowing in the circuit.

Of course, in the case of mobile x-ray machines, the mains switch is replaced by the plug which fits in the electrical outlet.

The on-off switch is situated in the control panel of the machine. Turning it on energizes the autotransformer and many auxiliary circuits, such as those for meters, filaments, electric brakes, the table-tilting motor, etc. The type of switch varies widely: It may be a push button which works directly, or one which operates an electromagnetic relay, or perhaps it may be a single-blade, spring-type switch, rather like the mains switch but operating on one circuit wire only.

The exposure switch, which is a simple push button or toggle switch, is of the dead-man type. That is to say, it requires constant pressure in order to keep it in the on position. If you remove your finger from the switch, it automatically springs into the off position. This feature is a safety device which makes it impossible to leave the x-ray tube operating accidentally.

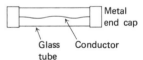

FIG. 8.26. A fuse. This device is connected in series with an electrical circuit.

Fuses and Circuit Breakers

A *fuse* is a safety device that is included in a circuit to prevent the passage of currents larger than those for which the circuit is designed. The fuse is a deliberate weak link in the chain of the circuit. Fuses may be included in many parts of the circuit; for example, within the casing of the main switch, and in the x-ray circuit immediately before the autotransformer.

The fuse itself may take the form of a thin wire encased in a glass tube with sealed metal ends. These ends are in electrical contact with the ends of the wire through the tube. The arrangement is shown in Fig. 8.26. During normal operation of the machine, current passes through the fuse wire. But if for some reason the current becomes larger than that for which the fuse is rated, the thin wire of the fuse becomes so hot that it melts, thus opening the circuit.

One should always investigate the reason for a blown fuse before replacing it, and one should never replace the fuse with a fuse that has a rating higher than that called for by the design of the circuit. Fuses are rated in accordance with the maximum current they will carry without melting, for example, 3 amp. On no account should a fuse be replaced by some other conductor, such as a safety pin or an odd piece of wire. If for some reason the gap which is normally bridged by the fuse is filled with a link able to carry more current than the fuse, there is danger that the circuit may be loaded with large currents which may heat the general wiring and perhaps cause fire by burning the insulation.

Some forms of fuse are made in which the conducting wire through the center is surrounded by an opaque ceramic or other insulation material. Some others may have shapes that are other than cylindrical, but all operate on the same principle.

Electromagnetic *circuit breakers,* which were discussed in Section 4.1, are often used instead of fuses between the mains supply and the input to the autotransformer. Their purpose is the same as that of fuses: to avoid overloading the circuit. If the current should rise to a value greater than designed, the circuit breaker will open and the x-ray machine is thereby effectively switched off.

Grounding

We have amply referred to grounding of a part of a circuit earlier, in connection with the location of the mA meter. In this case, the actual circuit is grounded in such a way that the potential of the circuit at the mA meter is ground potential, or zero potential, by definition. Even if the meter were not insulated, it would be safe for the technician to touch the circuit at this point, since he is presumably also at ground potential.

In addition to the actual circuit, many other parts of the x-ray machine which are normally insulated from the circuit itself may be grounded. A good electrical connection between a part of the machine and ground is often provided by a large copper wire which somehow is ultimately connected to a conductor of relatively large area. This conductor is buried in the earth at sufficient depth to ensure that, regardless of weather conditions, sufficient moisture is at hand to facilitate conduction to the surrounding earth. As an alternative grounding procedure, the grounding cables are sometimes simply connected to the water pipes. This latter procedure is the one commonly employed in the grounding required in the electrical wiring of homes.

In many cases, the ground connection serves only as a secondary precaution. During normal operation of the machine, even without the ground wire, a person touching the component could not get a shock because the currents within the apparatus flow through wires that are covered with insulation. But then, due to age, overheating, or mishandling, or even normal wear, the insulation may become cracked or damaged so that there is an electrical connection in some place other than that intended. The case of the equipment may, for example, act as a conductor. This new current pathway is called a *short circuit,* or simply a *short.* This term implies a pathway of negligible resistance. It is then that a shock may be received by a person touching the equipment, unless a ground connection has been provided. If a ground wire exists, because of its low resistance a larger current will travel through it than through any person who is providing a parallel pathway; the person provides a high-resistance pathway, compared with the ground wire. Therefore the current through the person, and the attending hazard, consequently will be much smaller. In effect, if the ground wire is not broken, the danger to the operator is nil.

Those parts of the x-ray machine which are commonly grounded are as follows: all casings and containers—such as the control panel and the high-tension transformer tank—the tube housings, and the outer metal casing of high-tension cables.

Shockproofing

Shockproofing, in the x-ray field, generally refers to the insulating and proper grounding of electrical components, particularly the x-ray tube housing and the high-tension cable, so that they may be safely touched while the circuit is switched on. (However, touching is not recommended in the case of the tube housing because of the associated radiation hazard.)

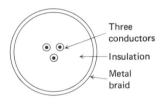

FIG. 8.27.   A high-tension cable.   This cross section shows three conductors for a dual-filament tube.

As mentioned above, one conductor of special interest, as far as shock-proofing is concerned, is the high-tension cable from the high-tension transformer to the x-ray tube.   Figure 8.27 gives a cross-sectional view of this cable, showing three conductors for this example of the cathode high-tension cable of a dual-focus tube. (The anode cable is usually the same, so as to be interchangeable with the cathode cable, but has connection made through one wire only.)   We see that the three wires are not very thick.   This is because the currents to be carried are quite small, up to perhaps 10 amp.   Also the insulation between the three wires is relatively thin because, as we know, the potential difference between the ends of the x-ray tube filament is only something in the order of 10 volts.   However, all the leads to the filaments may be at a potential of 50,000 volts, or more, with respect to ground.   So the insulation surrounding the trio of conductors is very thick and forms the major part of the cable.   Around the outside of the cable is a metallic braid sheath which covers the cable from one end to the other.   The sheath is connected electrically to the tube housing, the transformer tank, and then to ground.   Sometimes the metal braiding is covered with a cloth or plastic covering which forms the outer surface of the complete high-tension cable.

Interlocking Controls

We have already alluded to interlocking controls in Section 7.4, pointing out that intelligent use of the x-ray machine and its tube-rating chart is a necessity, even if such interlocking controls form part of the machine. Figure 8.28 shows, in outline, something of the function of the interlock-controls circuit in question.

Each of the three variables on the control panel—mA, kV, and time—is in some way connected with an electromagnetic relay. Each relay operates a switch in the timer circuit so that, until these three switches, A, B, and C in the figure, are closed, no exposures are possible. Each switch is designed to close when the control to which it is mechanically or otherwise connected is set at some value below the value which is critical for the x-ray tube. Moreover, these three interconnections are so arranged that each takes account of the settings of the other two. This interconnection is necessary because it is the product of the three settings, which is of prime importance with regard to tube ratings. We shall not discuss this last consideration, that is, the interdependence of the three controls, any further here. The student who wishes to find out how this is accomplished is referred to the book by Jaundrell-Thompson and Ashworth, listed at the end of this chapter.

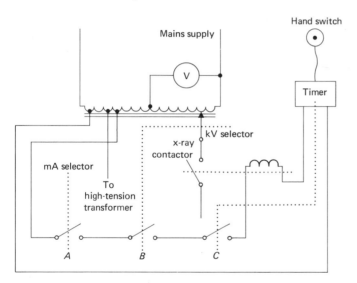

FIG. 8.28. An interlock circuit. The three switches, A, B, and C, ganged (as indicated by the dotted lines) respectively to the mA selector, the kV selector, and the timer, will not close unless these variables are set below certain values.

8.7 THE COMPLETE CIRCUIT

Now that we have dealt separately with the components of a typical x-ray circuit, it is time for us to put them all together. This we have in part done already, of course, in very simplified form in Fig. 8.2. We now go to Fig. 8.29, which introduces a few more complexities. You will see that, as promised, the figure looks formidable indeed, but closer study reveals

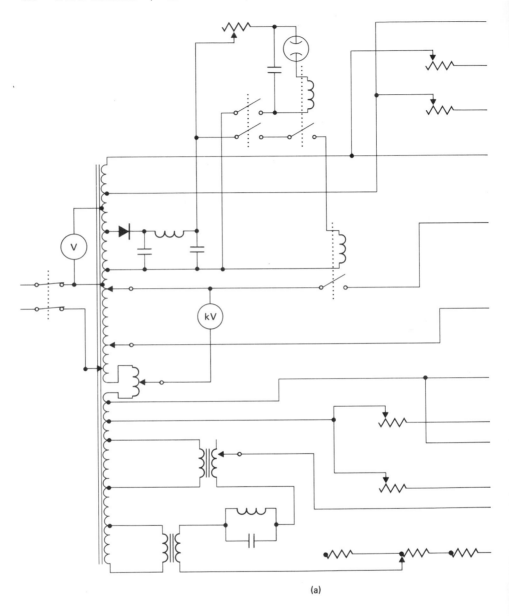

(a)

that it consists only of those parts which we have already discussed in this chapter. In fact, even some of those components we have discussed have been omitted for the sake of clarity.

When you have finished studying Fig. 8.29 carefully, we suggest that you try to construct your own circuit diagram from an understanding of the contents of this chapter. We warn you yet again: Do not try to memorize the diagram! Try to understand it, bit by bit.

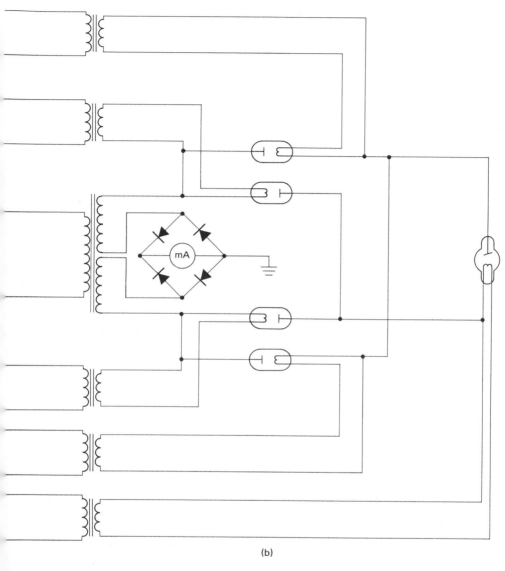

(b)

FIG. 8.29. The complete x-ray circuit.

8.8 THREE-PHASE X-RAY GENERATORS

Three-phase high-tension x-ray generators are finding more widespread use as the demand for shorter exposure times becomes greater. In angiographic radiography, very short exposure times, 0.01 sec or less, are essential. The three-phase generator makes its contribution by being able to produce an almost constant voltage and current through the tube. Without

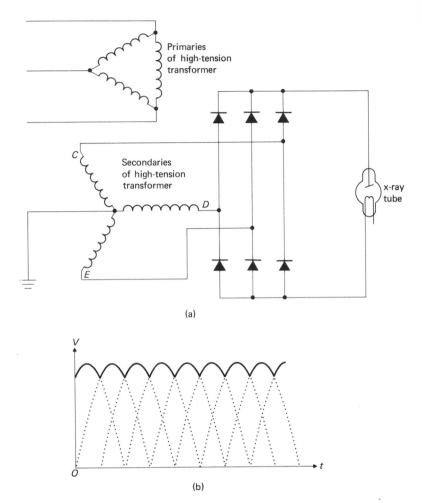

FIG. 8.30. A three-phase x-ray generator. (a) The H.T. primaries are delta connected and the secondaries are star connected. (b) The voltage waveform across the x-ray tube.

the addition of further components in the circuit, such as capacitors, there is a ripple voltage which may be as much as 20% of the peak value, but this is much nearer constant potential than the pulsating DC of the common single-phase generator.

We have already seen in Section 6.7 how a three-phase supply is produced. From the source to the x-ray room, the current is conveyed along either a three- or a four-wire system.

At the x-ray machine each phase requires a separate autotransformer, kV selector, and other important controls. From each autotransformer two conductors are taken to each winding of the three H.T. transformer primaries. These may be connected in a three-wire delta pattern, as shown in Fig. 8.30(a). In this type of connection, of course, although the windings have their ends connected as shown, the windings do not occupy this shape in the machine.

Each H.T. primary is wound on a separate limb of a common core, which limb also contains a single secondary winding. But now the three secondary windings are connected in a star pattern, as shown in the figure.

By means of this circuit and the six rectifiers shown in Fig. 8.30(a), we obtain three-phase full-wave six-valve rectification. Follow the current pathways to check. As the voltage in each secondary winding varies from zero to maximum, the other two will be 120° and 240°, respectively, out of phase. So when C is at a higher potential, that is, positive with respect to E, current will flow from C, through the diode to which it is connected, to the anode of the tube, back through the center diode in the figure, and so to E. A similar circuit can be followed for any other combination of polarities. The somewhat idealized voltage waveform across the tube, which is produced by this x-ray generator, is shown in Fig. 8.30(b). The dotted lines show the rising and falling voltages for the individual phases. The solid lines show the resultant total voltage of the three phases. It is this total voltage which appears as a ripple across the x-ray tube. The current waveform will of course be somewhat similar. (We previously saw this waveform in Fig. 6.27.)

The three-phase x-ray generator is more expensive than its single-phase counterpart because of the controls and auxiliary circuits required for all three phases. On the other hand, because of the system's approximation to a constant potential supply to the tube, the effective values of voltage and current are much higher (for sinusoidal three-phase voltage, $kV_{RMS} = 0.95$ kVp). This means a greater output of radiation per unit time. Also, although the exposure to the patient may be the same, nevertheless the absorbed dose will be smaller, due to the high effective kV, which results in a lower percentage of easily absorbed low-energy x-ray photons. With the addition of capacitors in the high-tension circuit, exposure times and absorbed doses may be made even smaller.

QUESTIONS

1. Discuss mains voltage compensation.

2. Draw and label a circuit diagram of a prereading kV meter compensator. Briefly explain how the compensator works.

3. Considerable insulation is required between the primary and secondary windings of an x-ray tube filament transformer, even though this transformer steps down mains voltage, which is relatively low, to an even lower voltage. Explain.

4. Explain what is meant by space-charge compensation. Describe, with the aid of a circuit diagram, how space-charge compensation is effected.

5. a) Why is it so important to maintain a constant AC voltage across the filament transformer?

     b) What circuit components are employed to achieve this end?

6. a) Draw and label a circuit diagram of an inverse voltage suppressor. Describe the operation of the circuit.

     b) In what type of equipment is such a suppressor necessary?

7. Draw a simple, complete, full-wave-rectified x-ray machine circuit and include all filament supplies.

8. Draw and explain circuit diagrams for the following:
     a) four-valve, full-wave rectification,
     b) two-valve, half-wave rectification.

9. An mA meter requires its own rectification circuit when used in a full-wave-rectified x-ray machine, but does not in a self-rectified unit. Explain.

10. With the aid of a circuit diagram and a brief text, explain how a phototimer operates. How is the exposure time changed?

11. a) Describe the spinning-top method of timer testing.
     b) Would it be possible under some conditions to get seven spots with a 60-cycle full-wave-rectification machine operation for $\frac{1}{20}$ sec without the timer being wrong? Explain.

12. Explain the principle and purpose of an impulse timer.

13. What would be the evidence, if any, on radiographs if one valve tube in a Graetz-bridge circuit became inoperative?

14. Discuss the rationale of grounding the casings of electrical equipment.

15. a) What is the function of a fuse?
     b) How is a fuse constructed?
     c) What other device is frequently employed to serve the same function as a fuse?

16. a) By means of a cross-sectional diagram and a brief text, describe an x-ray high-tension cable.
     b) In use, such a cable may be expected to be connected to supply voltages as high as 100,000 volts. However, the conducting wires within the H.T. cables are quite thin. Explain.

17. Sketch a diagram such as Fig. 8.31, and then:

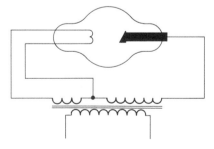

     a) indicate the conventional current direction through the tube;

     b) indicate the direction of electron migration in the tube;

     c) label all parts of the tube and the circuit;

     d) mark the place in the circuit in which you would place a control affecting the tube current (mA), without significantly affecting the kV of the tube;

FIG. 8.31. Simple x-ray circuit.

     e) indicate where the most advantageous place to ground the secondary circuit would be;

   f) redraw the transformer arrangement to show the best place to insert the mA meter;

   g) indicate the usual placement of the kV meter;

   h) sketch a time-voltage (time on abscissa) graph of current in the tube circuit.

   i) What type (if any) rectification is involved?

18. Find the timer circuit in Fig. 8.29. This circuit is energized by a DC supply, shown also in Fig. 8.22. Explain how such a DC supply is obtained. (You should be able to work this out from what you already know about diodes, capacitors, and inductors.)

19. a) Describe a three-phase x-ray generator circuit. Include a circuit diagram of the H.T. transformer connections.

   b) What is the main advantage of a three-phase x-ray machine over a single-phase machine?

SUGGESTED READING

FILES, G. W. (original editor), *Medical Radiographic Technic.* Springfield, Ohio: Charles C. Thomas, 1962 (second edition). Chapters 3 and 4 deal with basic x-ray generating circuits and x-ray apparatus, at about the same level as our book, but with less detail. The book is written with considerable authority, as it has been prepared by the Technical Service, X-ray Department of the General Electric Company.

GIBBS, J. B., *Transformer Principles and Practice.* New York: McGraw-Hill, 1950 (second edition). For those students who are interested in some of the further details of transformer construction and connections than are touched on in our book, we recommend the text by Gibbs.

JAUNDRELL-THOMPSON, F., and W. J. ASHWORTH, *X-ray Physics and Equipment.* Oxford: Blackwell Scientific Publications, 1965. Especially useful in Chapters 13 through 21 as a detailed reference for the discussions in our Chapter 8. Chapter 21 is concerned with interlock circuits, which we have touched on briefly in our Section 8.6. This book is the most complete reference available on x-ray circuits.

SCHALL, W. E., *X-rays, Their Origin, Dosage and Practical Application.* Bristol: John Wright and Sons, Ltd., 1961 (eighth edition). Chapters 3 and 4 include considerable material given in our Chapter 8, specifically timers, switch gear, and complete high-voltage generators for x-ray work. A notable feature of this book is the many excellent photographs of x-ray equipment.

VAN DER PLAATS, G. J., *Medical X-ray Technique.* The Netherlands: Philips Technical Library, 1965 (second edition). Professor Van der Plaats' Chapter 16 deals with "Apparatus for X-ray Diagnosis" and includes circuit diagrams. The book is intended particularly for medical radiographers in training.

YOUNG, M. E. J., *Radiological Physics.* London: H. K. Lewis and Co., Ltd., 1967 (second edition). Chapter 3, "The Production of X-rays up to About 400 keV in Energy," includes a discussion of x-ray circuits.

CHAPTER 9

X-Rays: Their Nature and Production

Now that we have seen how x-rays are produced, we shall take a closer look at the actual physical processes involved in the creation of x-rays. We shall look at the relevant affairs more on the microscopic level, and delve a little into the nature of x-rays.

Radiography was not only initiated but quite well established in the medical field before there was any precise understanding of Röntgen's x-radiation. The hypothesis that x-rays are transverse electromagnetic waves, similar to visible light but of shorter wavelength, received strong support from the phenomenon of polarization first noted in 1904 by the English physicist, C. G. Barkla (1877–1944). The crucial experiment in support of accepting x-rays as part of the family of electromagnetic radiations was suggested by the German theoretical physicist, M. T. F. von Laue (1879–1960) and performed by his students, W. Friedrich and P. Knipping, in 1912. Consequently one might consider 1912, the year that the diffraction of x-rays was demonstrated by these scientists, the key date in the development of an understanding of the x-rays which had been used in medicine since 1896. Von Laue was awarded the 1914 Nobel prize in physics for this work.

Next the father-and-son team of Sir William H. Bragg (1862–1942) and W. L. Bragg (1890–) took the diffraction of x-rays one step further and worked out methods for determining x-ray wavelengths by crystal diffraction. This research resulted in these English physicists receiving the Nobel physics prize in 1915. The Braggs are the only father-and-son combination ever to have been so honored.

With x-rays now firmly established as electromagnetic waves having measurable lengths, albeit much shorter than those of visible light, the American physicist and educator, Arthur Holly Compton (1892–1962), enters the picture with a discovery which won him the Nobel prize in physics in 1927. The Compton effect, reported in 1923, demonstrates that in some interactions x-rays behave like particles. That is, it appeared that the x-ray photons in striking electrons behaved like particles, the photon-electron interaction being much like the collision of billiard balls. The wave-particle nature of radiation was again evident, just as it had been earlier in the realm of ordinary visible light. We shall come back briefly to this matter shortly.

The x-rays produced with an x-ray machine are not all of the same wavelength. There is a spectrum of radiation, from some minimum wavelength to longer wavelengths. Moreover, there are also certain particular x-ray wavelengths which appear, depending on the nature of the x-ray target. These latter x-rays are called *characteristic x-rays*. They were first noted by Barkla, who was mentioned earlier in connection with the polarization of x-rays. The observation and explanation of the definite minimum wavelength was the work of the American physicists, W. Duane (1872–1935) and F. L. Hunt (1883–). The relationship, involving the tube kV, which can be employed to calculate the minimum wavelength of an x-ray spectrum, is known as the *Duane-Hunt law,* or *equation.*

9.1 SOME PRELIMINARIES

What are x-rays? We want to say that they are both waves and particles. Or rather, to be more correct, sometimes we can best explain their behavior by considering them as consisting of a stream of "particles," photons, and sometimes their behavior requires a description in terms of waves. Now everyone is quite familiar with what is meant by particles. And we have previously dealt with the photon concept, photons being the "particles" involved in dealing with radiation like light and x-rays. But the idea of waves perhaps requires a little elucidation.

Wave Phenomena

Everyone is acquainted with the disturbance created when a stone is thrown into a pond. A disturbance, a wave, is propagated outward from the point at which the stone strikes the water.

If, instead of throwing one stone into the pond, one were to throw similar stones into the water at the same point and at regular intervals, the disturbance in the water would be continuous. A continuous train of waves would be set up. Such waves are said to be *periodic*. In Fig. 9.1 we see such periodic water waves, in a duck pond.

FIG. 9.1. Waves in the duck pond.

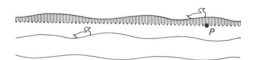

FIG. 9.2. A periodic wave. The point *P* here represents the point *P* in the duck pond.

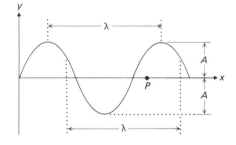

In order to establish clearly what is meant by the various terms important in a discussion of wave phenomena, we must now ask you to employ your imagination. Imagine that at a given instant in time we could take a vertical slice of the pond, as indicated by the shaded portion of Fig. 9.1. Now we redraw this slice, removing the freer aspects of art, including the duck. This is done in Fig. 9.2. The slice of water in this sense could then be taken as a graph of the height of the waves, y, as a function of their horizontal displacement, x.

In this representation of waves, the high points are usually called *crests* and the low points *troughs*. The distance from any given point on a crest or a trough to the corresponding point on the immediately succeeding crest or trough is called the *wavelength,* λ. (Note that λ now has an entirely different meaning than the one it had in Chapter 1, in which λ referred to the radioactive decay constant.)

The maximum height of a crest, or the maximum depth of a trough, as measured from the equilibrium position—which is the level the water has when there is no disturbance—is called the *amplitude.* Now think about the ducks of Fig. 9.1. We shall assume that, before the stones were dropped in the pond, the pond was calm, flat, and that the ducks were motionless. When the stones struck the water, a disturbance was propagated. This disturbance caused the ducks to go up and down. Work was done on the ducks. The ducks were recipients of energy. In other words, wave motion propagates energy. Moreover, when the amplitude is zero and there is no disturbance, no energy is expended on the ducks. However, when there is a large amplitude the ducks obviously have a lot of energy expended on them. We note that the amplitude of a wave is related to the energy of the wave motion. The bigger the amplitude, the greater the energy involved.

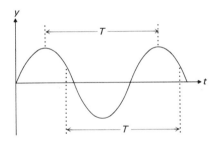

FIG. 9.3. Time graph of a periodic wave: the ups and downs of the duck at point *P* of Fig. 9.1 as a function of time.

Next we use our imagination again. Let us stand in the water at the point *P*, as indicated in Fig. 9.1, and observe the duck going up and down. Let us graph our observation. This time our graph will be *y*, the height of the wave, as a function of time. This gives us a second representation of a wave as shown in Fig. 9.3.

The time the duck takes to go from one height all the way up (or down), then all the way down (or up) and back to its original position is called the *period.* We have already met this term in our discussion of AC. It means the time for a complete cycle of any periodic behavior. At present it means specifically the time for one complete wave motion.

At this point we should recall Eq. (6.2) relating period and frequency. If the period is small, then the duck makes its up and down trips in a hurry: The frequency is high. (As an aside, we might note at this point that the unit for frequency, being the reciprocal of time, although previously referred to as cycles/sec, is simply sec⁻¹, and that it is now becoming common practice to use the unit *hertz* for 1 cycle/sec.)

Now for a third and final stretch of the imagination. Suppose that we again stand at point *P* in Fig. 9.1, but that no stone has yet been thrown. Then when the stones are dropped somewhere to the left of us, a wave comes along and lifts the duck at *P*. A moment later, as the duck is going back down, the water somewhere to the right is rising to a crest; in other words, the disturbance, the wave motion, is being propagated from left to right. We show this schematically in Fig. 9.4. Note how the crest, noted first at *P*, travels to the right. In the small time interval Δt_1, the disturbance has moved very little. In the interval Δt_2, it has moved considerably further to the right. In the time interval corresponding to one-half a period, $\frac{1}{2}T$, the crest has moved one-half a wavelength to the right. And in time *T* it has moved a whole wavelength.

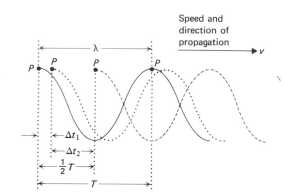

FIG. 9.4. A periodic wave propagating to the right at speed *v*.

Let us assume that the propagation takes place at a speed *v*. Then, from our knowledge of what is meant by speed (that is, distance per unit time), we can see from Fig. 9.4 that for our waves we get

$$v = \lambda/T. \tag{9.1}$$

More frequently this relationship is expressed in terms of frequency. If we use Eq. (6.2) to substitute for *T* in Eq. (9.1), we have

$$v = f\lambda. \tag{9.2}$$

Although we arrived at this expression by our imaginative pursuits in the duck pond, the expression is true for all wave motion. In the case of electromagnetic waves, like light and x-rays, the speed *v* is the speed of light, usually indicated by the symbol *c*, where $c = 3 \times 10^8$ m/sec. Equation (9.2) then becomes

$$c = f\lambda. \tag{9.3}$$

Finally, note that although the wave motion was propagated from left to right—that is, horizontally—the ducks and the actual water particles were disturbed or moved *up and down*. That is to say, the actual disturbance was at right angles to the direction of propagation of this disturbance. Waves with this characteristic are called *transverse waves*. The waves of interest to us are electromagnetic waves. They are transverse waves.

On the other hand, compressional waves, such as sound waves, are longitudinal. In sound waves the air molecules are displaced in the same direction as the direction of the propagation of the wave. The disturbance and its propagation are in the same direction, not at right angles to one another, as is the case with transverse waves. We shall have no further concern with longitudinal waves, although we should point out here that such waves, in the ultrasonic region of 2 megacycles/sec or more, are finding medical use in both diagnosis and therapy. In fact, ultrasonography may be used for certain diagnostic purposes in which radiography is not entirely effective.

Electromagnetic Waves

Ordinary visible light is a wave phenomenon. Moreover, it is a transverse wave phenomenon. Let us see what supports these contentions. Then, if x-rays exhibit similar behavior, we have support for the idea that x-rays are wave phenomena like light. And this is the present view.

We start by describing an experiment first performed in England in 1801 by a leading figure in many areas, the physician, linguist, and scientist, Thomas Young (1773–1829). A schematic plan of Young's so-called double-slit experiment is shown in Fig. 9.5. Here we have, on the left, a source of monochromatic light (all the rays of which are of the same color, that is, of the same wavelength). If a particle view of light were accepted, this source, passing light through the single slit on the right of it, should not permit any light to strike the screen on the far right. We assume, of course, that the particles, as one would intuitively expect, travel in a straight line; then they certainly cannot get from the source to the screen. The observation, however, shows something different. Not only does light strike the screen to the right of the double slit, but more surprising, the screen shows evidence of a series of light and dark striations.

We explain this effect as follows. Light behaves like a wave traveling outward from the source, the wave-front pattern being represented by the semicircular lines of Fig. 9.5. (This pattern is quite similar to the way that wave fronts move out from a disturbance such as that caused by throwing a stone into our duck pond.) Let us now assume that the white semicircular lines of part (b) of the figure represent the location of crests, and therefore halfway between the white lines, in the dark region, would be the troughs. When the waves from the source strike the first narrow slit, part of each wave emerges from the slit. In a way, we can now think of the slit as being itself a source of light. This light strikes the next two slits, each of which behaves like the single slit before, thus giving rise to two sources of light. But these two sources have a very important characteristic.

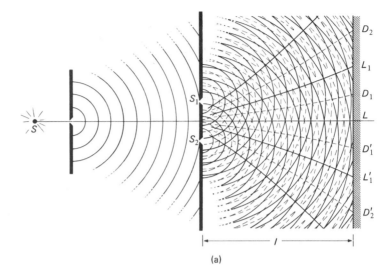

(a)

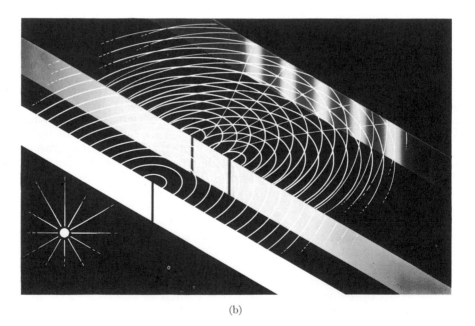

(b)

FIG. 9.5.   Schematic plan of Young's double-slit experiment; not to scale.   For the waves from either slit, S_1 or S_2, the distance between adjacent crests is grossly exaggerated.   This distance, the wavelength, is actually about 5×10^{-5} cm for green light.   Also, the distance l to the viewing screen has to be much larger than the separation between the double slits. In (a) the dashed semicircles represent troughs, while in both (a) and (b) the solid semicircles represent crests.   (Courtesy Holton and Roller, *Foundations of Modern Physical Science,* Addison-Wesley, 1958.)

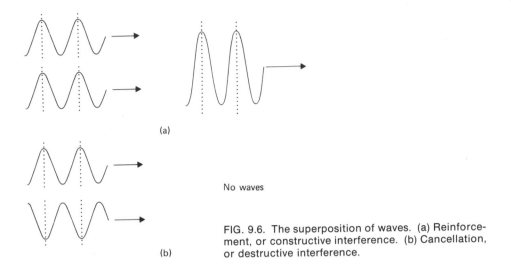

No waves

FIG. 9.6. The superposition of waves. (a) Reinforcement, or constructive interference. (b) Cancellation, or destructive interference.

FIG. 9.7. Photograph of an interference pattern of light from a double slit. (By permission, from Sears' *Optics,* Addison-Wesley, 1949.)

Since they both originate from the same source, these new sources provide waves which are in phase. That is, when a crest leaves the slit S_1, so does a crest leave the slit S_2. The light emerging from the slits is said to be *coherent.* Now observe the screen, which is struck by two sets of waves, one from each source slit. When the waves arrive in phase, that is, when a crest from one slit arrives with a crest from the other slit, the waves reinforce each other, as shown in Fig. 9.6(a). The light is bright because the wave amplitude, and hence the associated energy, is large. This effect is called *constructive interference.* Between these bright areas there are regions in which the crest from one slit arrives with the trough from the other. The waves cancel each other, as shown in Fig. 9.6(b). This latter effect is called *destructive interference.* Figure 9.7 shows a photograph of an actual interference pattern as achieved with Young's double-slit method.

Note that in our discussion we have freely indulged in the wave concepts discussed earlier. In fact we could study this interference phenomenon using our duck pond. If we started waves with stones at two different locations on the pond, then the waves would interact as discussed above. Wherever a crest of one set of waves appeared at the same time as the trough from the other set we would have no disturbance of the water. In fact, water waves are frequently used to study wave behavior in physics. By setting up waves in a shallow tray with a transparent bottom and shining a light through the water, one may readily see the various degrees of disturbance created in terms of gradations of shadow on a white paper placed below the transparent water-wave tray. This type of experimental apparatus has been given the appropriate name of *ripple tank.*

In summary, we can explain these bright and dark striations of Fig. 9.7 only by employing the ideas of constructive and destructive interference of waves. No particle theory of light has been found to offer a tenable alternative explanation.

The double-slit experiment just described actually involves two phenomena: First, *diffraction.* Diffraction is the property of waves of being able to bend around the edge of an obstacle in their path. Were it not for diffraction, the viewing screen of Fig. 9.5 would be dark. Second, there is the phenomenon of *interference,* also a wave property. This property, as we have pointed out, explains the alternate dark and light pattern on the viewing screen. Sometimes these two effects in combination are loosely referred to as *diffraction effects.* In fact, an optical device consisting of a large number of equidistant narrow slits side by side is called a *diffraction grating.* Diffraction gratings can be employed to measure the wavelengths of light. We shall return to this matter shortly, in connection with the measurement of x-ray wavelengths.

So light is waves or, more correctly, light exhibits wave behavior in the situation described. But light is not just waves. It is a particular type of waves: *transverse waves.* The transverse character of light waves is established by polarization. Let us see what this means.

If we were to agitate a rope up and down at point P of Fig. 9.8, the rope particles would go up and down but the disturbance created at P would travel along the rope to the right. We have a transverse wave. Note that the wave generated at P can pass through the slots A, B, and C, but will be

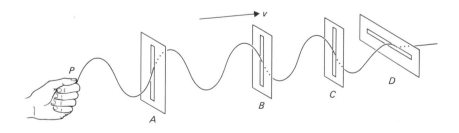

FIG. 9.8. A vibrating rope demonstrating transverse wave motion.

extinguished at slot D. On the other hand, were we to lay a spring through all four slots and then set up a compressional wave in the spring, this wave would pass through all four slots. Only a transverse wave can be extinguished simply by changing the orientation of a barrier.

The transverse wave we have so far considered has had its disturbance or deflection confined to a single plane. Such a wave is said to be *plane polarized.* A more complicated transverse wave in which the deflections are not confined to the same plane is said to be *unpolarized.* If an unpolarized disturbance were incident at barrier A, then only a vertically polarized wave would be transmitted.

Now light is normally unpolarized. The wave disturbances are every which way, in all planes, as indicated by the arrows in Fig. 9.9. However, for reasons which are understood but which will not be discussed here, certain crystals will readily transmit the disturbances, or waves, in one particular plane of the crystal and absorb or deflect waves striking at other angles, along other planes. Such crystals are called *polarizers.* Polarizers are now also made artificially. Polaroid is an example of an artificially made polarizer in wide use.

Once a light has passed through a polarizer, as shown at A in Fig. 9.9, it is plane polarized. If we now take a similar polarizer and place it at B, but rotate it by 90°, then no light gets to C. We have stopped light by using two transparent, but polarizing, materials. Light waves must be transverse. (Students who wish to pursue the concept of polarization further are referred to Chapter 36 of the book by Richards *et al.*, listed at the end of this chapter.)

At this point you might ask: If light is a wave, what is it that is waving? The answer is the electric and magnetic fields in the space in question. This answer is firmly established and dates to work done in the 1870's by James Clerk Maxwell, whom we introduced in Chapter 4. Maxwell showed that oscillating electrical charges should radiate electromagnetic waves which should have a velocity of propagation of very nearly 3×10^{10} cm/sec, or about 186,000 mi/sec. His predictions were confirmed. Moreover, the

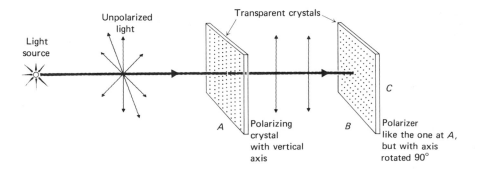

FIG. 9.9. Polarization of light rays. Both polarizers are transparent to unpolarized light.

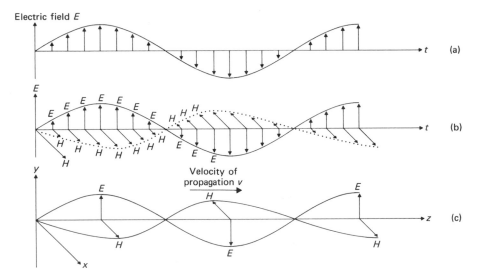

FIG. 9.10. Electromagnetic waves. (a) Variation with time of the electric field E at a given point in space. (b) The changing magnetic field, at right angles to the changing electric field, is added to the diagram of part (a). Here H is used to denote the magnetic field intensity in free space. Parts (a) and (b) are analogous to the water wave representation of Fig. 9.3. (c) Representation of electromagnetic waves traveling to the right. This diagram is analogous to the water wave representation of Fig. 9.2.

speed involved was the established speed of light, and so the electromagnetic nature of ordinary light came to the fore. Light was thereafter considered as an electromagnetic wave or, as is often abbreviated in the relevant literature, an EM wave.

As a preliminary to trying to clarify this notion of an electromagnetic wave further, we ask the reader to turn back to Fig. 9.3. We now draw a similar figure, Fig. 9.10(a), but for an electromagnetic rather than a water wave. Instead of watching a duck going up and down at point P, we now stand at point P with an electroscope, perhaps a pithball with a known electric charge on it, to detect the magnitude and direction of the electric field. We note the changes as time passes and record the results, thereby ending up with the graph of Fig. 9.10(a). Readers should, of course, realize that what has been described is rather idealized. In practice one could not achieve such a measurement because the rapid response required of the pithball would demand that it be inertialess. That means that we would need a pithball without mass. We don't have any.

Now, as a matter of fact, an electromagnetic wave has another component, a changing magnetic field which is always at right angles to the electric field. So we could have come up with a similar graph by employing a very sensitive, and inertialess, compass needle. Combining the two fields, we get a graph like Fig. 9.10(b). In Fig. 9.10(c) we show the conventional representation of an electromagnetic wave.

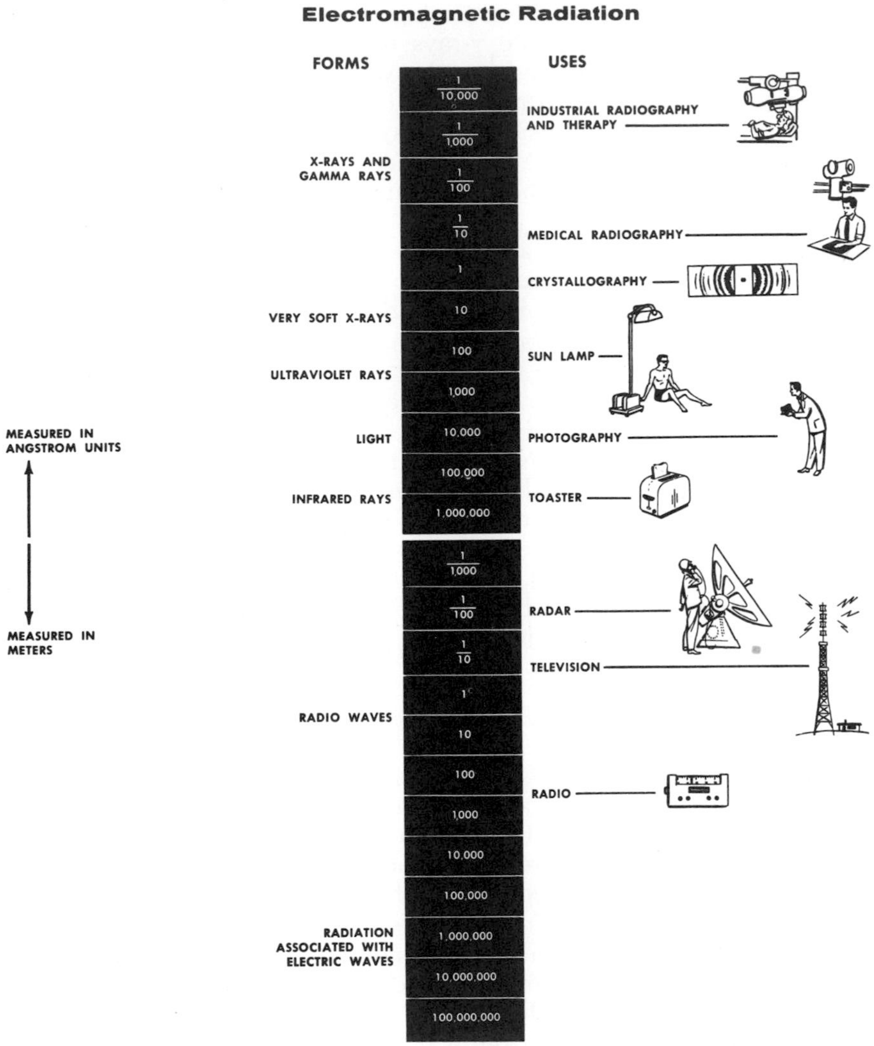

Electromagnetic Radiation

FIG. 9.11. Electromagnetic spectrum. (From *Fundamentals of Radiography*, published by Radiography Markets Division, Eastman Kodak Company.)

Again we might ask: How does all this relate to x-rays? It turns out that x-rays, like light, are part of the family of electromagnetic waves. Figure 9.11 shows the complete family, the electromagnetic spectrum. Note that there is no clear-cut division between one type of electromagnetic radiation and another. Precisely where x-rays start is entirely a matter of opinion, and whether radiation should be called γ-rays or x-rays is a matter of the source of the radiation rather than of energy or wavelength. It is usual to consider γ-rays as radiation arising in a radioactive decay process. It is thus actually true that some γ-rays have energies less than x-rays produced at only 15 kV, although on the whole γ-rays tend to be in the higher energy region, as shown in Fig. 9.11.

As a rough rule, one might say that x-rays lie in the wavelength region of 0.01 to 100 angstrom units. Most diagnostic work employs x-rays from 0.1 Å to 1 Å. Visible light, on the other hand, lies in the region of 4000 Å (violet) to 7000 Å (red).

Thermography (mentioned again in Section 12.1), which is a method of diagnosis depending on differences in body temperature, employs wavelengths even longer than those of visible light: heat radiated from the body. This heat radiation is in the infrared region, around 40,000 Å to 200,000 Å. Temperature differences of 0.5 C° can be detected with a thermograph, and since the skin temperature over a breast cancer may be about 1 C° higher than that of the surrounding tissue, thermography is proving to be a useful diagnostic technique. Note that this technique employs radiation almost at the opposite end of the electromagnetic spectrum from x-rays.

Although electromagnetic radiations may have all kinds of wavelengths, these waves all have the same speed in vacuum (3×10^{10} cm/sec), and even the same speed in air, to all intents and purposes. Hence from Eq. (9.2) it is easy to see that the longer the wavelength the lower the frequency. Now from the earlier relation

$$E = hf, \tag{1.1}$$

we see that the photon energy is higher as the frequency gets higher. In other words, the short-wave x-rays have a much higher energy than the long-wave radio waves. In that sense, in the electromagnetic spectrum the various radiations are ordered from the lowest energy to the highest energy, this order being reversed to that of shortest wavelength to longest wavelength.

At this point some readers are perhaps objecting to the sudden inclusion of Eq. (1.1). After all, a photon is a chunk, a particle or corpuscular concept, while up to now we have been blithely talking waves. True. We have given some evidence of the wave behavior of light. But there is other behavior, such as the photoelectric effect, which needs a quantum or corpuscular description. From such a viewpoint Eq. (1.1) enters the picture, the corpuscular concept of the discrete chunk of energy merging nicely with the wave concept of frequency. This wave-particle duality in nature bears further consideration.

Before we take a look at this wave-particle duality, however, we might just mention that although electromagnetic waves all have the same speed in vacuum—usually given the symbol c—their speeds in material media depend on their wavelengths. It is for this reason of the difference of the speeds of the various components of ordinary white light in glass that white light can be broken into its constituent color components by a glass prism, as shown in Fig. 9.12.

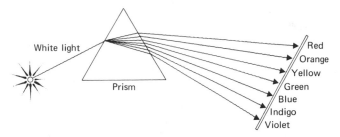

FIG. 9.12. Ordinary white light (such as from the sun) passing through a glass prism is separated into the spectral colors indicated. Note the mnemonic device for remembering the spectral order: Mr. Roy G. Biv.

The Wave-Particle Duality

In spite of what we have been saying, one might be tempted to ask at this point, is light a wave, or is light corpuscular in nature? Modern physics suggests that this is not the proper question. The proper question is: How does light *behave?* And the answer is that sometimes it behaves like a wave as evidenced by diffraction phenomena, and sometimes its behavior is best described in terms of a corpuscular character, as was employed, for example, in the discussion of the photoelectric effect in Section 7.8.

In the world of the very small, waves and particles appear to be simply different aspects of one and the same thing. These at first glance seemingly contradictory aspects were first implied in Einstein's work on the photoelectric effect in 1905. The "particle" associated with the "wave" of light was the photon. In fact we already mentioned in Chapter 1 that, as a consequence of the fact that atoms appear to absorb and emit radiation in definite discrete amounts—called *quanta* or *photons*—it became evident that, the success of the wave theory notwithstanding, one had to regard light, from some points of view at least, as if it were of a particle nature. This was the idea involved in the photoelectric effect as introduced by Einstein.

From Chapter 1 we again recall the equation:

$$E = hf, \tag{1.1}$$

where E is a quantum of energy or the photon energy, h is Planck's constant, and f the frequency of the associated waves. Since in relativistic mechanics the momentum p (mass × velocity) of a particle can be expressed by

$$p = E/c,$$

where c is the speed of electromagnetic radiations, we see that

$$p = h/\lambda.$$

This expression definitely relates the particle and wave concepts, in that p, the momentum, is characteristic of a particle and λ, the wavelength, is characteristic of a wave.

As we shall shortly see, x-rays themselves lend support to this wave-particle duality, in that von Laue's experiment demonstrated a wave behavior and the Compton experiment gave further support to the corpuscular character.

The important point to note now is that, although electromagnetic radiations exhibit both wave and particle aspects, they do not exhibit both aspects in the same experiment. As Niels Bohr pointed out in 1928, the two viewpoints are therefore not contradictory, but complementary. Our knowledge of electromagnetic radiations is partial—is incomplete—unless both the wave *and* the particle aspects are known.

Again: The wave and particle aspects are not exhibited in one and the same experiment. When radiation travels from one place to another without losing energy, that is, in such phenomena as reflection, interference, and diffraction, the wave aspect appears. But when radiation interacts with matter and gives up energy, then the particle aspect comes to the fore.

Those who still find the above duality a bit difficult to accept might meditate a moment on the following analogy. Consider a female x-ray technician, for example. She is a woman. She is an x-ray technician. She may be a wife. She may be a mother. She may be a bargain hunter. She may be a committee chairman. Surely she does not behave to her husband like an x-ray technician. Nor is it expected that she will exhibit her wifely traits on the job. And all the other traits we have described are likely to be exhibited only under the appropriate circumstances. She behaves differently in the different circumstances, and yet she is one and the same woman.

Although it seems difficult enough for some people to accept this viewpoint—that light can be explained either in terms of a wave or in terms of a particle, depending on the interaction to be studied—they find it even more difficult to accept an idea by de Broglie: that with any particle, such as a pingpong ball for example, one may associate a wave. In 1923, the year before he obtained his doctorate, the French physicist, Louis de Broglie (1892–   ) showed that with any "particle" there ought to be associated a "wave." He accomplished this brilliant piece of reasoning by combining the Einstein formula, which related mass and energy ($E = mc^2$), with that of Planck, which related frequency and energy ($E = hf$). The de Broglie relationship for material particles is

$$\lambda = h/p,$$

where λ is the wavelength of the "matter waves," h is Planck's constant, and p is the momentum of the particle with which the "matter wave" is associated. These "matter waves" are not electromagnetic in nature: Their explanation is in probabilistic terms relating to the localizing of the particle in space, an approach which is fundamental to quantum mechanics but beyond the scope of this book.

That this wavelike behavior of material particles is not a figment of the imagination was first proved experimentally by C. J. Davisson and L. H. Germer in 1927 at the Bell Telephone Laboratories. Davisson and Germer demonstrated that a stream of electrons under certain conditions exhibits diffraction effects like ordinary visible light, effects which cannot be explained except by recourse to a wavelike interpretation. The electron microscope, which has found wide use in medicine as well as other areas, depends on the fact that the waves associated with the fast-moving electrons are much shorter than light waves and thus permit "seeing" things too small to be observed with light.

Now again, what has all this to do with x-rays? We are preparing ourselves for the fact that we cannot understand x-rays except by treating them as wavelike under certain circumstances and particle-like under others, that is, as both waves and photons.

9.2 X-RAYS: WAVES AND PARTICLES

X-Ray Diffraction

One point that we neglected to mention in our earlier discussions of diffraction and interference phenomena is the relation between the size of the obstacle, or the spacing between the slits of a diffraction grating, and the wavelength of the light involved. Suffice it to say that if the effects are to be noticeable the spacing between the slits must be of about the same size as the wavelength of light. This is the reason diffraction effects were not readily observed with x-rays, whose wavelengths are very short, of the order of 1 Å. Actually, prior to the experiment suggested by von Laue, it was not generally agreed that x-rays were electromagnetic waves. However, there did exist the opinion that should x-rays be electromagnetic waves their wavelengths should be of the order of an angstrom unit. X-ray wavelengths were thus assumed to be of the same order as interatomic distances in solids.

Incidentally, we shall no longer distinguish between diffraction and interference phenomena. From now on we shall simply speak of diffraction (which results in interference), as is the common practice in x-ray work. And, as is also common practice, when we say *diffracted beam,* we shall mean one composed of a large number of individual scattered x-rays mutually reinforcing one another.

Now then, since diffraction could not readily be shown with standard diffraction gratings because of the difficulty of producing fine enough slits, close enough together, von Laue realized that if the atoms in a crystal were arranged in a regular way they might be close enough together to serve as scattering centers for x-rays. That is, a crystal might serve as a three-dimensional diffraction grating.

As we mentioned earlier, Friedrich and Knipping performed the appropriate experiment, using a crystal to diffract the x-rays, as shown in Fig. 9.13(a). The result, shown on the photographic plate of Fig. 9.13(b), confirmed the fact that x-rays exhibit diffraction. Now this diffraction pattern hardly looks like Fig. 9.7, but the fact that there is a symmetrical pattern indicating where x-rays strike (dark spots on negative) and where x-rays don't strike can be explained in the same terms we used to describe

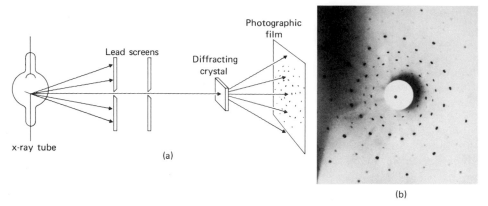

FIG. 9.13. Von Laue pattern. (a) The experimental setup. (b) Laue diffraction of NaCl taken with radiation from a tungsten-target tube operated at 60 kV. The faint radial streaks emanating from the center are due to continuous radiation; most of the spots are due to the characteristic radiation of tungsten. The white central disk is due to a small metal disk, cemented on the paper film cover, to prevent blackening of film by the nondiffracted transmitted beam. The dark patch to the right of the disk is due to x-rays scattered by the disk, while the patch at upper left is probably due to difficulty in film processing.

Fig. 9.7 (the double-slit experiment). In the more precise language of physics which we have now acquired, the dark spots are regions in which x-rays scattered by different atoms arrive in phase. The remaining areas are regions in which x-rays arrive out of phase, thereby resulting in destructive interference: The film emulsion "sees" few or no x-rays here. The reason that in this von Laue figure we see dark spots where constructive interference takes place, while on Fig. 9.7 the constructive interference of in-phase wave arrivals is shown by bright bands, lies in the fact that the von Laue pattern is presented as a negative, like medical diagnostic x-ray films, while Fig. 9.7 is a positive print.

The analysis of a von Laue pattern, and the pattern itself, are more complicated than that of the Young double-slit pattern because there are not just two atoms, as there were two slits, to scatter x-rays. Moreover, the scattering centers in the crystal diffraction case are arranged in a three-dimensional lattice, whereas the two slits of Young's experiment presented only a two-dimensional scattering mechanism. The important point, however, is that we cannot explain Fig. 9.13(b), the von Laue pattern, except by attributing a wavelike nature to x-rays. After all, we showed earlier that diffraction and related interference effects require a wave explanation.

Although von Laue and his colleagues were also able to employ this diffraction experiment to determine that the wavelengths of the x-rays they had employed were of the order of tenths of angstrom units, the Braggs in England, when they heard about the von Laue work, conceived of a simpler way to employ these newly confirmed ideas to measure x-ray wavelengths. Von Laue passed x-rays through a crystal, but the Bragg idea was to obtain the diffraction by "reflecting" x-rays from successive planes of a

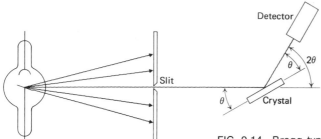

FIG. 9.14. Bragg-type crystal x-ray spectrometer.

crystal, and thereby to obtain a diffraction pattern. We put the word re-flecting in quotation marks above because we are using it in a way that is slightly different from the usual. In the usual sense, by reflection we mean a process taking place only near the surface of a material. But at the mo-ment we wish also to consider what happens with x-rays being scattered or reflected by atoms deep in the reflecting crystal.

Figure 9.14 shows the essential features of an x-ray spectrometer, as employed by the Braggs. The crystal and the detector are rotated and the intensity of the signal received by the detector is noted.

Before we go any further with the Bragg explanation of the observa-tions which can be made with such a spectrometer, we should dwell for a moment on what we mean by *intensity*. In general, what is meant by the intensity of radiation is whatever is recorded by a radiation-detection de-vice, such as a Geiger counter. This means that intensity is a measure of energy per unit time per unit area received by the detection device. That is, the intensity of radiation is the energy carried by the radiation in a unit of time through a small unit area of surface, perpendicular to the direction of the radiation. We may write this definition succinctly as

$$I = \frac{\text{energy}}{\text{time-area}}, \tag{9.4}$$

or, using Eq. (2.4), the definition of power, we may write it as

$$I = \frac{\text{power}}{\text{area}},$$

which implies that the units used to express it could be watts/m². (Inci-dentally, note that the symbol I here has an entirely different meaning from the previous use, where I meant electric current.)

Obviously, if the radiation is homogeneous, that is, if the photons are all of the same energy, then intensity could also refer to the number of photons per unit area per unit time. Further, from the definition expressed in Eq. (9.4), we see that a change in intensity might be brought about either by changing the actual individual photon energy or by changing the num-ber of photons. The latter way of changing intensity is particularly signifi-

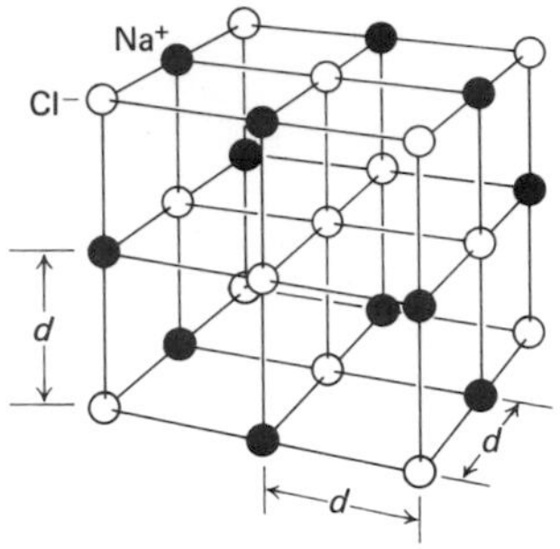

FIG. 9.15. Crystal lattice. Model of the arrangement of ions in NaCl. The lattice constant d is about 3 Å.

cant with respect to photographic effects, that is, x-ray film exposures, since it is the *number* of x-ray photons rather than their energies which primarily controls the changes in the film emulsion.

We now look at what has become a well-known optical principle known as Bragg's law, although Sir Lawrence Bragg himself reputedly suggested that the only novelty he supplied was the application of the principle to crystals and x-rays. Be that as it may, the Bragg law has proved a powerful tool both in the study of crystal structure and in the study of x-rays. For the sake of simplicity in our discussion, we shall assume a homogeneous x-ray beam, that is to say, all the x-rays are to be of the same wavelength. Then we must recall how one conceives the structure of a crystal. An example is shown in Fig. 9.15.

Now let us look at two layers of one plane of a crystal structure, as shown in Fig. 9.16. When is the signal received by a detector looking at x-rays scattered by the atoms of Fig. 9.16 greatest? When the x-rays scattered by the various atoms arrive at the detector in phase, when constructive interference takes place. When is the signal least? When the x-rays arrive completely out of phase so that they completely cancel each other; when there is perfect destructive interference.

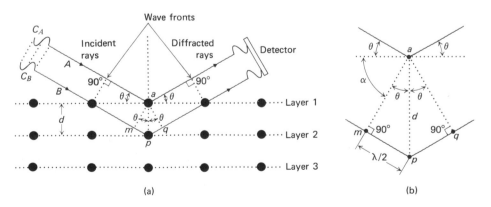

(a)   (b)

FIG. 9.16. Deriving the Bragg law: x-ray diffraction at different crystal layers.

With reference to Fig. 9.16, we shall now establish that the x-rays will arrive at the detector in phase, and thus give a strong signal, at a particular angle. We must perforce indulge in a little geometry and trigonometry.

First we suppose that a wave front, indicated by the dashed lines of Fig. 9.16(a), approaches the crystal from the upper left. A fraction of this wave is reflected by the first layer of atoms, and another fraction from the second layer. Since x-ray B has further to travel than x-ray A, the two rays will arrive at the detector out of phase, even though they started in phase, unless ray B has exactly one wavelength farther to go than ray A. Then, although the crests, paired off in the incoming beam of two rays, will not arrive at the detector together, there will nevertheless be crests arriving in phase at the detector. The crest from ray B will be C_B, the one which was exactly one wavelength ahead of crest C_A of ray A; C_A and C_B will arrive simultaneously, that is, x-ray A and x-ray B will indeed arrive in phase.

Now let us work out the proper angle of incidence to achieve this in-phase reception, or maximum signal. We refer now to Fig. 9.16(b). From our previous discussion, we recall that for the required in-phase relationship, the distance $\overline{mpq}$ has to be one wavelength, hence we require $\overline{mp} = \lambda/2$.

Next we need to show that the angle θ that the incident ray makes with a crystal layer is equal to the angle $\angle map$. This is so because $\angle\theta + \angle\alpha = 90°$, and also $\angle map + \angle\alpha = 90°$. Thus labeling $\angle map$ in the triangle map simply as $\angle\theta$ is truly correct.

Directing our attention to the right-angled triangle map, we now see that

$$\sin \theta = (\lambda/2)/d,$$

or

$$\lambda = 2d \sin \theta. \tag{9.5}$$

Thus we have established a relationship between λ, the x-ray wavelength, and d, the crystal lattice spacing.

Of course our earlier statement that for in-phase arrivals at the detector, the path taken by ray B had to be just one wavelength longer than the path taken by ray A, is not quite correct. It is too restrictive. Obviously we could still achieve the same in-phase relationship if the path of ray B were two wavelengths longer, or three wavelengths longer, or n wavelengths longer, where n is any positive whole number. With this fact in mind, we could rewrite Eq. (9.5) in the more general form

$$n\lambda = 2d \sin \theta. \tag{9.6}$$

Equation (9.6) is the Bragg law, to which we referred previously. If we know the lattice constant d, this relationship permits us to determine x-ray wavelengths and thus supports the hypothesis that the x-rays are electromagnetic waves. Of course, we need not restrict the use of this idea to homogeneous x-rays, as we did to simplify our discussion. If we investigate a *heterogeneous* beam, that is, one having x-rays of many different wavelengths, by this Bragg-type spectrometry, then we could obtain the

relative intensities of the different wavelengths present in the heterogeneous beam.

Now, on the other hand, if we know the x-ray wavelength λ, then we
can employ the Bragg law to gather information about crystal structures.
Certainly x-ray diffraction by crystals has been extensively used to determine the arrangement of atoms in crystals. For example, one of the
relatively few substances presently known to be effective against viral
infections is chlortetracycline, $C_{22}H_{23}O_8N_2Cl$, known as Aureomycin. The
structure of this substance has been precisely determined by the method
of x-ray diffraction. This knowledge will no doubt someday help to lead
toward a solution of the as-yet-puzzling problem of the action of drugs,
and the nature of disease, at the molecular level.

At this point we leave the wave behavior of x-rays with the note that
x-rays, in addition to exhibiting diffraction and interference effects, have
also been shown to exhibit polarization, as well as refraction and reflection
in the ordinary sense, so that there is every reason to include x-rays in the
electromagnetic spectrum with such similar radiations as ordinary visible
light and radio waves.

The Compton Effect

In a way, at this point we are jumping the gun, because the present chapter
is concerned with the nature of x-rays and the following chapter concerns
itself with the interaction of x-rays with matter. And the latter is more
properly the realm for a discussion of the Compton effect. However, this
particular interaction of x-rays with matter—the Compton effect—shows
that x-rays also exhibit a particle behavior, so that we must also talk about
x-ray photons. For this reason we look at the Compton effect now, although
we shall pursue the matter further in the next chapter.

The essence of Compton's discovery is that when x-rays are scattered
some of the incident radiation may undergo a change in wavelength. No
tenable wave theory can account for a change in wavelength in such an
interaction. Compton's explanation of this phenomenon is based on quantum theory and the theory of special relativity. The former decrees a
photon and the latter assigns a momentum to this photon. That is, the
photon is visualized as a particle to which can be assigned a momentum,
just as a billiard ball's velocity times its mass gives the billiard ball's
momentum.

With these ideas in mind, let us trace the complete event of a Compton
scattering process, as shown in Fig. 9.17. The incident photon has an
energy given by hf_1, as we might recall from Eq. (1.1). This frequency
f_1 is, of course, related to the wavelength of the incident x-ray by Eq. (9.2).

The incident photon now comes into collision with a loosely bound
outer electron of an atom. The photon bounces off in one direction and the
electron in another, quite analogous to a collision of two differently sized
billiard balls. The photon is found to have lost some energy from the interaction, while the electron has gained energy. The amount of energy is
the same in each case; the photon's loss has become the electron's gain.
In fact, the kinetic energy of this Compton recoil electron added to its

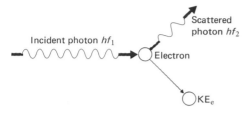

FIG. 9.17. Compton scattering. The scattered photon energy hf_2 is less than hf_1, the energy of the incident photon; KE_e is the kinetic energy gained by the electron in the interaction.

binding energy will equal the difference in energy between the incident and the scattered photon. But since the binding energy of an outer electron is negligibly small relative to the photon energies involved, we simply write

$$KE_e = hf_1 - hf_2,$$

where KE_e is the acquired kinetic energy of the electron and f_1 and f_2 are the frequencies of the incident and scattered photons, respectively. This is no more than a statement of the conservation of energy.

Since the scattered photon's frequency f_2 is less than f_1, the wavelength of the scattered x-ray should be greater than that of the incident x-ray. And that is observed.

Moreover, still considering the interaction analogous to a billiard-ball collision, we can apply the principle of the conservation of momentum and obtain theoretical results relating incident and scattered wavelengths to the angle of scatter. Such results agree entirely with experimental observations.

Thus indeed x-rays, like other electromagnetic radiations, on the basis of the Compton effect, do have to be treated sometimes as particles. The wave-particle duality is upheld with x-rays. That is, for example, on the one hand we might speak of x-rays of a wavelength of 0.3 Å, while on the other hand such x-rays may be considered as a stream of photons each having an energy of 40 keV. These related values of wavelength and photon energy are established by employing Eq. (9.8), the origin of which we shall discuss in Section 9.3.

9.3 X-RAY SPECTRA

The two most important distinguishing features of a beam of x-rays are its *intensity* and its *quality*. The first term, of course, refers to how much radiation, to the *quantity* of radiation. The second term, the *quality*, refers to the kind of radiation, that is, how penetrating the radiation is. This latter characteristic is often expressed in terms of wavelengths. Consequently, we shall discuss some of the details of the production of x-rays by considering some x-ray spectra, the spectra being presented as graphs of intensity as a function of wavelength.

Continuous Spectrum

In the previous section we saw one way that we may obtain this spectral information: The intensity, as given by Eq. (9.4), is measured in terms of the ionization produced in the detector of Fig. 9.14 and the corresponding wavelength is calculated from Bragg's formula,

$$n\lambda = 2d \sin \theta. \tag{9.6}$$

Employing this procedure with a given element as the x-ray tube target, one obtains a spectral curve of the type shown in Fig. 9.18. Such a spectrum is called a *continuous spectrum*. It is interesting to note, incidentally, that recent developments in solid state radiation detection devices have led to the possibility of gathering the data for such a spectrum in one fell swoop, eliminating the stepwise procedure described above.

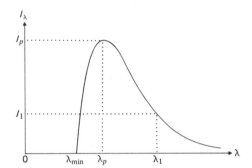

FIG. 9.18.   Continuous x-ray spectrum. As a rule, the peak intensity occurs for a wavelength $\lambda_p \approx 1.5\lambda_{min}$.

The essential features of this spectrum are a continuous distribution of wavelengths, a well-defined minimum wavelength, λ_{min}, a sharp rise to a maximum intensity at a wavelength about 1.5 times λ_{min}, and a gradual falling away of intensity at the long wave end. At the long wave end the intensity is said to approach a zero value asymptotically; that is, it never quite gets to zero. But for practical purposes the actual total x-ray energy produced at this end of the spectrum is negligible.

Before we consider the various possible interactions of high-speed electrons with a target material in order to see what kind of mechanism might bring about a continuous x-ray spectrum, let us dwell for a moment on the quantities represented in a graph such as that of Fig. 9.18. The ordinate is labeled intensity, which we have earlier defined by Eq. (9.4) as energy per unit area per unit time; that is to say, power per unit area. Actually, however, the various intensity values represented in the x-ray spectrum refer to intensities at specific wavelengths; that is to say, the I on the ordinate really refers to intensity per specific wavelength. The ordinate might thus be calibrated in actual units such as watt/m²/Å. Or else the axis might simply give the relative intensity per unit wavelength without assigning any actual numerical values. For this reason—that the ordinate refers to intensity per unit wavelength—the ordinate is generally labeled I_λ. Then, by I, one means the total beam intensity due to the contributions of the intensities at all the wavelengths present in the particular spectrum.

The abscissa is calibrated in units of length, usually angstrom units. From our earlier discussion, we thus see that λ_{min} implies photons of maximum frequency, that is, maximum energy. The graph tells us that there is zero energy/area/time at wavelengths less than λ_{min} and it specifically tells us the intensity of each part of the x-ray beam having a given wavelength. For example, the intensity of the beam due to x-rays of wavelength λ_1 is I_1.

To understand the mechanism which results in the continuous spectrum, we need to visualize again the essential happening in the production of x-rays, as discussed in Section 7.1: In the x-ray tube, high-speed electrons strike a target material. These electrons penetrate the surface layers of the target and interact with the atoms of the target, thereby giving up energy. The electrons may undergo two basically different energy losses: (1) radiation losses, involving the nuclei of the target atoms, and (2) collisional losses, involving the atomic electrons, most frequently electrons in the outer orbits. Let us look at some typical examples.

Case A. The electron loses all its energy by a series of collisions, possibly thousands of collisions, with outer atomic electrons. This excitation of the target atom may result in the emission of visible light, as discussed in Section 1.4. More frequently, the energy appears as increased vibrational energy of the atom, that is, as heat. This type of interaction is the most common. It is for this reason that, as we recall from Chapter 7, the problem of possible overheating of the x-ray tube target arises.

Case B. The electron undergoes many collisional losses, but finally emerges from the target as a back-scattered electron. This process also contributes to target heating.

Case C. The electron collides with and ejects an electron from the K-shell of the target atom. The process by which the target atom so excited returns to the ground state is the emission of a photon of sufficient energy to qualify as an x-ray. This is the so-called *characteristic x-ray*, which we shall shortly consider further.

Case D. The electron has a radiative collision, giving up a part, or sometimes all, of its kinetic energy. This process results in x-rays of the various wavelengths which constitute the continuous spectrum. Another way of saying the same thing is that radiative collisions yield photons of various energies.

We shall now describe this x-ray-producing mechanism, referring to Fig. 9.19. The electron is slowed down, is deflected from its original path by the electrical attraction force between it and the positively charged target nucleus. Classical electromagnetic theory predicts that radiation will occur whenever an electric charge undergoes a change in its velocity (acceleration, deceleration, or even just change in direction), and that

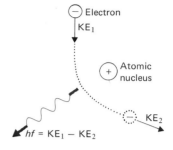

FIG. 9.19. Bremsstrahlung, a radiative "collision" of a high-speed electron of original kinetic energy KE_1 with a target nucleus.

the rate that energy is radiated is proportional to the square of the change in velocity; that is, it varies as the square of the acceleration. From this fact we can see, by recalling Coulomb's law, Eq. (2.2), that a heavy target element with a large charge on the nucleus should result in greater x-ray production than a target of a relatively low atomic number. Why? Because the greater the charge on the nucleus the greater the Coulomb force, and hence the greater the change of the electron's velocity. For this reason, as we already know, tungsten ($Z = 74$) is a more efficient x-ray tube target than, for example, aluminum ($Z = 13$).

Since this radiative collision process involves the slowing down of the incident electron, the German word *bremsstrahlung* (braking radiation) is employed to denote this x-ray-producing mechanism.

At this point students sometimes ask whether or not bremsstrahlung is a process which is the private domain of the electron, whether or not x-rays could also be produced by interactions that are similar but that involve charged particles heavier than electrons. The answer is that indeed other charged particles could produce bremsstrahlung, but not as readily as electrons. This is so because analysis shows that the charged particle's acceleration varies inversely as its mass, and hence its radiation varies inversely as the square of its mass. For this reason, electrons yield more than a million times as much bremsstrahlung as protons of comparable initial speed.

Minimum Wavelength

Quantum theory demands that the energy given up by the electron in bremsstrahlung be emitted in the form of one or more photons. Depending on the magnitude of the photon, various wavelengths are possible. And a maximum-energy photon, corresponding to a minimum wavelength (as shown in Fig. 9.18), must exist. This is the case when the electron has a head-on collision with the nucleus and gives up all its kinetic energy in one glorious moment, giving birth to one high-energy photon.

Professor William Duane and F. L. Hunt investigated this matter of the minimum wavelength in 1915, showing that λ_{min} depends solely on the voltage across the x-ray tube. From our previous discussion we can see the sense of this conclusion.

We assume that the electron acquires essentially all its kinetic energy from the electric field in the x-ray tube. The voltage V across the tube gives the work per unit charge done on a charge by the electric field. Thus the total work done on a single electron of charge e would be Ve. This then is the amount of kinetic energy gained by the electron in its trajectory from the filament to the target. If it gives up all this energy to a single photon, whose energy is hf (Eq. 1.1), we get

$$Ve = hf.$$

As an example, if the tube voltage is 60 kV, then the maximum x-ray photon energy, that is, the maximum value of hf, would be 60 keV.

We now employ Eq. (9.2) in order to substitute wavelength λ for frequency f, thus obtaining

$$Ve = hc/\lambda.$$

Rearranging this latter result and marking the wavelength as λ_{min}, since this corresponds to the greatest photon energy (V being the peak value of the voltage across the tube), we get

$$\lambda_{min} = hc/Ve, \tag{9.7}$$

where h is, of course, Planck's constant, c is the speed of light, V is the tube voltage, and e is the charge of the electron. Equation (9.7) is known as the *Duane-Hunt equation* ($h = 6.63 \times 10^{-34}$ joule-sec).

For purposes of application in x-ray work, it is convenient to reduce all the constants in the Duane-Hunt equation, that is, h, c, and e, to a single number, in a manner such that simply inserting the tube voltage in kV yields the minimum wavelength in angstrom units:

$$\lambda_{min} = \left[\frac{12.4}{kV}\right] \text{Å}. \tag{9.8}$$

Let us see what the minimum wavelength would be with a kV of 70:

$$\lambda_{min} = \left[\frac{12.4}{70}\right] \text{Å} = 0.18 \text{ Å}.$$

Now, using the approximation quoted earlier, relating λ_{min} to the wavelength with the greatest or peak intensity in the continuous spectrum, we see that a setting of 70 kV yields the highest x-ray intensity at a wavelength

$$\lambda_p \approx (1.5 \times 0.18) \text{ Å} \approx 0.27 \text{ Å}.$$

Now if the minimum wavelength is solely determined by the tube voltage, changing the tube target material should not alter λ_{min}. And it does not, as is shown in Fig. 9.20.

On the other hand, increasing the kV should yield a decreased minimum wavelength. This is shown in Fig. 9.21.

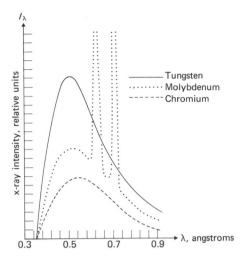

FIG. 9.20. X-ray spectra of three target metals at 35 kV. [C. T. Ulrey, *Phys. Rev.* **11**, 405 (1918)]

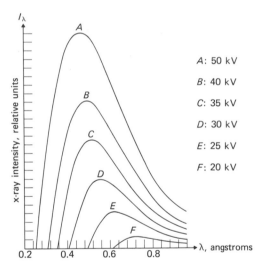

FIG. 9.21. X-ray spectra of a tungsten target, showing the effect of changing the kV. [C. T. Ulrey, *Phys. Rev.* **11**, 407 (1918)]

At this point we reemphasize that stating a minimum wavelength is equivalent to stating a maximum photon energy. In fact, it is quite common to find x-ray spectra plotted in terms of photon energy instead of wavelength. Figure 9.22 shows the spectrum of the same x-ray beam plotted in these two different ways.

The Characteristic Spectrum

Some readers, studying Fig. 9.20, may have wondered about the spikes sticking up in the region of 0.6 to 0.7 Å. These spikes are due to so-called characteristic radiation. Leaning heavily on our discussion of optical spectra in Section 1.4, we describe characteristic x-radiation in pictorial fashion

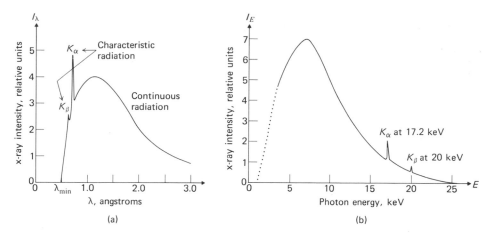

FIG. 9.22. Two ways of plotting the x-ray spectrum of molybdenum at a peak tube voltage of 25 kV. (a) Relative intensities at various wavelengths as a function of the wavelengths. (Line widths of characteristic radiation not to scale.) (b) The same information as in (a), plotted with relative intensities at various photon energies as a function of the photon energies. The dashed part of the curve is for photon energies lower than available from the data of curve (a).

only by reference to Fig. 9.23. Note that this x-ray process is just like that described in the case of optical spectra. The difference is only in the size of the energy level differences involved. We see from this figure that for these major characteristic x-rays of tungsten to appear, the tube voltage must be set at about 60 kV ($L \rightarrow K$ transition possible), or higher. In practice, the tube voltage needs to be probably around 80 kV for the characteristic radiation to make a noticeable appearance in the x-ray spectrum. Above this voltage the percentage of the total x-ray energy due to characteristic radiation gradually increases, and then decreases again. In the diagnostic voltage region, the contribution of x-ray energy by characteristic radiation may be as much as 10% or more, depending on the actual tube voltage and the filtration. As an example, we cite results by Epp and Weiss:[*] at 105 kV, with 2 mm Al added filtration, 7.5% of the total number of photons are due to the tungsten characteristic radiation. Since these photons are on the high-energy side of the spectrum, they therefore contribute more than 7.5% of the total x-ray beam energy. The remaining beam energy is, of course, as indicated before, due to bremsstrahlung.

Note that in Fig. 9.23 we have shown only the so-called K-series characteristic x-rays, where K_α refers to the particular photon emitted in an electron transition from the L- to the K-shell, while the K_β refers to the photon of an M-to-K transition. But it is also possible to produce x-rays by a transition from the N- to the L-shell. Such a characteristic x-ray would

---

* Epp, E. R., and H. Weiss, "Experimental Study of the Photon Energy Spectrum of Primary Diagnostic X-Rays," in *Physics in Medicine and Biology*, **11**, 235 (1966).

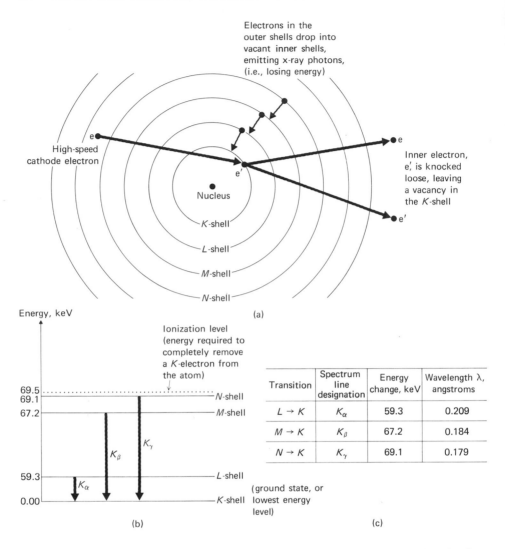

FIG. 9.23. The story of the characteristic x-rays of tungsten. (a) Mechanism of production. (b) Energy-level diagram of electrons going into K-shell. (c) Approximate wavelengths of some K-characteristic x-rays.

be called an L_β ray, while the photon due to a transition from M to L would be labeled L_α. Since it is common practice to record these x-rays on photographic plates in which different wavelengths produce differently placed lines on the plate, one often speaks of the L_α or the K_β lines, etc.

The fact that specific atomic energy levels are characteristics of a given element suggests that x-ray emission from an element could be used to identify the element. This is so. Each element, for example, has its own special K_α line in a spectrum. In 1913 H. G. J. Moseley embarked on the first comprehensive study of characteristic x-rays. This study first established clearly the significance of the atomic numbers of the elements.

X-Ray Intensity

In discussing the mechanism of bremsstrahlung, we showed why x-ray production might be expected to be more efficient with a target material of a high atomic number than with one of a lower atomic number. Moreover, in Section 7.4 we pointed out that this efficiency was approximately directly proportional to the atomic number (Eq. 7.2).

Can we see that this fact is supported by experimental evidence? By results such as shown in Fig. 9.20, for example? Yes. But to do so we need to realize what is represented by the area under the spectral curve. Tungsten ($Z = 74$) has a larger area under its curve than molybdenum ($Z = 42$), and molybdenum in turn has more area under its curve than chromium ($Z = 24$). Since each of these curves is produced at the same kV and mA, that is, produced with the same power input, we may expect the area under the curves to represent power output in the form of x-rays. That would show tungsten as more efficient as an x-ray target than molybdenum.

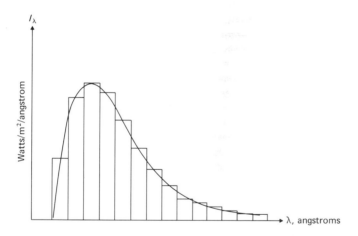

FIG. 9.24. The area under the spectral curve is equal to the total intensity of the x-ray beam in watts/m².

Without proving anything, we now simply state that it can be shown that the area under such an experimentally determined spectral curve is directly proportional to the x-ray power output per unit area, that is, the total x-ray intensity. A quick dimensional check using the facts stated in our earlier discussion of the meaning of the quantities assigned to the axes of a spectral graph shows the plausibility of this categorical assertion. Let us refer to a spectrum in which the area under the curve is broken into rectangular segments, such as shown in Fig. 9.24. To get the total area under the curve we would just add the areas of the various rectangular segments, which we would in turn choose to be very, very narrow in order to fit the curve. The height of one such rectangle is a certain number of watts/m²/Å, while the width is some small number of Å. Hence the area of one rectangle is the product [(watts/m²/Å) (Å)]. That is, the rectangular area represents watts/m², which is a unit of intensity, on the basis of the definition of intensity by Eq. (9.4). Thus we can see that the sum of the areas of the various rectangles is indeed intensity, the total intensity of the beam. To repeat then: For a given power input, the area under the curve for tungsten is much greater than for chromium, thus demonstrating the fact that the power output per unit area, that is, the x-ray intensity, is much greater for tungsten than for chromium. Tungsten is a more efficient target.

Calculations involving the area under spectral curves can be made quite precisely. Such calculations yield the fact, stated earlier, that with a tungsten target operated in the diagnostic voltage region, up to 30% of the total power output may be due to characteristic radiation, the remainder being bremsstrahlung; provided, of course, that the kV is set at 69 or higher.

Moreover, certain calculations based on the areas under these curves may also be employed to determine the total x-ray power output which, we may recall, is of the order of 1% of the power input.

Since we have suggested that the area under a spectral curve yields the x-ray power output/area, that is, the x-ray intensity, we might look to

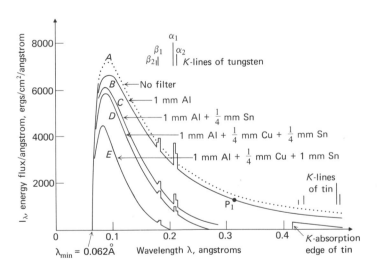

FIG. 9.25. The effect of filtration on a heterogeneous x-ray beam. Beam *A* is the unfiltered beam from a tungsten target. The other curves show the effect of successively heavier filtration. (From Johns, H. E., *The Physics of Radiology,* second edition, 1964. Courtesy of Charles C. Thomas, publisher, Springfield, Ill.)

see if kV affects this output. Turning back to Fig. 9.21, we see that the area under the spectral curve gets larger as the kV is increased. Again this is in accord with what we stated on this matter in Section 7.4.

Another factor that would alter the area under the spectral curve of the radiation reaching a patient would be the insertion of a filter between the x-ray tube and the patient. Since the filtering material attenuates the radiation beam, we might expect the filtered spectrum to have a smaller area. Moreover, since the low-energy photons are more readily stopped than the high-energy photons, we would expect the filter to decrease the x-ray intensity more pronouncedly at the long-wavelength end of the spectrum. We see the effect of filters on a tungsten x-ray spectrum in Fig. 9.25.

Finally, we might ask what would be the effect on a spectrum of an increase in mA. Increasing the mA increases the power input to the tube, but does not increase the maximum photon energy. Only increasing the kV can achieve the latter. So the effect of an increase in mA is reflected only in an increase in the number, but not the energy, of the photons. That is, an increase in the mA is reflected in an increase in the intensity, shown on a spectrum diagram as an increased area under the spectral curve.

· 9.4 SUMMARY OF X-RAY PROPERTIES

It must be understood that this summary of the properties of x-rays is not all-embracing. Further, in providing the summary we draw upon our previous discussions and suggest some areas to be investigated in later chapters.

First of all, x-rays belong to the class of *electromagnetic radiations.* They are located at the low-wavelength end of the electromagnetic spectrum, the x-rays in the diagnostic region having wavelengths of the order of 0.1 to 1 Å.

By saying the above we have summarized a lot. We have implied that x-rays are propagated with a speed of nearly 3×10^{10} cm/sec; that they are unaffected by electric or magnetic fields; that they may be refracted, reflected, diffracted, and polarized; that when we consider the fact that their interaction with matter involves an energy exchange, we must treat them as a stream of discrete energy bundles, photons, the relation between the wavelength and the photon being given by

$$E = hf = hc/\lambda,$$

which combines Eqs. (1.1) and (9.2). All this is implied when we state that x-rays are electromagnetic waves.

Then we recall that x-rays are produced when electrons strike any solid body, and that the x-rays are emitted in a continuous spectrum, the short-wavelength limit of which is determined by the tube voltage.

In this connection we must remember that, in medical work particularly, we are generally working with a heterogeneous beam of x-rays, while many effects of interest are calculated on the basis of assuming a homogeneous (one wavelength only) beam of x-rays. Two approximations are therefore sometimes useful. The first we have already stated in Section 9.3: The maximum beam intensity occurs at about 1.5 λ_{min}. The other approximation is that for some matters one may roughly consider a heterogeneous beam to have about the same effect as a homogeneous beam of energy about 30% to 50% of the maximum beam energy of the heterogeneous beam. The important point to remember here is that an x-ray beam at 90 kV does not produce photons all of 90 keV energy, but rather produces a beam which in some respects resembles a homogeneous beam of, say, 30-keV photons.

A study by E. R. Epp and H. Weiss suggests that in the case of diagnostic x-rays the mean photon energy is almost one-half the maximum photon energy.* Of course, the fact that a heterogeneous and a homogeneous beam have the same mean photon energy does not mean that the beams have the same HVL (see Section 10.2); and it is comparable half-value layers that are generally implied when two x-ray beams are said to be equivalent.

We conclude by enumerating some of the properties of x-rays that are of particular interest to the radiographer.

1.   In view of their extremely high energy (high frequency or short wavelength), x-rays are able to penetrate materials which readily absorb and reflect visible light. In this property lie at once the usefulness of x-rays for radiography and also their potential danger.

2.   X-rays are differentially absorbed by matter. Whereas all substances are to some extent transparent to x-rays, in general the thicker and the denser the material the greater the absorption and scattering of the x-ray beam. Since the rationale of radiography is based on differential absorption, we shall discuss this matter of absorption and scattering more fully in Chapter 10.

3.   X-rays travel in straight lines and are not readily refracted or reflected. The straight-line propagation is, of course, of prime importance in the forming of a useful x-ray picture.

4.   X-rays are able to produce ionization in gases and to influence the electrical properties of liquids and solids. The ionizing property forms the basis of many commonly found radiation meters. Such meters will be discussed in Chapter 11.

5.   X-rays affect photographic film in much the same way as ordinary visible light.

6.   X-rays produce fluorescence in certain materials. That is to say, x-rays cause certain materials to emit radiation in the visible region.

---

* E. P. Epp and H. Weiss, "Experimental Study of the Photon Energy Spectrum of Primary Diagnostic X-Rays," in *Physics in Medicine and Biology*, **11**, 236 (1966).

We shall discuss this property further when we deal with intensifying screens and fluoroscopy screens in Section 10.6.

7.   X-rays are able to damage or kill living cells. The ability to kill biologic cells is the basis of radiation therapy. But we have a two-edged sword, in that damage may also accrue to normal tissue, thereby resulting not only in somatic damage but also in biologic changes of a genetic nature. Radiation hazards will thus bear further consideration, which we shall give it in Section 11.5.

QUESTIONS

1. a) Explain briefly what is meant by wavelength and frequency.
    b) Give the relation between wavelength and frequency.

2. Give a brief explanation of why there is no inherent contradiction in the wave-particle duality of matter. [*Hint:* When is a wave description employed and when is a particle description employed?]

3. The hypothesis that x-rays are transverse EM waves, similar to visible light but of shorter wavelength, has received powerful support from certain phenomena. Name and describe these phenomena.

4. Name and describe a phenomenon which supports the idea of the particle-like behavior of x-rays.

5. Arrange the following electromagnetic radiations in order, with the longer wavelengths at the left going to shorter wavelengths on the right: visible light, gamma rays, ultraviolet, infrared, diagnostic x-rays.

6. What is the photon energy, in keV, associated with x-rays having a wavelength of 1 Å?

7. List the essential requirements for the production of x-rays.

8. What is the effect on the x-rays produced when the kilovoltage across the x-ray tube is increased?

9. Sketch a graph of the relative intensity as a function of the wavelength for x-rays produced with a tungsten target at 90 kV. On this sketch indicate the effect of increasing the kV to 100 and also the effect of filtering the beam with copper.

10. With reference to Fig. 9.26:
    a) Name all the parts indicated by the letters A through F.
    b) Describe how and for what this device is used.

11. Sketch the graph of a continuous x-ray spectrum to show the effect on the spectrum of increasing the mA while keeping the kV constant.

12. Employ the Bohr concept of the atom to explain the production of the characteristic x-rays of an element.

13. What happens to the x-ray spectrum of the tungsten target if radiation from this target is filtered by aluminum?

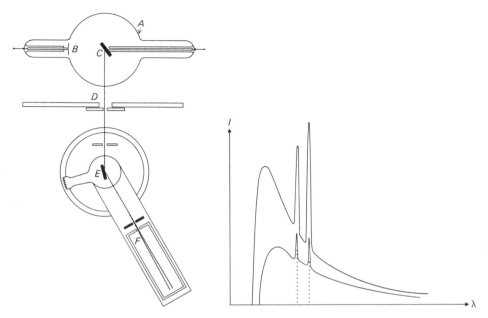

FIG. 9.26. A Bragg x-ray spectrometer.   FIG. 9.27. X-ray spectra.

14. List any four properties of x-rays of particular significance to the x-ray technician.

15. Refer to Fig. 9.27:

   a) Are the two spectra produced at the same kV? Comment.
   b) Are the two spectra of the same target element? Comment.

16. Consider a heterogeneous beam of x-rays produced at a setting of 90 kV.

   a) What is, to all intents and purposes, the maximum energy, in keV, of an electron striking the target?
   b) What is the maximum photon energy in the x-ray beam in keV?
   c) What is the energy of the photons in a homogeneous beam approximately equivalent to this heterogeneous beam for radiographic purposes?

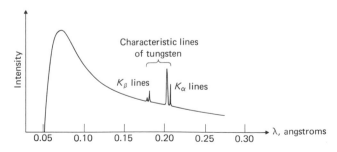

FIG. 9.28. X-ray spectrum of a tungsten target. (Courtesy of H. K. Lewis and Co., from Young, M. E. J., *Radiological Physics*)

17. Refer to Fig. 9.28:
    a) Using your knowledge of characteristic x-ray spectra, as summarized in Fig. 9.22, explain why the K_α spike or line in the tungsten spectrum of Fig. 9.28 appears at a higher wavelength than the K_β line.
    b) What was the approximate kV employed to produce this spectrum?
    c) What, if anything, would happen to the K_α and K_β spikes if the tube voltage were reduced to 40 kV? Explain.

18. Substitute the appropriate values for the constants in Eq. (9.7) and show how this equation can then be rewritten in the form of Eq. (9.8).

SUGGESTED READING

CLARK, G. L., *Applied X-Rays*. New York: McGraw-Hill, 1955 (fourth edition). Having progressed this far in our book, the reader may well find it enjoyable and profitable to read Part I of Professor Clark's book. In Part I, "General Physics and Application of X-Radiation," there is an excellent summary of the properties of x-rays. Another profitable aspect is that acquaintance with *Applied X-Rays* will broaden the x-ray technician's outlook on the x-ray world by indicating fruitful pursuits with x-rays outside the medical arena.

JOHNS, H. E., *The Physics of Radiology*. Springfield: Charles C. Thomas, 1964 (second edition, revised second printing). Chapter II on the production and properties of x-rays provides considerable information, in a relatively brief presentation, covering matters discussed in our Chapters 7, 8, and 9.

RICHARDS, J. A., JR., F. W. SEARS, M. R. WEHR, and M. W. ZEMANSKY, *Modern University Physics*. Reading, Mass.: Addison-Wesley, 1960. Chapter 40, "X-Rays," is recommended for those readers who wish to have a closer look at x-ray diffraction and characteristic x-ray spectra than provided in our book, but yet wish to avoid the more advanced detail of the monograph by Worsnop and Chalkin.

WEIDNER, R. T., and R. L. SELLS, *Elementary Modern Physics*. Boston: Allyn and Bacon, 1960. Chapter 4, which deals with x-ray and electron diffraction, provides a very readable treatment of the complementarity aspect of waves and particles. No mathematics beyond algebra required.

WORSNOP, B. L., and F. C. CHALKIN, *X-Rays*. London: Methuen, 1950 (third edition). This 122-page monograph is for those seeking authoritative details on the nature and production of x-rays. Although a sound mathematical background is presumed, much of this little book is comprehensible to those having access only to elementary algebra and trigonometry.

CHAPTER 10

The Interaction of X-Rays With Matter

We have been occupied, up to the end of the last chapter, with the fundamentals that lead to an understanding of what x-rays are and how they are produced. We now turn to a consideration of how x-rays interact with matter, since their interaction with the patient and with the x-ray film form the essence of medical radiography.

During his long life the English physicist J. J. Thomson (1856–1940), later knighted, made many discoveries which brought him fame. Although photon scattering is not his most-often quoted work, as is his discovery of the electron, he was able to show by classical reasoning (that is, without the use of quantum mechanics) the probability with which x-ray photons of low energy may be scattered by electrons and, although altered in direction, maintain their original energy. This type of scattering is now known as *unmodified, classical,* or *Thomson scattering.*

Other important interactions between x-rays and matter to be considered in this chapter involve the work by A. H. Compton, already discussed in Section 9.2, and Einstein's explanation of the photoelectric effect described in Section 7.8.

We shall now go on to look at these various interactions more closely, and from a viewpoint different from that in our earlier encounters. But before we begin our discussion proper, it would be well to define a few terms which need to become part of the x-ray technician's vocabulary.

10.1 ATTENUATION OF X-RAYS

Some Definitions

Attenuation means reduction in intensity. And intensity has been defined in Section 9.2. Hence material which interacts with radiation in such a way as to decrease the intensity of the beam in a given direction is called an *attenuator*. Sometimes the term "absorber" is loosely employed to mean "attenuator."

Absorption refers to any process by which the intensity of a beam of radiation is attenuated due to radiation energy being given to the absorber through ionization. In other words, absorption in the true sense, or *real absorption* as it has been called in the past, involves energy transfer from the radiation beam to the absorbing material. In the new parlance real absorption is now referred to as *energy transfer.*

Secondary radiation is radiation arising from any and all processes in which the primary beam energing from the x-ray tube interacts with matter. Secondary radiation may include charged particles, such as electrons, as well as photons.

Scattered radiation refers to radiation which is changed in direction as a result of interaction with some medium. Scattered radiation includes both the primary radiation, which is changed only in direction, and the modified radiation, which is changed in wavelength as well as direction. Scattered radiation is one form of secondary radiation.

We should note at this point that there has been, and still is, a certain amount of variety in the way the above and related terms are used in the literature. The International Commission on Radiological Units and Measurements (ICRU), in a report issued in 1962, attempted to clarify the situation by recommending a system of concepts and a set of definitions. We have tended to follow the ICRU recommendations. Nevertheless, the reader should be aware that much of the literature, including some of our Suggested Reading, uses different terminology, in part at least. For example, usage of the terms "apparent absorption," "real absorption," and "absorption coefficient" in lieu of the ICRU recommended "attenuation," "energy transfer," and "attenuation coefficient," respectively, is quite common.

There is another concept which we should mention at this stage. In the literature regarding the production of x-rays and their interaction with matter, you are likely to encounter the term "cross section." This term is precisely defined by physicists, but for our purpose the precise definition is not really required. What is important is the realization that this term indicates the *probability* with which a certain process takes place. An example will make this clear.

It is found that σ, the cross section per atom for photoelectric attenuation, in the region of x-ray energies which are greater than the K-shell binding energy of the atoms of the material in question, may be given by

$$\sigma \approx \frac{kZ^4}{(hf)^3},$$ (10.1)

where σ is the cross section, k is a constant, Z is the atomic number of the attenuating material, h is Planck's constant, and f is the frequency of the incident radiation. This means that the probability of a photoelectric interaction taking place on the part of photons with the given energy, hf, increases with the atomic number of the attenuating material, or more precisely, as the fourth power of Z. Further, the probability decreases as the energy of the incident radiation increases; more precisely, the probability varies inversely as the cube of the energy of the incident photon.

Exponential Attenuation

Suppose that we have a beam of radiation, all the photons of which have the same energy. As mentioned before, such a beam is called *homogeneous,* or *monoenergetic,* or *monochromatic.* There are several ways in which we might study what happens when this beam interacts with matter. One way is to set up an experiment to see according to what apparent rules the radiation is affected by the interaction.

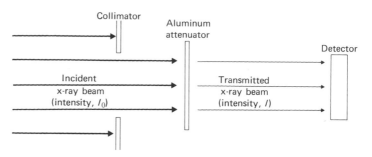

FIG. 10.1. The attenuation of a homogeneous beam of x-rays by means of an aluminum attenuator. A decrease in beam intensity is shown by the use of lighter lines.

If we were to pass a homogeneous beam through a certain thickness of aluminum, for example, we would find the intensity of the transmitted beam to be less than the intensity of the incident beam. Figure 10.1 shows the essence of the experimental arrangement for making such measurements of the attenuation of radiation.

Now let us suppose that the original layer of aluminum is 1 cm thick. We then add another centimeter of aluminum. The transmitted radiation will have an even lesser intensity. Were we to go on adding thicknesses of attenuator in this way, then for each added layer the intensity of the transmitted beam would be further diminished. When we tabulated the findings from such an experiment, we might obtain results similar to the rather idealized ones shown in Table 10.1.

Note how each successive thickness of aluminum produces a transmitted beam with the same fractional decrease in intensity as that produced by a similar preceding thickness. There is a constant fractional decrease in transmission per unit of attenuator thickness. Now any de-

Table 10.1

ATTENUATION OF X-RAYS

Thickness of attenuator (arbitrary units of thickness, x)	Intensity of transmitted beam as a fraction of the original incident beam, I/I_0
1	0.5000
2	0.2500
3	0.1250
4	0.0625
5	0.0313
6	0.0156

crease is termed attenuation, and this particular mode of decrease is called *exponential attenuation*. That is to say, the transmitted beam decreases exponentially in intensity with increasing attenuator thickness.

In our particular imaginary experiment, this fractional decrease per unit thickness of attenuator is 50%, or simply 0.5. It could very well have been some other percentage, such as 35%, for example. The actual figure depends on the chosen unit thickness of attenuator, the material of the attenuator, and the energy of the incident beam. However, whatever the fractional decrease is, it is always constant for homogeneous radiation in an isotropic attenuator.

When we plot the variables of Table 10.1, that is, the relative intensity of the transmitted beam (I/I_0), and attenuator thickness (x) on a graph, we get the type of curve shown in Fig. 10.2. The equation for a curve of this shape can be given as follows:

$$I = I_0 e^{-\mu x}, \tag{10.2}$$

where e is the base of natural logarithms, x is the thickness of the attenuator measured from $x = 0$, where $I = I_0$, I is the intensity of the radiation transmitted through the stated thickness of attenuator, and I_0 is the

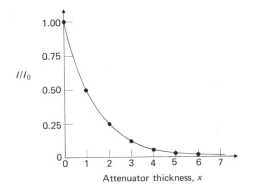

FIG. 10.2. The exponential attenuation of homogeneous radiation.

intensity of the incident radiation. At the moment we may simply say that μ is a constant depending on the wavelength of the radiation and the material of the attenuator.

Note that again we encounter a now-familiar exponential equation. The same mathematics does seem to be useful in many applications. Let us compare: Equation (10.2) is identical in form to Eq. (1.4), which refers to the exponential character of radioactive decay. In that instance, instead of I, the intensity of radiation at a given distance through the attenuator, we used N as the number of atoms present at a given time; in place of the thickness x, the second variable was time t.

When we look at Fig. 10.2, what do we see? Essentially, of course, we see whatever information we can get from Table 10.1, but this time displayed in a different and perhaps more informative manner. In the first place, as the thickness of attenuator is increased, we find that the amount of transmitted radiation decreases. This is not unexpected, of course. However, when we look closer we find that the absolute rate of decrease becomes progressively less. The curve is less steep as the thickness of attenuator is increased. The same fraction is attenuated each time through each unit thickness of attenuator but the absolute quantity attenuated each time becomes smaller.

As in any exponential process, the curve will never reach zero: Theoretically, this type of radiation will never be completely attenuated, although eventually it will become so attenuated that present-day instruments are unable to detect it. What happens, in effect, is that the photon counting rate of concern becomes small compared to the background counting rate due to cosmic rays and other natural radiation activity.

Linear Attenuation Coefficient

In the imaginary experiment just described, we found that a constant fraction of the radiation was attenuated for each unit thickness of attenuator. As previously indicated, exactly how much is attenuated will depend on the energy of the radiation and the material of the attenuator, as well as its thickness. This fact is expressed numerically by the index μ in Eq. (10.2).

This index μ is a constant, known as the *linear attenuation coefficient*, defined as the fractional decrease in intensity per centimeter thickness of attenuating material as determined for a thin layer of attenuator. That is,

$$\mu = \Delta I / I \, \Delta x.$$

The reason for the "thin" layer of attenuator specified in the definition above is that it can be shown that μ is not a constant unless one considers a value of Δx infinitely thin. This fact is not readily shown without recourse to the calculus.

[*Note:* Students who have calculus at their disposal should realize that the precise definition of μ is $\mu = dI/I \, dx$.]

For homogeneous radiation, μ is numerically equal to the fractional number of photons removed from the beam per cm of attenuator.

Table 10.2

SOME ATTENUATION COEFFICIENTS (APPROXIMATE VALUES)*

Material	Linear attenuation coefficient, μ	Mass attenuation coefficient, $\tau(= \mu/\rho)$
Water	0.2 cm⁻¹	0.2 cm²/gm
Aluminum	1 cm⁻¹	0.4 cm²/gm
Calcium	1.5 cm⁻¹	1 cm²/gm
Lead	7 cm⁻¹	6 cm²/gm

* Photon energy: 50 keV

The reason μ is called an attenuation coefficient, in accord with ICRU recommendations, as opposed to the commonly employed term absorption coefficient, is that not all of the beam attenuation is due to absorption. Some radiation is simply scattered. Table 10.2 shows some values of μ.

When we look at Table 10.2, we see a new term: mass attenuation coefficient, τ, where μ is the familiar linear attenuation coefficient and ρ is the density of the attenuating material in gm/cm³. The attenuation properties of matter may be expressed in a number of coefficients other than μ, such as electronic attenuation coefficient, atomic attenuation coefficient, as well as the mass attenuation coefficient referred to above. We do not intend to go into detail on these various coefficients in this text. They obviously all have their specific uses. Readers who wish to know more on this subject are referred to the section on suggested reading, at the end of this chapter. We might, however, state at this point that the cross section σ of Eq. (10.1) is quite simply related to the linear attenuation coefficient μ as follows: $\sigma = \mu/N$, where N = number of atoms/cm³.

The mass attenuation coefficient is probably the one most quoted in tables of attenuation coefficients. In a way, it is more fundamental than μ because, unlike μ, it is independent of the attenuator density. Note also that the mass attenuation coefficient is given in cm²/gm. It is thus also easy to relate this type of coefficient to the cross section σ, defined in Section 10.1, since the unit for cross section is one of area. Of course, it obviously makes sense that attenuation coefficients and cross sections for attenuation processes should be related, in that they may both be employed to indicate the relative likelihood of much or little attenuation with a given attenuator.

A graphical representation of the attenuation effect with two different materials having different μ's is shown in Fig. 10.3.

And finally, the fact that, as stated earlier, attenuation varies with the photon energy is shown in Fig. 10.4.

So far we have been concerned with the attenuation of homogeneous radiation. The reason for this is that a description of the attenuation process with this restriction of beam homogeneity is relatively simple and there-

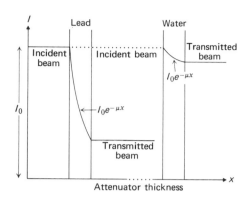

FIG. 10.3. The attenuation effect of two different materials, lead and water, with the same energy of incident radiation. Lead has a large value of μ and water has a small value of μ.

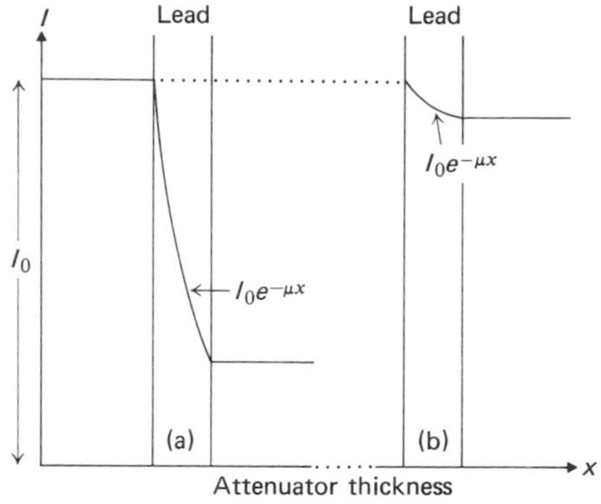

FIG. 10.4. The attenuation effect of the same attenuator material on two beams of different energies. The beam of lower energy, (a), has a large value of μ. The higher energy beam, (b), has a smaller value of μ.

fore provides a useful basis for the understanding of more complicated situations of the heterogeneous beam. But we already know from our discussion of the production of x-rays in the previous chapter that the beam used in medical radiography is heterogeneous rather than homogeneous. We shall look into this state of affairs in the next section.

10.2 QUALITY OF RADIATION

As we stated in Section 9.3, the *quality* of a beam refers to the kind of radiation in the beam, more specifically to the penetrating ability of the beam. Let us see.

Attenuation of Heterogeneous Radiation

For an experiment similar to the previous one, but this time with a beam having a mixture of wavelengths, we are likely to produce a graph as shown in Fig. 10.5, curve A. Here we find that each succeeding centimeter of attenuator does not remove the same fraction of radiation in each case; but rather, as the attenuation continues through several thicknesses, the fraction removed from the beam becomes smaller. Now note that curve B is obtained with homogeneous radiation. This curve is like the one in Fig. 10.2. Both curves, A and B, however, were produced under similar experimental circumstances.

If we compare the two curves, we find that the curve for the heterogeneous beam has a shape slightly different from that of the homogeneous beam. Note particularly that at the beginning curve A, heterogeneous beam, is steeper than curve B, homogeneous beam. Next we see the two curves cross and the attenuation of the heterogeneous beam proceeds at a lesser rate.

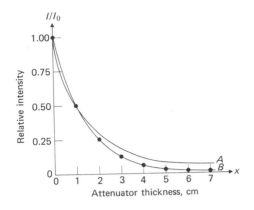

FIG. 10.5. The attenuation of heterogeneous radiation, curve *A*, and homogeneous radiation, curve *B*.

The reason for the steepness of curve *A* at the beginning is that the first layer of attenuator will remove from the heterogeneous beam, in fairly large quantities, those rays which have longer wavelengths, that is, those that have less energy. But later, after the low-energy components of the beam have been removed, the beam will consist of x-rays having a higher average energy than was the case at the beginning: The beam is said to be *harder*. Therefore the next centimeter of attenuator will remove a smaller fraction of the beam than the previous centimeter. After each successive layer of attenuator the beam will become progressively greater in average energy, that is, harder, so that the next fraction removed will be smaller. Obviously in this case, as with the homogeneous radiation, it will be theoretically impossible to remove all the radiation from the beam by attenuation processes.

Now, what does this mean in the x-ray department? First of all, we have a very useful coefficient of attenuation which tells us quite a bit about the attenuation process in terms of the beam and the attenuator. But we find that the usefulness of the coefficient is somewhat less than perfect in the case of the heterogeneous beam. For any particular real (that is, heterogeneous) beam and attenuator, the coefficient will not be constant, but will become smaller as the attenuator is made thicker.

Half-Value Layer

Although it is impractical to try to specify the nature of a heterogeneous beam (since it has a multitude of attenuation coefficients, as implied above) by means of the linear attenuation coefficients, some method of specification which makes use of the beam's attenuation by a material still has much to recommend it. Such a method involves the *half-value layer*, and we shall shortly see the true extent of the half-value layer's practicality.

The half-value layer, sometimes called the *half-value thickness*, is defined as the thickness of a given material required to reduce the intensity of a beam to half its original value.

In any discussion of the quality of radiation, it is not always sufficient to give a value to the minimum wavelength in the beam, that is, to discuss the beam in terms of kilovoltage. The effect of a beam on a radiograph, a protective barrier, or a patient, for example, depends not only on the voltage at which the beam is produced but also on the spectral distribution of its component wavelengths below the minimum set by the voltage. Since the spectral distribution of wavelengths may differ greatly from beam to beam, we require some criterion other than the voltage by which we may describe the beam. The criterion employed is the half-value layer, generally abbreviated as HVL. Radiation that has a relatively large HVL is said to be *hard*. Radiation easily attenuated, that is, having a small HVL, is said to be *soft*. The method of determining the half-value layer for any particular beam is relatively simple, and it is this fact which makes the half-value layer particularly useful. Although the half-value layer certainly does not give full information regarding the quality of a beam, experience has nevertheless shown that it has a wide utility.

Whenever the half-value layer of a beam is given, the material with which the figure was obtained should be clearly stated. This material, usually a metal, is that which is most convenient for the type of beam under consideration. For example, in the usual diagnostic energy range aluminum is a useful material, but at higher energies, up to 3 MeV, copper may be used because the thickness of aluminum would become rather large. At still higher energies the half-value layer is usually quoted in terms of lead.

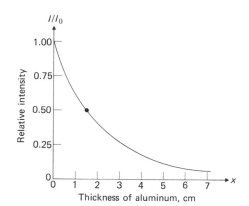

FIG. 10.6. Determination of the half-value layer of an x-ray beam by means of aluminum.

Referring now to Fig. 10.6, we see a curve obtained by measuring the transmission of a beam of radiation through various thicknesses of aluminum. On this graph we see that it requires 1.5 cm of aluminum in order to decrease the beam intensity to 50% of its initial value. This particular beam may therefore be described in terms of its quality or penetrating ability by saying that it has a half-value layer of 1.5 cm of aluminum. We could just as well have given a half-value layer (at some other figure of course) in terms of another material, such as copper; but at the energy involved in the case at hand we would probably have found that the copper had to be inconveniently thin for a practical experiment.

Referring back to Fig. 10.5, we can see that both beams of radiation, heterogeneous and homogeneous, have the same half-value layer, even though some of their other properties are different: The heterogeneous beam is at first softer and after a certain amount of attenuation becomes harder than the homogeneous one.

In summary, let us note two points before we go further. *First:* For homogeneous radiation, the half-value layer will be valid whether or not it is quoted for a filtered or unfiltered beam. That is, the beam will have the same half-value layer as the initial beam even after it has been attenuated by several centimeters of material. In other words, if the linear coefficient of attenuation is constant, so is the half-value layer.

Second: In the case of the heterogeneous beam, as the linear coefficient of attenuation varies and diminishes after successive attenuations, so will the half-value layer vary and become greater after any previous attenuation of the beam. Thus, as previously implied, despite its practicality the half-value layer does not uniquely describe a beam any more than the linear coefficient of attenuation does.

Since the HVL and μ may both be used to describe radiation characteristics, we must necessarily be able to relate these two quantities:

$$\text{HVL} = 0.693/\mu. \tag{10.3}$$

This relationship is derived as follows: First of all, we take the equation in which the coefficient first appears,

$$I = I_0 e^{-\mu x} \tag{10.1}$$

Dividing both sides of Eq. (10.1) by I_0 and then taking the logarithm to base e, we get

$$\ln (I/I_0) = -\mu x.$$

Now if $I = \tfrac{1}{2}I_0$, then $x = \text{HVL}$. Thus

$$\ln \frac{\tfrac{1}{2}I_0}{I_0} = -\mu(\text{HVL}) \qquad \text{or} \qquad \ln 0.5 = -\mu(\text{HVL}).$$

Rearranging the last equation, we obtain

$$\text{HVL} = -\frac{\ln 0.5}{\mu}.$$

Then, using the value of $\ln 0.5$ as found in a table of natural logarithms, we finally arrive at

$$\text{HVL} = -\left(\frac{-0.693}{\mu}\right) \qquad \text{or} \qquad \text{HVL} = \frac{0.693}{\mu}. \tag{10.3}$$

We now draw the reader's attention to the fact that the mathematical gymnastics performed here are identical to what was done in Section 1.6, where the radioactive decay constant was related to the half-life, which quantities are analogous to the linear attenuation coefficient and the HVL in the present development.

10.3 ATTENUATION PROCESSES

Now that we have some general idea of the exponential nature of attenuation of radiation by matter, we might naturally ask the question: What happens inside the attenuating material? Although there is much that is of practical importance to the medical radiographer in a general discussion of the attenuation of x-ray beams, a detailed look at the actual attenuation processes themselves is of even greater significance, both from the standpoint of radiographic technique, and from the standpoint of protecting the patient and the technician.

Summary of the Various Attenuation Processes

The more important of the attenuation processes are as follows:
  a) unmodified scattering
  b) photoelectric attenuation
  c) Compton effect
  d) pair production
  All these processes may in due course give rise to scatter, that is, radiation whose direction is changed from that of the primary beam.

The first-mentioned process, *unmodified scattering*, although it is an attenuation process, does not involve any actual transfer of energy from the beam to the scattering material. The remaining processes, (b) through (d), all involve transfer of energy to the attenuating medium. These processes are termed *real absorption* or, as is the trend in current literature, energy-transfer processes, while unmodified scattering is often referred to as *apparent absorption* or, again, simply attenuation.

Of the energy-transfer processes listed, pair production, as will be shown shortly, has little significance in medical radiography.

Unmodified Scattering

Scattering in its general sense in the context of electromagnetic radiation means the bringing about of a less orderly arrangement of the photons' directions due to the deflections caused by charged particles interposed in the electromagnetic radiation beam.

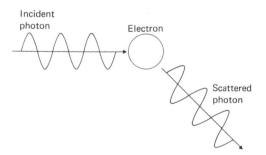

FIG. 10.7. Unmodified scattering: The electron is relatively free, perhaps in the outer shell of an atom. The incident photon is scattered without any loss of energy; therefore the electron is left unchanged.

Unmodified scattering of electromagnetic radiation refers to the scattering of this radiation chiefly by relatively free charged particles, such as the outer electrons of atoms (see Fig. 10.7). This scattering effect may be computed classically, as J. J. Thomson did, or it may be computed according to quantum theory.

The classical interpretation assumes that as an electromagnetic wave passes near an electron the transverse electric field of the radiation (see Section 9.1) sets the electron oscillating with the same frequency as that of the incident electromagnetic wave. The electron then, due to its acceleration during the oscillations, radiates energy of the same frequency as the incident radiation energy. This process is entirely analogous to what is involved in the emission of radio signals and the energy loss by radiation in the case of high-frequency AC. In the case of radio, the electrons are caused to move back and forth in the transmitter antenna and thus radiate electromagnetic waves, which have, of course, a much greater wavelength than x-rays.

Although such scattering causes an attenuation of the x-ray beam in the forward direction, there is, as stated before, no energy transfer involved. The energy of the incident photon is immediately reradiated, unchanged in frequency although changed in direction. The scattered photon is said to be *coherent*, that is, "in step," with the incident photon.

The fact that this scattering process gives rise to attenuation seems obvious. Certainly if this process were the only one involved in interactions between radiation and matter, measurements would nevertheless show a lower value of intensity for the transmitted beam than for the incident beam. Some scattered photons will be so scattered as not to reach the far side of the medium subjected to radiation, and therefore will not be measured.

Photoelectric Attenuation

Photoelectric attenuation, as shown in Fig. 10.8, takes place when an incident photon interacts with an inner atomic electron and has sufficient energy to eject the electron from its shell. All the energy of the photon,

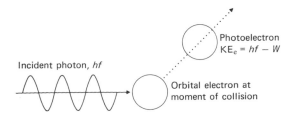

FIG. 10.8. Photoelectric absorption. The incident photon ejects an electron from an inner shell of the atom. This electron is called a *photoelectron*. Its kinetic energy, KE_e, is equal to the energy of the incident photon, *hf*, minus the energy which bound the electron to the atom, *W*. The energy of the characteristic photon depends on which shells were involved in the subsequent movement of another electron within the atom. (See Fig. 10.9.)

which energy must equal or exceed the binding energy for the particular electron, is transferred to the electron. Any energy in excess of the binding energy is given to the ejected electron as kinetic energy.

This fact may be expressed as

$$KE_e = hf - W,$$

where KE_e is the electron's kinetic energy, hf is the energy of the incident photon, and W is the work function, that is, the energy required to remove the electron from its constituent system. This equation is the Einstein photoelectric equation referred to in Section 7.8.

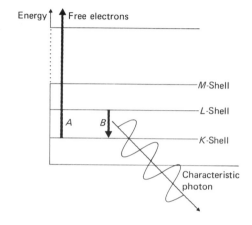

FIG. 10.9. Photoelectrons and characteristic radiation. *A* represents an electron from the *K*-shell raised to such a high energy level that it becomes independent of the atom. It is now called a photoelectron. An electron, *B*, from the *L*-shell falls to the *K*-shell to fill the vacancy. Energy, equal in quantity to the difference in energy between the two shells, is emitted as a photon of characteristic radiation. Its wavelength will depend on the atom and the shells concerned in the process.

The ejected electron is known as a *photoelectron*. After an electron has been ejected from the inner shell, that is, lower energy level, the most probable event is for another electron from an outer shell, that is, higher energy level, to fall in to fill the inner vacancy. In so doing, the electron radiates a photon of energy equal to the difference in energy between the two energy levels represented by the shells involved, (e.g., the *K*- and *L*-shells). See Fig. 10.9. Since, as pointed out in Chapter 1, the various energy levels and consequently their differences are characteristic of the atoms of a given element, this radiation is known as *characteristic radiation*. We met a similar mechanism in Chapter 9 when we were discussing characteristic x-rays, but in those cases the characteristic radiation was originated not by incident photons but by electrons incident upon the x-ray tube target. Of course, all the characteristic radiation itself may not be absorbed near its point of origin. Some of it may escape from the attenuator in such a way that even the photoelectric effect may in some cases give rise to some scatter.

The probability per unit thickness of material of photoelectric attenuation occurring in the material varies approximately as the cube of the wavelength of the incident photons. That is to say, if the wavelength is doubled the probability of photoelectric attenuation becomes eight times greater. Also the probability of photoelectric attenuation per unit thickness increases approximately as the cube of the atomic number of the material. For example, lead has an atomic number approximately ten times greater than that of oxygen. The probability of photoelectric attenuation in lead is therefore about a thousand times greater than it is in oxygen. These statements may be succinctly summarized:

$$\tau_{PE} \propto \lambda^3, \qquad \tau_{PE} \propto Z^3,$$

where τ_{PE} is a measure of the probability of photoelectric attenuation, the mass attenuation coefficient in this case; λ is the wavelength of the incident photon; and Z is the atomic number of the attenuating material. The above information is, of course, also contained in Eq. (10.1) of the cross section for photoelectric attenuation.

Readers might wonder why we have just given a Z^3-dependence for photoelectric attenuation while Eq. (10.1) gives a Z^4-dependence. We may use the answer to this apparent inconsistency as a vehicle for clarifying some of the seeming confusion in the relevant literature due to the usage of the various coefficients mentioned earlier. First of all, the probability of photoelectric attenuation per atom varies as Z^4. And cross sections are generally interpreted as meaning cross sections per atom. Now since there are Z electrons in an atom, the probability per electron would be only Z^3-dependent. Next we use the fact, which is not difficult to show, that all materials except hydrogen have essentially the same number of electrons per gram. Thus the probability per gram, that is per unit mass, would, as the electronic probability, also vary as Z^3.

The photoelectric process transfers only very little energy permanently to the atom directly concerned in the process. This small energy transfer is just enough to conserve momentum in the interaction. Thus almost all the energy of the incident photon is transferred to the ejected photoelectron. But energy is transferred to the attenuating material in the subsequent collisions and ionization events involving the photoelectron. If the kinetic energy of the photoelectron is high, then the amount of ionization the electron produces will be greater than if its kinetic energy were low. In soft tissue, such as the abdomen, the length of a photoelectron track is relatively short and the actual range or distance from the point of origin of the electron's zigzag track is even shorter. But the number of ion pairs produced may nevertheless be quite large. For example, a photoelectron ejected from tissue by a 100-keV photon has a range of a fraction of a millimeter, but produces almost 3000 pairs of ions.

Because of the dependence of photoelectric attenuation on the atomic number of the attenuator, this process assumes considerable importance in medical radiography. The higher atomic number of the elements in bone (for example, Ca: $Z = 20$; P: $Z = 15$; bone: effective $Z = 13.8$), as compared with soft tissue (for example, C: $Z = 6$; O: $Z = 8$; H: $Z = 1$; soft tissue: effective $Z = 7.4$), leads to greater attenuation in bone. This fact is largely responsible for the contrast between bone and soft-tissue areas in a radiograph.

The Compton Effect

The Compton effect is also known as *modified scattering* or *Compton scattering*. Like unmodified scattering, this process occurs most probably when a photon interacts with an outer, loosely bound atomic electron.

By loosely bound we really mean that the electron's binding energy is small relative to that of the x-ray photon. In the interaction, not all the energy of the incident photon is given to the electron. Part of the original photon energy remains as photon energy: A photon of less energy than that of the incident one consequently originates at the site of the interaction. (See Fig. 9.17.)

As mentioned in the previous chapter, this process may be thought of as a collision between an incident photon and an electron, resulting in the electron being ejected from its orbit and the photon bouncing off from the collision with diminished energy. The electron and the photon may travel in any directions, providing that in the interaction momentum is conserved. For a more detailed review of this interaction the reader is referred back to Section 9.2.

The probability per unit mass of a Compton collision in the region of diagnostic x-ray energies varies slightly with the wavelength of the incident photon. As the wavelength is increased, that is, as the energy of the photon is decreased, the probability very slowly decreases. Since this process involves the outer or relatively loosely bound electrons of an atom, the likelihood of a Compton interaction is substantially independent of the atomic number of the material.

Absorption of energy by this process in tissue is brought about via both the Compton electron and the scattered photon. The Compton electron behaves similarly to the photoelectron previously discussed, traveling about the same distances, depending on its energy, of course, and producing a similar number of ion pairs. The scattered photon may in some instances be nearly as energetic as the incident photon, as is the case in a glancing collision. In many cases the scattered photon will have sufficient energy to leave the tissues and/or in the meantime undergo any one of the attenuation processes summarized earlier.

As implied in our discussion of photoelectric attenuation, when scattered photons leave the tissue the energy actually absorbed by the tissue is obviously less than it would be if the scattered photons were not to leave; moreover, the scattered radiation may reach the film and produce fog. In fact, these unabsorbed photons account for a significant proportion of the scatter produced in medical radiography.

Pair Production

Pair production can occur only if incident photons have energies of at least 1.02 MeV. If a photon of this energy, or more, approaches a nucleus, the photon may disappear, and in its place two particles—one electron and one positively charged electron, or *positron*—may appear, as shown in Fig. 10.10. In other words, there is a conversion of energy into matter. The two particles move away from their point of origin with a total kinetic energy equal to the difference between the energy of the incident photon and the minimum or threshold value of 1.02 MeV at which these events can occur. It should be noted that 1.02 MeV is the energy equivalent of the masses of the two particles produced, calculated from the Einstein expression $E = mc^2$, which we first met in our discussion of the chemical law of definite proportions in Section 1.2.

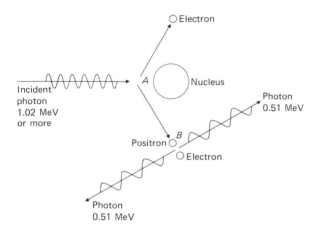

FIG. 10.10. Pair production. The incident photon is converted to matter, an electron and a positron, at *A*. The positron sooner or later meets another electron, *B*, and these two particles undergo mutual annihilation. In their place two photons are produced in opposite directions. If the positron and the electron at annihilation have no kinetic energy, the resulting photons will have exactly 0.51 MeV each. The fact that the particles have kinetic energy increases the energy of the resulting photons.

The newly created electron will in due course be captured by a positive ion and become part of a neutral atom. On the other hand, the positron will soon collide with another electron in the attenuator in a process of mutual annihilation, giving rise to two photons of equal energy, of minimum value 0.51 MeV each. This process is no more than the inverse of the pair production discussed above. There is reason to believe that the electron-positron pair, prior to annihilation, often exists for an extremely short time as a hydrogenlike atom, the positron taking the role of the proton in an ordinary hydrogen atom. The "element" of these temporary atoms, which have a very transitory existence (half-life of about 10^{-7} sec), is called *positronium*.

As we said before, the electron has a mass of 9.1×10^{-28} gm, and it is known that the energy required to create this mass is 0.51 MeV. Consequently, the probability of pair production occurring below the threshold energy of 1.02 MeV goes to zero. Above this energy of 1.02 MeV the probability, as you might reasonably suppose, becomes increasingly larger.

Sometimes three particles may be produced: That is, triplet production may take place. And at higher energies, 8 MeV and greater, other attenuation processes occur which involve nuclear reactions but, as the energies involved are much greater than those met with in diagnostic radiography, we shall not consider them here.

We may express the probability of pair production per unit mass as follows:

$$\pi \propto \frac{1}{\lambda},$$

where π is a measure of the probability of pair production and λ is the wavelength of the incident photon.

Pair production is also proportional to the atomic number of the material in question, which fact may be represented thus:

$$\pi \propto Z.$$

That pair production is more probable with materials of high atomic number is due to the fact that in the pair-creation process momentum cannot be conserved unless some heavy nucleus is nearby to participate in the process simply to the extent of absorbing the appropriate amount of momentum. There is to date no knowledge of any physical process taking place in which the momentum of the system involved is not conserved.

Since pair production cannot occur with the photon energies used in conventional medical radiography, we shall not discuss the process further here, except to say that transfer of energy occurs along the ionization tracks of the positron and the electron and via the further attenuation of the annihilation radiation.

Some Summary Comments

The processes we have so far described, together with the primary radiation which has been transmitted unchanged by the attenuator, are summarized in Fig. 10.11. It must be realized, however, that this figure and the accounts of the processes of attenuation, although they seem to imply that any attenuation process occurs alone, may in reality be extended to the nth degree. Each process gives rise to various products, which may then in turn undergo the same or other processes of attenuation, and so on. Hence, wherever we have used the term "incident photon" in the descriptions of the attenuation processes, we might equally well have meant a photon arising from a previous process in the attenuator but now incident upon a new atom.

In biological tissue, about a quarter of the energy absorbed from an x-ray beam produces damage, as typified by electron bond disruption in molecules. The rest of the absorbed energy, three-quarters of the total

FIG. 10.11

	Process	Products
	Unmodified scattering	Scattered photons
Incident x-ray photons	Photoelectric absorption	a) Photoelectrons b) Characteristic photons
	Compton effect	a) Compton electrons b) Scattered photons
	Pair production	a) Electrons b) Positrons c) Annihilation photons

FIG. 10.11. Summary of processes of interaction between x-rays and matter. This represents only the first-order processes but, of course, may be extended to the *n*th degree. Photons and particles from the "products" column may then become incident agents in further interactions with matter.

absorbed (that is, transferred from the beam to the tissue), is finally dissipated as heat, which raises the tissue temperature. However, the temperature increases involved are extremely small. For example, let us consider a primary x-ray beam giving an exposure of 1000 roentgens. Although we shall define the roentgen in Section 11.1, in the meantime it suffices perhaps to indicate that this exposure of 1000 roentgens represents approximately the total exposure involved in some 5000 mass miniature chest radiographs. Now then, assume that a single tissue cell is exposed to 1000 roentgens: The temperature of the cell would rise no more than 10^{-3} to 10^{-2} C°.

To sum up then, what are the things that may happen when x-rays meet matter? The x-rays may be transmitted unchanged, be scattered, or undergo true absorption, that is, transfer their energy, in whole or in part. The linear attenuation coefficient μ of Section 10.1 thus really consists of several components, which depend mainly on the four attenuation processes summarized earlier. Since considerable attenuation involves scattering of one kind or another, and since scattering is so important to the radiographer, we shall discuss it more fully in Section 10.5.

10.4 THE RATIONALE OF RADIOGRAPHY

Now we begin to see the reasons why medical radiography is possible. We see that, due to certain interactions between x-rays and matter, the transmitted beam emerging from the patient contains information. Although before the attenuation processes took place the x-ray beam had a more or less uniform intensity, now, when it leaves the patient, this is no longer true; the beam now contains an "image" made up of regions of different intensities. The beam intensities in these regions depend on the atomic number of the part the beam has traversed and the energy of the photons of which the beam consists.

We also see that the "image" we refer to is to some extent made less clear by the presence of random information in the transmitted beam, because the transmitted beam also contains scattered photons arising from the various interactions within the patient. The amount of scatter also depends on Z and kV. This problem of scatter obviously does not completely thwart medical radiography, but it does make it more difficult.

Finally, we realize that if energy transferred from x-rays to body tissue constitutes a hazard, then there is some hazard in medical radiography. From a study of the attenuation processes we can obtain some estimate of the amount of this energy absorbed by the tissue, and thus of the size of the hazard.

Relative Importance of Various Attenuation Processes in Soft Tissue

Table 10.3 shows the relative importance of three attenuation processes. Unmodified scattering is not included because it forms only about 10% of the total energy loss of the incident beam at energies of approximately 50 keV. Throughout the diagnostic range of photon energies this process is of very little importance, except that it adds to the number of scattered photons arising from within the part x-rayed. Some of these photons may reach the film and fog it. The results given in Table 10.3 refer to water, as this has about the same average atomic number as soft tissue.

Let us now look at Table 10.3 and talk about the information summarized there. First of all, we should recall that a photon energy of 50 keV does not imply a tube voltage of 50 kV. Rather, as pointed out in Section 9.4, with a heterogeneous beam such as used in medical x-ray work, a tube voltage of 150 kV would give a beam with about the same effect as a homogeneous beam somewhere in the region of 50 kV to 60 kV.

Now then, up to 50 keV: Photoelectric attenuation appears to be of most importance; by this we mean important with respect to energy absorption. Although at this energy photoelectrons account for only about 10% of the electrons produced by the interaction of the x-ray beam with water, nevertheless the energy carried by these electrons is about 60% of the total energy of all the electrons produced by the attenuation processes. Only at about 10 keV do the photoelectrons represent about 95% of the total number of electrons produced and also carry nearly all the energy. The characteristic radiation produced by this process is of a very low energy in soft tissue and in general does not travel more than, at most, the diameter of a few cells within the tissues of the patient. Therefore, in diagnostic radiography this secondary radiation is of little account in terms of its effect on the radiograph.

Next, 60–90 keV: In this energy range more than 90% of the electrons produced by incident photons are Compton or recoil electrons, although photoelectrons still account for about one-third of the total energy transfer. In soft tissue this energy range will therefore produce many scattered photons of a wavelength sufficiently short to permit them to leave the tissue and radiate into the surrounding air. Many of these photons will

Table 10.3

RELATIVE IMPORTANCE OF DIFFERENT TYPES OF ATTENUATION IN WATER[*]

Photon energy	Relative numbers of electrons as % of total electrons produced by the three processes listed			Percent of total energy carried by total electrons produced by all three processes		
	Photo-electrons	Compton electrons	Electron pairs (and triplets)	Photo-electrons	Compton electrons	Electron pairs (and triplets)
Common diagnostic energies						
10 keV	95	5	0	100	0	0
20	70	30	0	99	1	0
26	50	50	0	96	4	0
30	39	61	0	93	7	0
40	20	80	0	80	20	0
50	11	89	0	61	39	0
57	8	92	0	50	50	0
60	7	93	0	43	57	0
80	3	96	0	20	80	0
100	1	99	0	9	91	0
150	0	100	0	2	98	0
200	0	100	0	1	99	0
400	0	100	0	0	100	0
1 MeV	0	100	0	0	100	0
2	0	99	1	0	99	1
4	0	94	6	0	93	7
6	0	88	12	0	86	14
8	0	83	17	0	79	21
10	0	77	23	0	72	28
15	0	65	35	0	59	41
20	0	56	44	0	50	50
24	0	50	50	0	43	57
50	0	29	71	0	24	76
100	0	16	84	0	13	87

[*] Adapted from H. E. Johns, *The Physics of Radiology,* second edition, revised second printing, 1964. Courtesy of Charles C. Thomas, publisher, Springfield, Illinois.

reach the x-ray film and, because of their random direction and distribution, will produce a more or less even fogging of the film. When relatively large body parts are to be x-rayed, the considerable quantity of this scattered radiation will necessitate the use of Potter-Bucky grids (see Section 10.5) or other similar devices.

Now 150 keV–1 MeV: Compton attenuation alone is present. We are now outside the range of normal diagnostic radiography.

Finally 50 MeV–100 MeV: Pair production predominates in this energy range, which is out of the diagnostic region.

Note that throughout these considerations radiographers must think of two aspects as being of prime importance: (1) How much scatter will be produced and will reach the film to fog it, and (2) how much radiation the patient will absorb. In the first case, a poor-quality radiograph is obviously not to the patient's advantage; in the second, absorbed x-ray energy of any amount constitutes a hazard.

Differential Values of Attenuation Coefficients

Now that we have seen by what processes radiation is attenuated, let us look again at Table 10.2. We are now in a position to realize how important differential values of attenuation coefficients are in medical radiography. We see that the mass attenuation coefficient of water is approximately 0.2 cm²/gm. This value is about the same as for soft tissue. For calcium the mass attenuation coefficient is 1 cm²/gm. This figure, we can say, is very approximately the same as that for bone. If we compare these two figures it is clear that, gram for gram, bone will remove five times more radiation than soft tissue at the energy quoted, that is, 50 keV. It is important to note that, in this energy region, which is that of medical radiography, radiographic contrast results from differences in atomic number (because the mass attenuation coefficient is Z-dependent) as well as differences in subject density. Note that by the term *density* we mean here the mass per unit volume (gm/cm³). Elsewhere in the literature, and in this book, the term density is also employed to refer to the darkness, or lightness, of a film; in this latter sense density is a photographic density, as measured by a photometer.

Contrast Media

A certain part of the body, for example the stomach, may attenuate radiation to no greater or lesser extent than the tissues surrounding it. For this reason, no separate visualization of the organ is apparent in the radiograph. To overcome this problem, the body cavity (kidney, stomach, or blood vessel) may be filled with a contrast medium. Such a medium consists of a material with an atomic number and density different from the surrounding tissues.

Contrast media may have atomic numbers and densities less than surrounding structures. Air and carbon dioxide are in this category. Or materials with higher atomic numbers and densities than body tissues may be used. Examples of these are salts of barium and iodine. The increased attenuation of these high-atomic-number media is due largely to increased photoelectric attenuation. This is what we might expect from our discussion of the probability of this interaction with respect to Z.

Some contrast media are introduced indirectly into the organ to be examined. The material of high atomic number is combined with another substance so as to produce a compound which the organ will absorb from the bloodstream and thereafter concentrate. This is the case with the gall bladder in cholecystography. Sodium tetraiodophenolphthalein is the contrast medium often used. After the patient is given it by mouth, it is excreted by the liver and is then concentrated by the gall bladder.

Other media, such as barium sulfate suspensions used in the x-ray examination of the alimentary canal, may also be given by mouth to reach the part of the body in question directly. Still other contrast media may be injected into veins and arteries or body cavities such as the lungs or bladder.

Besides having a different mass attenuation coefficient, contrast media must of course have one other essential feature: They must be nontoxic.

10.5 SCATTERED RADIATION IN RADIOGRAPHY

As implied before, the problems associated with scattered radiation in medical radiography intrude themselves to a considerable degree into the technical considerations of nearly all radiographic examinations. For those parts of the body thicker than the knee or the upper arm, scatter may quite easily be responsible for more than 50% of the film blackening in the finished radiograph if some method is not adopted to prevent the scattered radiation from reaching the film.

Now that we have examined the attenuation processes which may give rise to scattered radiation, we look at scatter from a slightly different viewpoint: where it originates in the x-ray room; its various energies, directions, and intensities.

The Effect of kV and Z on the Intensity of Scattered Radiation

In our discussion of the relative importance of various attenuation processes in soft tissue, we have seen that for photons between 20 and 30 keV, that is, x-rays produced at settings of, say, 60 to 100 kV, it is the Compton effect that accounts for about 50% of the electrons produced. And associated with these electrons there is a similar number of scattered photons of wavelength sufficiently short to penetrate through to the outside of the patient.

Reflection on the interactions which occur between a beam of radiation and a particular attenuator leads to the obvious conclusion that some of the radiation is transmitted unchanged, some is absorbed, and some is scattered. Figure 10.12 demonstrates the relationship between the energy of the primary beam and the relative percentages of absorbed and scattered radiation.

In the figure the two curves shown refer to materials having different atomic numbers. Curve A refers to copper ($Z = 29$) and curve B refers to water (average $Z \approx 7$).

If we examine the copper curve first, we see that at very low peak kilovoltages (25 kV to 45 kV), nearly all of the radiation removed from the primary beam is absorbed and very little is scattered. However, as the energy of the primary beam is increased, this ratio of absorbed to scattered radiation changes and we see that at about 110 kV, about 50% of the radiation removed from the beam is absorbed and about 50% is scattered. At 165 kV only 25% of the radiation removed from the beam is absorbed by

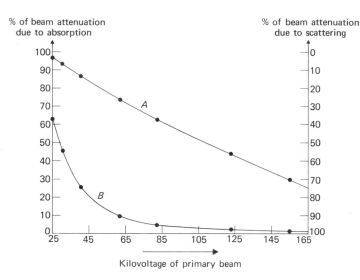

FIG. 10.12. The attenuation of radiation by two different materials, copper (curve A) and water (curve B). These curves show how the proportions of scattered radiation and absorbed radiation vary with the attenuator material and with changes in the kilovoltage of the primary beam. A curve for bone would lie between curves A and B and would have a curvature between the extremes shown in curves A and B. (Adapted from W. E. Schall, *X-rays, Their Origin, Dosage, and Practical Application*, Bristol, England: John Wright and Sons, 1961)

the attenuating material and 75% is scattered. Incidentally, these figures are relatively easy to obtain for copper; and note that the Z of copper, 29, is similar to that of calcium (Z = 20), a constituent of bone (Z ≈ 13.8).

In the case of curve B, for water, we see a different state of affairs. Water has, of course, been chosen in this instance because of its similarity to soft tissue in its atomic-number and radiation-attenuating characteristics. Here we see that, of the radiation removed from the primary beam at a low kV, for example 30 kV, half of it is absorbed by the water and half of it is scattered. But as the kV of the primary beam is slowly increased up to about 65 kV, we see that the production of scatter relative to absorption increases sharply. For example, at 60 kV only 10% of the radiation removed from the primary beam is absorbed and 90% of it is scattered. Above 80 kV the proportions change much more slowly, and even at 165 kV we still find a small proportion absorbed.

So we see that in the case of these two materials the trends are the same, but for the material of lower atomic number the change from absorption, that is, energy transfer, to scattering takes place much more rapidly with a rise of kilovoltage.

All this means two things to the x-ray technician: First, with the use of higher kilovoltages the amount of radiation absorbed by the patient becomes progressively less; that is, radiation hazard to the patient becomes smaller. This is obviously a most desirable feature. On the other hand, we can also see that for materials such as soft tissue or water, at the higher kilovoltages, say 80 kV and above, the amount of scatter produced becomes greater, and this may lead to fogging of the film. The technician will therefore have to decide whether it is better to produce a radiograph without fog or to minimize the radiation hazard to the patient. Usually the decision is a compromise between these extremes. And it is at this point that one might say that radiography as a science becomes so subjective that it may be called an art. Moreover, the decision regarding kV may be further complicated if the technician chooses a higher kV while at the same time using a radiographic grid of some sort to remove the scatter from the beam of radiation after it emerges from the patient and before it can reach the film. But by doing this the technician decreases the photographic effect on the film, and the film may appear underexposed. So, to counteract this, one increases the exposure to the patient so that the radiograph will be properly exposed. Also, of course, the use of high kV tends to diminish film contrast, for reasons which are distinct from reasons having to do with the obliteration of contrast by fogging.

From what we have said here about the effect of kilovoltage and atomic number on the intensity of scattered radiation and from what we have said elsewhere in this text, one can readily see that medical radiography is by no means a simple matter. But, we hope, one can also appreciate that the choice of technical factors may be made more intelligently and in the best interests of the patient and the radiologist if the radiographer has a basic understanding of what is involved in each alternative.

The Energy of Scattered Radiation in Different Directions

Obviously the way in which a primary beam is scattered within the patient is of great importance to the medical radiographer. Whether more radiation is scattered forward toward the film than in any other direction and whether the energy of this radiation is great or small will determine the degree to which the finished radiograph may be fogged.

In the case of unmodified scatter the energy of the scattered photons in different directions is, to all intents and purposes, the same in all directions because of the nature of the scattering process. But in the case of modified scattering arising from the processes of the Compton effect, the energy of the scattered photon will depend on how much of the energy of the incident photon has been transferred to the Compton electron. During the Compton collision a greater or smaller amount of energy may be transferred from the incident photon to the electron; whatever is left may be different from case to case. (At this point we would emphasize that most of the scatter in medical radiography arises from the Compton effect.)

Experiment has shown that the difference in energy between the incident photon and the scattered photon is related to the angle at which the photon is scattered. As this angle becomes greater, the energy of the scattered photon becomes less, so that radiation from this process scattered in a forward direction has greater energy than radiation scattered backward in a direction opposite to that of the incident photon. Scatter which forms an angle of less than 90° to the primary beam is called *forward scatter* and radiation which is scattered at an angle of greater than 90° is called *back scatter*. At 0°, radiation in the same direction as the primary beam has the greatest energy of all. In other words, in this instance there has been no scattering at all and the photon concerned is obviously the incident photon passing on unchanged.

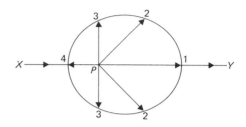

FIG. 10.13. The energy of scattered radiation. Each radial vector indicates the energy of photons scattered in a different direction. (Adapted from W. E. Schall, *X-rays, Their Origin, Dosage, and Practical Application*, Bristol, England: John Wright and Sons, 1961)

Figure 10.13 shows by means of a vector diagram, the relationship between angle of scatter and photon energy. (We use the term *vector* because the arrows in the diagram indicate by their orientation the direction of certain photons. The lengths of the various arrows are representative of the respective photon energies. And a vector is a quantity which is fully specified only if both magnitude and direction are given. Incidentally, we have already met quantities like this; for example, an electric field E and a magnetic field B.) The line XY represents an incident photon passing through a point P. In the case of XY there has been no scattering and the angle made by the "scattered" photon with respect to the incident photon is 0°; that is, the angle of scatter is zero. The other radial vectors arising from point P, the point of scattering, indicate the energy of scattered photons with respect to the direction of scattering. It can be seen that scatter directed at increasingly large angles with respect to the primary beam becomes progressively less energetic. We may think of the lengths of the vectors 1, 2, 3, 4, etc., as representing frequency or energy. Where the frequency is greatest the vector is longest, the represented energy is greatest.

Another way of representing photon energy is, of course, in terms of wavelength, where short wavelength means high energy. It is therefore common practice to express the differences in energy between incident and scattered radiations by means of their relative wavelengths. In Compton scattering the difference in wavelength is determined only by the angle of scatter and not by the wavelength of the incident photon nor by the material of the scatterer. The formula which is used to calculate the difference is quite simple:

$$\Delta\lambda = [0.0243(1 - \cos\,\theta)]\text{Å}, \tag{10.4}$$

where θ is the angle which the scattered ray makes with the primary beam and $\Delta\lambda$ is the difference in wavelength in angstrom units.

Table 10.4

THE ENERGY OF RADIATION SCATTERED IN DIFFERENT DIRECTIONS

Primary		Scatter					
		45°		90°		180°	
Å	kV	Å	kV	Å	kV	Å	kV
0.2000	62	0.2075	60	0.2243	55	0.2486	50
0.1550	80	0.1625	76	0.1793	69	0.2036	61
0.1240	100	0.1315	94	0.1483	84	0.1726	72

To see more clearly what this means, we might calculate a simple example. In a beam of radiation produced at 62 kV, the minimum wavelength within the beam will be

$$\lambda_{min} = \left[\frac{12.4}{kV}\right] \text{ Å}, \tag{9.8}$$

or

$$\lambda_{min} = \frac{12.4}{62} \text{ Å}, \qquad \lambda_{min} = 0.2 \text{ Å}.$$

Let this be the primary photon wavelength. Now assume that this photon is scattered within a material and that the scattered radiation emerges at an angle of 45° to the primary beam. From Eq. (10.4) we have

$$\Delta\lambda = [0.0243(1 - \cos 45°)] \text{ Å} = (0.0243 \times 0.2929) \text{ Å} = 0.0075 \text{ Å}.$$

This part of the calculation indicates that no matter what the energy of the primary beam, any radiation scattered at this angle will have a wavelength different from that of the primary by 0.0075 Å. In the case of the primary beam, at 62 kV and a minimum wavelength of 0.2 Å, the minimum wavelength of the scattered radiation will therefore equal

$$\lambda + \Delta\lambda = (0.2 + 0.0075) \text{ Å} = 0.2075 \text{ Å}.$$

Expressed in terms of kV, the above result means that the scattered radiation is approximately as produced with 60 kV. (Incidentally, note that to subtract energy we have to add to the wavelength!)

From this result we see that radiation scattered at an angle of 45° to the primary beam has an energy only slightly less than the primary beam itself. Yet this scatter will probably reach the film at some lateral distance from the primary beam and will therefore cause a random photographic effect, or fog.

To complete this discussion, let us tabulate the results from primary beams of three different energies and the energies of scatter in three different directions. Table 10.4 gives the kilovoltages to the nearest whole number. Note how primary beams at lower kilovoltages produce scatter more nearly like themselves, while the higher kilovoltages, for example

100 kV, produce scatter which is considerably less energetic than the primary beam concerned. Note, however, that this is a statement of the relative state of affairs; the energy of the scatter in all cases is still high enough to make it a problem in medical radiography.

The Intensity of Radiation Scattered in Different Directions

Not only does the energy of scattered radiation vary with the angle of scatter; the intensity of the scattered radiation varies with this angle too. In general, scattered radiation produced in a forward direction has a greater intensity than that produced in any other direction. Also the amount of this forward scatter increases with greater energies of primary beam. This is shown in Fig. 10.14, where XY is the direction of the primary beam and P is the point of scatter. The intensity of scatter is given by the vectors denoted by the angle at which the scatter occurs. The magnitude of the vector quantities is given by the two enclosed curves. The inner curve represents the case of a very energetic primary beam of about 550 kV, and the outer curve corresponds to radiation at about 90 kV. At the higher energy a much larger proportion of the scatter is in a forward direction.

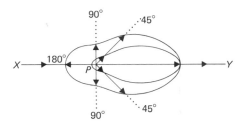

FIG. 10.14.   The intensity of radiation scattered in different directions. Each radial vector indicates the intensity of photons scattered in a different direction. (Adapted from W. E. Schall, *X-rays, Their Origin, Dosage, and Practical Application,* Bristol, England: John Wright and Sons, 1961)

Sources of Scatter in the X-ray Room

Among the origins of scatter in the x-ray room are the tube housing, cones, collimators, the table top, cassette and tray, and the floor. But by far the greatest portion of scatter arises in the patient. For this reason the patient has the greatest bearing on the problem of the protection of staff against radiation scattered during fluoroscopy, and on the problem of film fogging in radiography. In the case of fluoroscopy, suitable protection is arranged round about the patient to cut down to a safe level the amount of scatter reaching the radiologist and other members of the staff.

Of course, a factor which significantly influences the amount of scatter produced is the volume of the tissue irradiated. With a larger volume there is a greater quantity of scatter. This may be shown by taking two radiographs of the same area of the body, one with a small collimator aperture and one with a much larger aperture. The area x-rayed with the smaller aperture will give rise to a lighter film than the other. When the exposures have been suitably adjusted so that both films are of similar density, that film with the smaller field will show a greater degree of contrast, as there will be less fog due to scatter.

To prevent most radiation scattered from the patient from reaching the film, grids of various types, such as Potter Bucky and stationary grids, are used. A short aside is in order on grids: In general, a *grid* is a device which prevents x-rays other than those in the original direction of the primary beam from striking the film. A *Potter Bucky grid* is a secondary radiation grid which is made to move during the x-ray exposure so that its lead strips, while blocking out scatter, do not leave an image on the film.

Radiation which is scattered back from the floor, x-ray table, or from the wall in the case of a horizontal primary x-ray beam, is of lower energy than radiation scattered in other directions by the sources discussed earlier, and is therefore more readily attenuated. It is attenuated before reaching the film by a thin sheet of lead in the back of the cassette. In dental radiography, back scatter from the teeth beyond the film is attenuated to a considerable degree by a thin lead foil included in the film package.

10.6 LUMINESCENCE

Luminescence is an emission of visible light not due directly to incandescence and occurring at a temperature below that of incandescent bodies. The term includes phosphorescence and fluorescence evoked by the interaction of nonvisible electromagnetic radiations, such as x-rays, with certain materials.

The Process of Luminescence

Among semiconducting materials are certain particular ones called *phosphors.* Phosphors are materials that can in one way or another be made to emit visible light without being heated. One example of a phosphor is barium platinocyanide. We may recall that this was the material which Röntgen saw glowing and which thus led him to the discovery of x-rays.

It is perhaps justifiable to regard a phosphor simply as a crystalline semiconductor in which the outer orbital electrons are shared between neighboring atoms, which situation, under most circumstances, appears to be relatively stable. But when photons give energy to the crystal lattice (as they may do during x-radiation), some of the electrons become more energetic and free to move throughout the lattice. However, before one of these newly freed electrons has gone very far through the crystal, it may come to a place where an electron bond is missing (many such flaws exist in all crystals) and there the electron may occupy the vacancy, thereby assuming a lower energy state. When it does so, the difference in energy between the relatively free state and the relatively fixed one is given off as a photon of energy; in this case a photon of visible light. The energy of the photon, and therefore its wavelength or color, depends on the material of which the phosphor is made and the nature of its impurities (that is, the energy or type of the electron bonds).

Figure 10.15 illustrates this situation. When the electrons are free they travel along the uppermost plateau, but when they fall to the lower energy positions they fall into the holes and become trapped, while at the same time emitting a corresponding amount of energy.

The emission of light by means of this process in many cases may persist for only 10^{-7} sec after the absorption of the incident energy, so that to the eye the two events seem to occur simultaneously. When this is the case, the emission is known as *fluorescence*.

When the emission or luminescence occurs for a somewhat longer time than in the case of fluorescence and continues after the incident energy has stopped, the process is known as *phosphorescence*. Such a light may persist for hours in some cases.

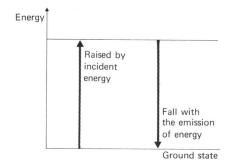

FIG. 10.15. Electrons within the crystal lattice are raised to a higher energy level by incident photons of various energies. (These photon energies must exceed the energy difference between the two levels.) The electrons may then return to their ground, or valence, level with emission of photons equal to the energy level difference. The fluorescence is usually less energetic than the incident photons.

Let us here point out that the incident energy necessary to produce luminescence does not always have to be radiation, such as light or x-rays or β- or α-particles. Many biological organisms produce luminescence by chemical reactions, but the process is still one of a molecular system changing from an excited (higher-energy) to an unexcited (lower-energy) state. Such organisms include certain bacteria, fungi, sponges, corals, clams, snails, fish, and insects.

Two things one should now note about luminescence: One is that there is no sharp dividing line between fluorescence and phosphorescence. There is always a time interval between the absorption and emission of energy, but in the case of phosphorescence this time interval, as mentioned before, is noticeable by an observer. The other point is that it is the materials which fluoresce that are called phosphors, and that this term is not to be confused in this context with the element phosphorus.

Intensifying Screens

A great deal of medical radiography is undertaken not by means of the direct interaction of x-rays with x-ray film but with the final image produced by means of visible light. This is done by having the x-ray film in

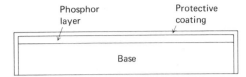

FIG. 10.16. The construction of an intensifying screen.

close contact with a sheet of material which fluoresces when struck by x-radiation. In practice, two sheets of fluorescent material are held inside a light-tight cassette with a sheet of x-ray film between them. When x-rays emerge from the patient they give rise to a light image on the two sheets, called *intensifying screens,* the active faces of which are toward the film. After suitable photographic processing, the image produced by this light is made visible on the film. This exposure process is much faster—that is, it requires smaller amounts of radiation to produce the same photographic effect—than that of direct radiography, as the film is more sensitive to visible light, particularly blue, than to x-rays. The blue light is easily stopped by the film emulsion, while x-radiation, on the other hand, passes unchanged through the film in considerable quantity. And, as you may suspect, only that energy which is actually absorbed is converted to a radiographic image.

Figure 10.16 shows the construction of a typical intensifying screen. The base consists of a sheet of cardboard or a polyester support which must be strong but flexible. Onto this is coated a layer made up of the phosphor in a suitable transparent binder. The phosphor crystals lie as close as possible to the front surface of the screen, which is covered by a very thin protective coating to resist abrasive wear and to permit easy cleaning. In use, the two screens lie on either side of the x-ray film within its cassette, as shown in Fig. 10.17.

Calcium tungstate and barium lead sulfate are used in intensifying screens for medical radiography. These phosphors emit radiations in the blue, violet, and ultraviolet regions. Film which is manufactured for use with screens of this type is more sensitive to the light from such screens than from x-rays alone. Film for use in direct radiography is more sensitive to x-radiation than to blue light. The two different types of film are known as *screen film* and *nonscreen film,* and each is more efficient from an exposure point of view when used under those conditions indicated by its type name.

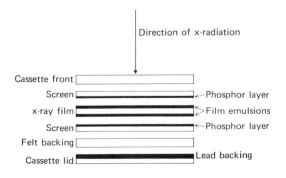

FIG. 10.17. Cross section of a loaded cassette.

In this chapter, we have said something about this question of film spectral sensitivity. The probability and type of absorption of blue light and x-rays by a silver bromide crystal may be roughly estimated by the use of the information we have given here.

The speed of intensifying screens is a measure of their ability to produce a given photographic effect by means of a greater or smaller exposure. The speed is controlled by the manufacturer by means of three factors: the type of phosphor used; the amount of phosphor included in the screens, in other words, the coating weight; and the size of the phosphor crystal.

As mentioned earlier, in high-speed, medium-speed, and high-definition screens, calcium tungstate is used almost universally. However, barium lead sulfate is also used as a phosphor, but for high-speed screens only.

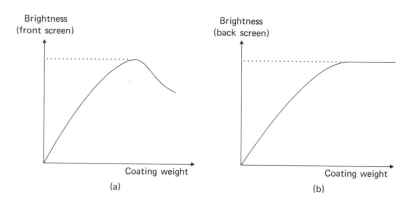

FIG. 10.18. The relationship between screen brightness and phosphor coating weight for (a) a front screen, and (b) a back screen.

Increasing the coating weight increases the speed, although there is a limit beyond which the addition of more phosphor material brings no increase in speed. This is illustrated in Fig. 10.18 by means of the two graphs, one for a front screen, the other for a back screen. In the case of the front screen, radiation will pass through the base of the screen and reach the phosphor layer from behind. At first, with the addition of more phosphor, the speed will increase, as shown, until it reaches a maximum. Beyond this point the addition of more phosphor crystals increases the depth of the phosphor layer so that radiation reaching the front layer of crystals is diminished in intensity. At the same time, light which is produced by the deeper layers of crystals in the screen cannot reach the surface and the film because of the overlying surface layers. The result is a decrease in the amount of light emitted from the surface of the screen. This is shown on the graph by the reverse slope of the curve.

In the case of a back screen, the addition of more phosphor increases the speed until a maximum is reached. But, because radiation to this screen reaches it from the front, the addition of more crystals produces a thicker layer to no purpose. Light which is able to reach the film is produced only from those crystals at the surface. The fluorescence of those crystals deeper in the layer is absorbed by those above. No matter how the coating weight is increased, the total number of crystals at the surface will remain the same, so the light output from this screen will remain constant at this maximum level. This is shown on the graph by the horizontal section of the curve.

Modern intensifying screens are often interchangeable with regard to position in the cassette. This means that the speeds of back and front screens are the same when tested individually.

The size of the phosphor crystals in intensifying screens varies from something like 10 microns ($= 10^5$ Å) to 15 microns, with barium lead sulfate crystals usually at the larger end of this range.

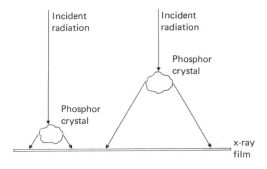

FIG. 10.19. The spread of light from phosphor crystals. The area of the light image on the x-ray film is larger from the phosphor crystal which is further from the film, even though both crystals are of the same size.

During exposure of the intensifying screen, each crystal of the phosphor will fluoresce, whether all or only a part of it is irradiated. Therefore the use of larger crystals leads to an increase in blur due to the transfer of light from the intensifying screens to the photosensitive emulsion of the x-ray film. However, the differences in blur between screens with different crystal sizes is minimal, due to the narrow range of crystal sizes used.

While we are on the subject of blur due to intensifying screens, we may add two other contributing factors: the thickness of the phosphor layer and the thickness of the supercoat. In both these cases, any increase in thickness will produce increased blur. As shown in Fig. 10.19, an increase in the distance of a phosphor crystal from the film emulsion produces a greater region of image on the film.

Of all the factors noted as contributing to screen blur, probably the greatest is the thickness of the supercoat.

The three common categories of intensifying screens in use in medical radiography are *detail screens, par-speed screens,* and *high-speed screens.*

Detail and par-speed screens are made of calcium tungstate, while high-speed screens are of either calcium tungstate or barium lead sulfate, as noted earlier. Par-speed screens are used for much general radiography, while the high-speed screens are used where small exposures and radiation hazards are of paramount importance, such as in the radiography of maternity patients. The use of detail or high-definition screens is most common in radiography of the chest. Here it is often desirable to be able to show very small structures in the lung fields. And since the chest is largely an air-filled cavity, it requires a much smaller exposure for its thickness than most other parts of the body; therefore the loss of speed can be tolerated in order to gain the advantage of fine detail.

The speed of intensifying screens is often quoted by means of the *intensification* or *intensifying factor,* defined for a given type of film as

$$\frac{\text{The exposure required without screens}}{\text{The exposure required with screens}},$$

for a given density. The intensification factor is quoted under some standard conditions of exposure, of which the only variable is the mAs. From the above definition, it follows that the intensification factor is always greater than unity.

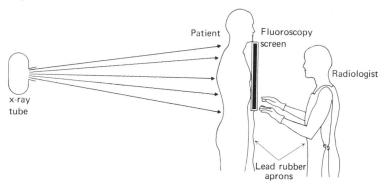

FIG. 10.20. The basic fluoroscope. The radiologist is protected by lead glass in the fluoroscope screen, by lead rubber aprons, and lead rubber gloves. Screen and tube move together.

Fluoroscopy Screens

Fluoroscopy screens are similar in construction to intensifying screens. But, because fluoroscopy screens are used for direct visual examination under x-radiation, the phosphor of which they are composed should fluoresce with a color in the maximum sensitivity range of the eye. Thus the chief difference between the two types of screens is in the wavelength of the emitted light. The phosphor most often used for fluoroscopy is zinc cadmium sulfide, which "converts" x-rays to a yellow-green light.

In order to obtain the brightest possible image, the designers of fluoroscopy screens use crystals that are quite large (approximately 30 microns in diameter) when compared with those used in intensifying screens. But, even with this modification, the image is very dim when produced by tube voltages and currents which are within the limits imposed by considerations of radiation hazard to the patient. Consequently, the fluoroscopy screen must be viewed in complete darkness after something like 20 to 30 min of dark adaptation on the part of the radiologist.

Figure 10.20 shows a typical fluoroscope arrangement. The fluoroscopic screen is covered on its viewing side by a sheet of lead glass. This glass is transparent to the light image and attenuates the x-ray beam. By this means, the radiation hazard to the radiologist and other personnel present is greatly diminished.

Because of the relatively high dose rate to the patient and the low level of brightness of the image in conventional fluoroscopy, much work has been done to make possible brighter images with lower dose rates. This work has led to the invention and development of image-intensifier systems. We shall discuss some of the principles of these in Chapter 12.

QUESTIONS

1. Define real absorption (that is, energy transfer); secondary radiation; scattered radiation.

2. What is meant by the "exponential attenuation" of radiation?

3. a) Explain what information is given by the linear attenuation coefficient.
   b) List the following materials in the order of increasing linear attenuation coefficient: water, lead, bone, copper.

4. With respect to linear attenuation coefficients, how does monoenergetic radiation differ from heterogeneous radiation?

5. What is meant by the half-value layer? Discuss the shortcomings of the half-value layer as a specification of heterogeneous beam quality.

6. Describe four important attenuation processes which occur as interactions between matter and radiation of energies up to 3 MeV.

7. What is the minimum photon energy required for pair production? Explain the reason for the minimum value.

8. a) Identify the attenuation processes indicated in Fig. 10.21.
   b) Which attenuation process is of chief importance in the energy region of diagnostic x-rays?
   c) How does the probability per unit mass of the above process vary with photon energy and atomic number?

9. Describe the effect of kV and Z on the intensity of scattered radiation.

10. What is the mathematical relationship between the wavelengths of the incident and scattered photons in Compton scattering with respect to the angle of scatter?

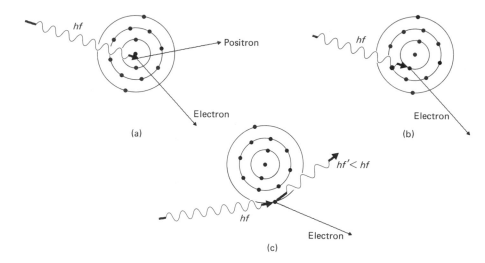

FIG. 10.21.   Some attenuation processes.

11. Discuss the intensity of scattered radiation with respect to the direction of scatter.

12. What is luminescence? Give a definition and outline a theory which explains luminescence in crystalline solids.

13. On the basis of the material discussed in this chapter, describe various methods by which you could decrease radiation to patients and staff.

14. a) What is meant by a contrast medium in medical radiography?
    b) How and where does such a medium produce contrast?

15. Why does a bone appear as a different photographic density in a radiograph, compared with the photographic density of surrounding soft tissues?

16. What is back scatter and what are its implications in medical radiography?

17. Draw and label a cross-sectional diagram of an intensifying screen. Describe the function of each part.

18. What is meant by "intensification factor," and how would you determine it in the x-ray department?

19. Discuss radiation protection with respect to fluoroscopy screen design and use.

SUGGESTED READING

ANDREWS, H. L., *Radiation Biophysics.* Englewood Cliffs, N.J.: Prentice-Hall, 1961. As the name implies, this is a text dealing entirely with radiation from the point of view of its effects on biological material. Chapter 5 covers photon absorption.

INTERNATIONAL COMMISSION ON RADIOLOGICAL UNITS AND MEASUREMENTS, *Radiation Quantities and Units, Report 10A.* Washington, D.C.: United

States Department of Commerce, National Bureau of Standards, 1962. This handbook, Number 84, contains the latest recommendations of the ICRU on the use of several terms to be found in this chapter and in Chapter 11.

JOHNS, H. E., *The Physics of Radiology.* Springfield, Ill.: Charles C. Thomas, 1964 (second edition). This authoritative text devotes two chapters, Chapters V and VI, to the absorption of radiation.

WEIDNER, R. T., and R. L. SELLS, *Elementary Modern Physics.* Boston: Allyn and Bacon, 1960. This book treats the fundamentals of modern physics fairly rigorously. For the more advanced student, we recommend reading Chapter 3, which covers the particle aspects of electromagnetic radiation and includes a derivation of the Compton-effect equation. Prerequisites are an understanding of elementary physics and introductory calculus.

CHAPTER 11

Photon Dosage and Dosimetry

Figure 11.1, which presents the results of the exposure of animals to x- or γ-rays, is a forceful reminder of the hidden danger inherent in the use of high-energy radiation.

The implication of Fig. 11.1 is that for safety's sake alone we need to know something about radiation doses and how they are measured. There are also, of course, other reasons for pursuing knowledge of radiation and radiation dosimetry. There are, in the hospital itself, a wide variety of diagnostic and therapeutic uses of radiation of various kinds. For example, the thyroid scan of Fig. 1.18 is dependent on relatively sophisticated dosimetry.

To promote and develop understanding and research in radiation at the international level, many special organizations have been set up. One of these international bodies convened in April, 1962, in Montreux, Switzerland, and discussed, among other matters, some new recommendations regarding terminology in the field of radiation measurements. We had occasion in Chapter 10 to refer to this international group, and we shall follow its recommendations in this chapter. We refer to the International Commission on Radiological Units and Measurements (ICRU).

The ICRU has been in operation, under the auspices of the International Congress of Radiology, since 1925. In 1928, at Stockholm, the second meeting of the International Congress of Radiology adopted the roentgen as the basic unit of radiation output from an x-ray source and from radioactive materials. Except for a slight alteration in definition effected at a 1937 meeting, the present definition of the roentgen is the same as that conceived in 1928.

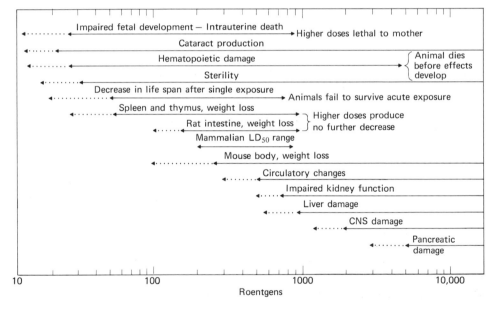

FIG. 11.1. Comparison of sensitivities of various organs and organ systems to single exposures of x- or γ-radiation. Solid lines represent the range of exposures over which effects
have been observed. Dotted extensions to the left of the solid lines indicate that the effects
might be detectable at lower exposure values. The symbol LD_{50} means that such an exposure
is lethal to 50% of a large group; that is, mammalian LD_{50} is the exposure that would cause
50% of the mammals so exposed to die of the immediate effects of the radiation. (From J. F.
Thomson and R. L. Straube, "Organ and Organism Response," from *Radiation Biology and
Medicine,* edited by W. D. Claus, Reading, Mass.: Addison-Wesley, 1958.)

11.1 EXPOSURE

Exposure and Absorbed Dose

Before we proceed with our discussion of radiological units and their measurements, we need to emphasize, in the light of experience, a point which became evident as time went by. After the concept of the roentgen as a measure of the quantity of radiation was adopted, it soon became obvious that it was being employed for two different concepts. With respect to x-ray work, the two concepts were roughly measures of (a) the energy emerging from the machine, or striking the patient, and (b) the energy absorbed by the patient.

Since concepts (a) and (b) are different, a new concept and unit were formulated in 1956. The new concept—having its own unit, the rad— was one which referred essentially to the energy absorbed by a body subjected to radiation exposure. In other words, *absorbed dose* refers to the energy transferred from the radiation beam to the body.

An analogy with education is apropos here. On the one hand there is the exposure: all the instruction, reading, viewing, hearing, etc., to which one is subjected. On the other hand, there is the absorbed dose: that which we understand, retain, and make part and parcel of our being. This is bound to be only a fraction of the exposure.

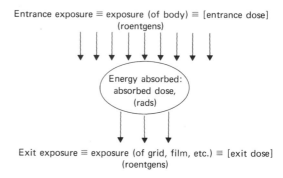

Entrance exposure ≡ exposure (of body) ≡ [entrance dose]
(roentgens)

Energy absorbed: absorbed dose, (rads)

Exit exposure ≡ exposure (of grid, film, etc.) ≡ [exit dose]
(roentgens)

FIG. 11.2. Exposure (measured in R) and absorbed dose (measured in rads). Variations of the current terminology are given, as well as the older terms, which are in square brackets.

Figure 11.2 represents these concepts pictorially, and also introduces the notions of entrance and exit exposure. The latter is, of course, the important radiation quantity with respect to radiographic effects on the film.

Incidentally, although *exposure* is the terminology most recently recommended, the reader is bound to find the earlier term *exposure dose* common, even in current literature. The present intent of the ICRU, however, is to keep the word dose linked only to the concept of absorbed radiation, that is, absorbed dose.

Keeping the above distinction between exposure and absorbed dose in mind, let us concern ourselves first with exposure.

The Roentgen

If we consider the radiation at a given point in space, say the radiation at a point exactly 14 in. below the center of the x-ray tube portal when the machine operates at 70 kV and 10 mAs, and compare this situation mentally with the case at the same point but at 70 kV and 50 mAs, we can visualize that more radiation energy has reached the point in question in the second case than in the first. The exposure at the point in question is greater in the second case.

More precisely: The exposure (or exposure dose) of x- or γ-radiation at a certain point is a measure of the quantity of radiation, based on its ability to produce ionization in air. The measurement of exposure is made at a given point in the radiation field without the presence of a scattering body.

In view of the fact that exposure refers to the ability to produce ionization, one could of course say that it refers to the amount of energy per unit area reaching a certain region. In that sense, we may think of exposure as being x-ray intensity (Section 9.2) times time. Thus exposure at a point will depend on five factors: the kV, the mA, the filtration of the beam, the length of time of the irradiation, and the distance of the point in question from the tube portal, since x-rays, like light, vary in intensity (in vacuum) as the inverse of the square of the distance from a (point) source.

The unit of exposure is the roentgen, abbreviated R. *One R is an exposure of x- or γ-radiation such that the associated corpuscular emission per 0.001293 gm of air produces, in air, ions carrying one electrostatic unit of quantity of electricity of either sign.*

Let us look more closely to see what this definition says. First of all, from our discussions in Chapter 10 we realize that the interaction of x-rays with air molecules results in the release of both photoelectrons and Compton electrons and, if the energy is high enough, in electron pairs. These high-speed electrons, or *corpuscular emission* as they are called in the definition of the R, in turn cause ionization along their tracks. In other words, positive and negative charges in the form of positive and negative ions, as well as electrons, make their appearance.

Under ordinary circumstances, of course, these positive and negatively charged particles, which appeared as the result of the x- or γ-rays, would recombine. To measure the charge produced by the radiation, we thus need to keep these charges separated and collect them, as indicated in Fig. 11.3.

Now it is possible to measure the total charge so collected. If the amount of air in question is 0.001293 gm (that is 1 cm^3 at 760 mm Hg and 0°C), and if the charge collected at the collecting plate is 1 electrostatic unit (1 esu = $\frac{1}{3} \times 10^{-9}$ coul), then the quantity of the radiation is said to be 1 R.

Thus, if we want to measure an exposure in roentgens, we must have a known mass of air and collect the ions produced in this air. The basic measuring device involved is the standard ionization chamber. We shall discuss this instrument in Section 11.4.

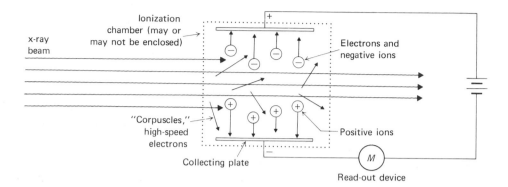

FIG. 11.3. Schematic of ionization produced by x-ray beam in air. The high-speed electrons are the "associated corpuscular emission" of the definition of the roentgen; *M* is a device which measures the total charge collected at the plates and so indicates the exposure. This *M* could also be a current meter and thereby indicate dose rate or, more properly, exposure rate, in R/min, for example. (See Section 11.4.)

As we shall see, it is the physical limitations of the ionization chamber which in effect impose this restriction on the definition of the roentgen: The roentgen is not defined for photon energies in excess of 3 MeV.

Since we have now emphasized that the roentgen is a unit of exposure, and not of absorbed dose, the reader may wonder how it is that the roentgen often appears in articles in which the context suggests that the author is referring not to exposure but to absorbed dose. The explanation is simple. In many cases, the absorbed dose may be readily calculated from the exposure in roentgens, and hence the roentgen has tended to remain in use in practical dosimetry, even in areas in which the biological effects of radiation, and hence the absorbed dose, are of prime consequence.

Sometimes it is desirable and/or convenient to measure not the total exposure, but the quantity of radiation per unit time, that is, the exposure rate. The instrument for making such a measurement is calibrated, not in roentgens, but in roentgens per unit time, say roentgen/min.

Back Scatter

We have already employed our knowledge of factors affecting x-ray intensity (Section 9.3) in our discussion relating to exposure dose. The question now is whether or not other factors besides kV, mA, time, filtration, and distance from the tube affect the exposure experienced by a patient. Yes, there is another factor: the patient himself.

Let us visualize the following experiment. We place a patient on the x-ray table for a given examination. We take the film, at the same time measuring the exposure in roentgens at the skin surface, using some kind of a small ionization chamber. Next we repeat the performance, but without the presence of the patient. We now observe that, even though we used the same technique and our ionization chamber was held at the same position as before, the reading went down. Without the patient present, the exposure was less than with the patient present.

The explanation of this observation is *back scatter*. The x-ray beam directed on a patient gives rise to scattered and secondary radiation within the patient, some of which increases the actual exposure of the skin surface. The additional radiation at the skin surface is called back scatter.

Back scatter is of particular significance in radiation therapy. In diagnostic work the most important point to keep in mind regarding back scatter is that it does contribute to radiation hazard for both patient and personnel, and that the back-scattering process also takes place beyond the film, when the scattering may result in fog (see Section 10.5).

The exposure, taking back scatter into account, is referred to as *skin* or *surface exposure*. The ratio of exposure with scatter to exposure in air is referred to as the *back-scatter coefficient*. This coefficient depends on the area of the field being x-rayed, the thickness of the part being examined, and the quality of the x-ray beam. Roughly back scatter, and consequently the back-scatter coefficient, increases with field size and thickness of part, but decreases with increasing HVL. The reader should now meditate on the plausibility of these dependencies of back-scattering, which should be readily apparent if he understands the interaction of x-rays with matter, treated in the previous chapter.

To summarize some of the preceding comments, let us use an example. A possible example of a back-scatter factor is 1.3. Employing this factor, what would be the skin (or surface) exposure if the exposure in air were 2 R? (We now draw the reader's attention to the important distinction between R, the roentgen, and italicized R, which henceforth refers to the exposure in roentgens. It should also be noted that X is coming into use as the symbol for exposure; that is, $R \equiv X$.

We let $R_S \equiv$ exposure at skin surface, $R_A \equiv$ exposure (in air), and $F \equiv$ back-scatter factor. Then

$$F = R_S/R_A.$$

Hence we obtain, for the exposure at skin surface,

$$R_S = R_A F = (2 \text{ R})(1.3) = 2.6 \text{ R}.$$

Some Typical Exposure Values

All people are exposed, in varying degrees, to background radiation of the order of 100 mR/yr.* This background radiation is primarily due to cosmic rays, radioactive minerals in the ground, and radioactive elements (such as potassium-40, carbon-14, and radon) within the body.

Other typical radiation exposure values are summarized in Table 11.1. As noted in this table, measurements made by the authors tend to confirm the diagnostic x-ray exposures reported by Duggan.

---

* The symbol mR stands for milliroentgens.

Table 11.1

SOME TYPICAL VALUES OF RADIATION EXPOSURE

Radiation source	Location	Exposure
Wrist watch (1) (1 μCi of Ra per watch)	Central body, including sex organs, at average distance of 1 ft	40 mR/yr
Luminous dials in airplane cabin (100 dials with 3 μCi of Ra each) (1)	Pilot at an average distance of 1 yd from the dials	1300 mR/yr
Phosphate rock (commercial fertilizer 0.01 to 0.025% U) (1)	Flat surface ground	280–700 mR/yr
People (1)	Packed in crowd	2 mR/yr
X-rays (2)	Lumbar spine, AP	1080 mR
	Lumbar spine, Lat.	4450 mR
	Chest, PA	65 mR
	Pelvis, AP	395 mR
X-rays, dental	Single film	0.05–5 R
Fluoroscopy without image amplifier (3)		3 R/min
with image amplifier (3)		0.3 to 0.6 R/min

(1) W. F. Libby, *Science*, 122, 3158, 57 (1955)
(2) H. E. Duggan, *Canadian Medical Association Journal*, 91, 894 (1964)
(3) G. M. Ardran and H. E. Crooks, *British Journal of Radiology*, 26, 352 (1953)

Regarding the x-ray exposures given in this table, let us make two observations: First, the values are for surface exposures. Second, these values are indicators only, and are not definitive unless one knows all the relative parameters, such as kV, mA, AFD, filtration, and details of patient. As a rough approximation, we might say that radiographic surface exposures fall generally in the region of 50–5000 mR, while the exposure rate for fluoroscopy is in the region of 3 to 5 R/min, 10 R/min being generally accepted as a maximum. Note also that the use of an image amplifier may reduce the exposure rate during fluoroscopy by as much as a factor of ten. On this topic it is also interesting to note that 100 mR is sufficient to cause x-ray film fogging dense enough to render the radiograph unsatisfactory for diagnosis of gross fractures.

One final point concerns the question of the relationship between the *curie* and the *roentgen*. The curie* is the unit of activity of a radioactive material. Hence one would certainly expect the intensity of radiation at a given point from a radioactive source to be higher when coming from a source with a high activity than when coming from a source with

---

* The abbreviation of the curie is Ci; the microcurie, which is one-millionth of a curie, is abbreviated μCi.

a relatively low activity. And the exposure rate is an indication of the intensity of radiation. Although there is no simple relationship which leads to the result coupling the activity of the radioactive watch dial to the exposure quoted in Table 11.1, it is possible to make exposure calculations if the activity of the radioactive material and various other parameters are known. For us the important point is that the curie and the roentgen are units of entirely different quantities. Moreover, experimentally one may establish such facts as, for example, that at one yard from an amount of I-131 having an activity of 1 curie, the exposure rate is 0.276 R/hr, while at the same distance the same activity of Co-60 yields 1.59 R/hr (Radiological Health Handbook, U.S. Dept. of Health, Education, and Welfare, 1957).

11.2 ABSORBED DOSE

Since the biological effects of ionizing radiation, such as x-rays, are due presumably only to energy imparted to matter, it seems that biological effects should be more closely correlated with absorbed dose than with exposure. For example, the energy absorbed per roentgen of exposure varies with the kind of tissue being irradiated and the quality of the radiation beam. For this reason, it behooves us to be somewhat familiar with the concept of absorbed dose. Also, for the same reason, radiation guides (Section 11.5) in the form of maximum permissible dose (MPD) are expressed in units of absorbed dose. However, as we said before, particularly with x-rays, there may be a ready relationship between the absorbed dose and the exposure, and thus the roentgen, the unit of exposure, is still found sometimes where one would expect the data to be stated in terms of the unit of absorbed dose (rad) or of dose equivalent (rem).

The Rad

The rad is the unit of absorbed dose. *One rad is approximately equal to the dose absorbed by soft tissue exposed to one roentgen of medium-energy x-rays.* Thus we see why rad and R are often used interchangeably, although to do so is not rigorously correct.

To define the rad precisely, we need first to define the term "absorbed dose" more carefully. The absorbed dose of any ionizing radiation is the energy transferred to matter by ionizing particles (exclusive of energy reradiated as the ionizing particles slow down) per unit mass of irradiated material at the place of interest.

The rad is the absorbed dose when 100 ergs (10^{-5} joule) of energy per gram is transferred to the absorbing material. That is, in short:

$$1 \text{ rad} = 100 \text{ ergs/gm.} \tag{11.1}$$

This is a very small amount of energy per unit mass, because although 1 gm is not much mass the erg is a quite small unit of energy (the electron volt is an even smaller unit, however). In terms of the foot-pound referred to in Section 2.3, the erg is indeed minute:

$$1 \text{ erg} \approx 74 \times 10^{-9} \text{ ft-lb}$$

And in terms of the energy unit employed when we were talking about heat (Section 7.4):

$$1 \text{ erg} \approx 2.4 \times 10^{-8} \text{ calorie.}$$

This amount of heat energy will not raise the temperature of a gram of tissue very much. In fact, if we assume that the specific heat of tissue is about the same as that of water, we can easily show that the effect of a therapy dose of 300 rad on 1 gm of tissue would be to raise the temperature of the tissue by about 7×10^{-4} C°.

Keeping the definition of the rad in mind, we now see why R is sometimes used to indicate what should be expressed in rad: the energy absorbed per R of exposure in the photon-energy region common to radiography is about 95 ergs/gm for soft tissue.

Quantitative Relationship Between the Rad and the Roentgen

We start with an aside regarding electronic equilibrium. By electronic equilibrium in a medium we mean that, during irradiation, for each electron leaving the region of concern another one of practically the same energy enters. This concept will now serve as a restriction on the relation between absorbed dose and exposure, and we shall again invoke it and clarify it when we discuss the ionization chamber in Section 11.4.

Now: Under conditions of electronic equilibrium, the absorbed dose D is proportional to the exposure R according to the relation

$$D = fR, \tag{11.2}$$

where f is a proportionality constant depending on both the composition of the irradiated material and the quality of the radiation beam.

If the absorbing material is air, then, since the average energy required to produce an ion pair in air is about 34 eV, f has the value 0.87 rad/R. (Some students who may wish to test their calculating skills might derive the above value. What one needs to recall is that the R results in one electrostatic unit of charge, which in turn indicates the number of electronic charges, thus yielding the fact that one R results in 2×10^9 ion pairs, assuming ions are singly ionized.)

Table 11.2 shows some typical values of f.

Students may wonder how f is related to the attenuation processes discussed in Chapter 10. The relationship is quite simple. But we do need first to backtrack to some notions regarding attenuation. Let us recall the linear attenuation coefficient, μ. This coefficient takes account of all attenuation processes and is therefore not quite what we are looking for because we want some index of actual energy absorption. So we need to exclude from the attenuation processes radiation which is scattered from the scene of the interaction. Consequently, we could consider a reduced coefficient, reduced by the fluorescent radiation arising from the photo-

Table 11.2

SOME AVERAGE VALUES OF ABSORBED DOSE PER ROENTGEN OF EXPOSURE*

kV	Filter, mm of Al	f in rad/R			
		Air	Water	Muscle	Bone
100	5.5	0.87	0.91	0.94	3.1
250	3.0	0.87	0.96	0.96	1.42
400	nil	0.87	0.97	0.97	1.11

* The values of f for materials other than air are from ICRU Handbook 62, U.S. Department of Commerce, National Bureau of Standards, 1956.

electric interaction, the modified radiation arising from the Compton process, and the unmodified scatter. This new coefficient is called the *energy transfer coefficient* (real absorption coefficient in some literature). One more restriction is yet required: What about the bremsstrahlung which may be produced as the electrons set into motion by the primary beam are slowed down? This radiation is not likely to be locally absorbed and thus also should be removed from any index purporting to give an indication of the actual energy absorbed from the primary beam at the locale in question. We must therefore consider a still smaller coefficient. This final coefficient is called the *energy absorption coefficient*, μ_{en}. It is the one of interest when we are considering f. Now we can show how f fits into the picture. We rewrite Eq. (11.2) as follows:

$$D_M = \left[D_A \frac{(\mu_{en})_M}{(\mu_{en})_A} \right] R = \left[0.87 \text{ rad/R} \frac{(\mu_{en})_M}{(\mu_{en})_A} \right] R,$$

where the subscripts M and A indicate the medium in question and air, respectively, and D and R are, as before, the absorbed dose in rads and the exposure in roentgens, respectively.

Now all the terms in brackets above are lumped together and called f, thus yielding

$$D_M = fR,$$

or simply

$$D = fR. \tag{11.2}$$

So indeed, as we would expect, our attenuation discussions of the past play a role in the concept of absorbed dose.

We shall not delve into any calculations involving Eq. (11.2), since the results obtained are of no immediate consequence in diagnostic radiology. In radiography, where the protection aspect is of consequence, two general observations suffice. *One:* For soft tissue, $f \approx 1$ rad/R, and hence the absorbed dose is numerically about equal to the exposure. *Two:* For bone, f is larger and, more important, it decreases significantly with increasing kV. The latter point might suggest to the radiographer that, as we mentioned before, insofar as contrast requirements permit, the patient absorbed dosage should be decreased by employing suitably high kV.

Patient Absorbed Dose in Radiography

As an aside at this juncture, we might note that very little of the patient exposure (entrance exposure) leaves the patient, because of scattering and absorption. The exit exposure is, of course, of considerable interest in that part of it, but only part of it, becomes the exposure for the x-ray film. Depending on a variety of factors—the thickness of the part being examined and the kV used are the key ones—the exit exposure (see Fig. 11.2) may be of the order of 10% of the entrance skin exposure of the patient. In fact, the actual exposure of the film may in some cases be as little as 1%, or even less, of the patient entrance skin exposure.

For example, a screen film which demands, say, one mR exposure, may require a patient skin exposure of 100 mR to achieve the one mR at the film. This suggests that in order to obtain this film the patient may have an absorbed dose,

$$D = fR \qquad\qquad (11.2)$$
$$\approx (1 \text{ rad/R})(0.1 \text{ R}) \approx 0.1 \text{ rad} \qquad \text{or} \qquad 100 \text{ millirad,}$$

f having been approximated from the values suggested in Table 11.2.

By comparison, the dosages required to destroy bacteria for purposes of sterilizing pharmaceuticals and surgical supplies are not in the millirad region, but in the megarad region (1 megarad = 1 million rads), say, 0.1–2.5 megarads.

The Rem

It has been known for some time that the energy transferred to a body, that is, in effect, the ionization produced by radiation is not a sufficiently good criterion of biological effect. The distribution of the ionization along the ionizing particle's track, that is, in how long or short a distance the energy is given up, turns out to be also significant. In other words, the biological damage done by one rad of x-rays turns out to be not the same as the damage done by one rad of alpha particles. The damage done by the latter is about 20 times that of an equal absorbed dose of x-rays.

In consequence of the above fact, more new terminology entered the radiation field. Of course, if diagnostic x-rays alone were of concern, no further dose quantities beyond the rad would have had to be devised. But, particularly from the viewpoint of protection, it was desirable to have a common language for all radiations. Therefore it became necessary to devise a quantity which, in the case of the alpha particles, takes care of the fact that they do more damage than x-rays. It became necessary to modify the rad.

The new concept is the *dose equivalent.* The dose equivalent *DE* is defined as the product of the absorbed dose *D* and the appropriate quality

Table 11.3
SOME APPROXIMATE NUMERICAL VALUES OF RBE

Radiation	RBE
X-rays	1
Beta rays	1
Protons	5
Neutrons	3–10
Alpha rays and heavy recoil nuclei	10–20

factor, as well as other modifying factors. We shall be concerned only with the quality factor, which in the case of alpha particles is about 20, if one chooses the quality factor for x-rays as unity.

In terms of symbols,

$$DE = (QF)\,D, \tag{11.3}$$

where DE is the dose equivalent in rems, QF is the qualifying factor, and D is the absorbed dose in rads.

In radiobiology this qualifying factor is generally given the name RBE, which stands for *relative biological effectiveness*. Some approximate values of RBE are given in Table 11.3.

Note that in Table 11.3 the RBE for beta rays is the same as for x-rays. This fact seems plausible. After all, the ionization produced by x-rays is essentially that produced by the liberated photo and Compton electrons, and "beta rays" is simply another term for a stream of electrons.

Since, as we said before, in the realm of radiation protection some common denominator is desirable, x-ray technicians find that even in x-ray work the rem appears as a unit of absorbed dose, the unit for dose equivalent, to be precise. For example, film badge readings and radiation guides in the form of maximum permissible dosages (Section 11.5) are now expressed in rem, or millirem, the unit of dose equivalent.

Note again the simplicity with respect to x-rays: A one-R exposure yields about a one-rad absorbed dose in soft tissue, which in turn means a one-rem dose equivalent in soft tissue. This is why one sometimes finds the terms R and rem used interchangeably (albeit incorrectly). For x-rays of moderate energy and for fleshy parts of the body, the R and the rem are numerically the same.

A qualitative way of considering the chief quantities encountered in this chapter so far is this: Roentgens give an indication of incident energy, rads tell how much of this incident energy is absorbed, and rems are a measure of the relative biological damage done.

Finally, let us point out that although instrumentation to measure either exposure (R) or absorbed dose (rad) is plentiful, to date there is not available any instrument which will measure the equivalent dose (rem) directly.

11.3 THE DETECTION OF RADIATION

Before we embark on a discussion of some of the chief radiation detection
and measurement devices of interest in radiography, we shall first look at
the various interactions of radiation with matter that might lead to detection and then perhaps also to measurement.

The Photographic Effect

Historically, of course, the chemical effect which results in the blackening
of a photographic film was of prime significance. The reader may recall
from Chapter 1 that this photographic effect led from the discovery of x-rays
to the discovery of radioactivity. The photographic effect is of course the
basis of radiography as well as the basis of the film badge generally employed as a protective control in the x-ray department.

The physics of the photographic emulsion is a very complex subject
in its own right and therefore cannot be satisfactorily treated here. Suffice
it to say that the series of events involving ionization produces a latent
image (Gurney-Mott Theory of 1937) which may then be made visible
by the chemical process called development. For further information, the
reader is referred to the photography texts listed at the end of this chapter.

Ionization

We have talked a good bit about ionization earlier in this book. The
ionizing effect of radiation is the basis of what is probably the commonest
class of radiation detectors, including, of course, the ionization-chamber
timer mentioned in Section 8.5. In the main, the difference between these
various detectors lies not so much in what gas, if any other than air, is
ionized by the radiation, as what voltage is applied across the electrodes
of the ionization chamber such as, for example, the collecting plates of
Fig. 11.3.

Actually, ionization as a detection mechanism is much more effective
with α-particles than with x-rays. Moreover, an ionization method is not
directly applicable with neutrons at all, because these electrically neutral
particles do not interact with atoms to produce ionization. The rela-
tive ionization effectiveness of the α-, β-, and γ- or x-radiation is about
10,000/100/1, respectively.

Since we shall deal fairly extensively with ionization-type detection
devices in the following section, let us review the basic mechanism involved in the ionization produced by x- or γ-rays:

a)   High-speed photoelectrons and Compton electrons are produced by
the interaction of the radiation with the medium in question (say air).

b)   These primary electrons thereupon lose their energy a step at a time
in successive contacts with molecules, knocking out other electrons,
called secondary electrons, thereby creating ions.

c)   Most of the secondary electrons in turn produce further ions.

d) The electrons are finally captured either by molecules, to form negative ions, or by positive ions, to form neutral molecules; unless, of course, the separated charged particles are kept separated by the application of an electric field.

We can calculate the energy of the incident photon only if we can somehow detect all the ion pairs produced by the primary and all the secondary electrons initiated by an x- or γ-ray photon. We must bear this fact in mind in our later discussion of radiation-measurement devices based on ionization.

Luminescence

The fluorescent effect must rule, of course, in the historical sense. It was the glowing in the dark of barium platinocyanide which put Professor Röntgen on the trail of x-rays. Fluorescent effects have since then been extensively employed to detect radiation. Fluorescence is obviously the basis of fluoroscopy, and the fluorescent effect is, as has been mentioned earlier, also employed in the phototimer and intensifying screens. However, our main concern here is that the fluorescent effect, as described in Section 10.6, is the basis of a radiation-measurement device known as a *scintillation counter*.

The commonest early scintillator was zinc sulfide. Presently the knowledge that not only certain inorganic crystals but also organic crystals, such as naphthalene (moth powder), could fluoresce has led to vast developments in the scintillation counter field. The advantage of organic crystals is that they are readily grown to relatively large sizes, whereas the growing of inorganic crystals is a formidable problem. And large single crystals are desirable for efficient detection. Now there are even liquid scintillators available.

Recently luminescence has again come more and more into favor for radiation detection. This is due to the fact that in some materials the electrons raised to higher energy levels by means of the energy imparted by radiation may require stimulation to drop back to their former ground-state level, during which process photons of visible light are emitted. One such phosphor, after irradiation, emits light when it is heated. This effect is the basis of *thermoluminescence dosimetry* (TLD), since the amount of emitted light is dependent on the amount of radiation energy that is absorbed by the phosphor. TLD-type dosimeters which are capable of measuring radiation exposure with a precision of ±3%, and yet which are only about 1 mm in diameter and 6 mm long, have already been produced and TLD is now in use in radiation therapy.

Another luminescence phenomenon employed is *radiophotoluminescence*. In this case, the irradiated phosphor emits visible light when it is stimulated by ultraviolet light. Radiation dosimetry that depends on this phenomenon is called *radiophotoluminescence dosimetry* (RPLD). Both this type and the TLD-type dosimeter are currently referred to as *solid-state detectors*.

Among other solid-state detectors are those that exhibit a change in electrical resistance on irradiation, ones that change color on irradiation, and the p-n junction detectors, to be discussed shortly.

Polymers are often employed for the first two types of these solid-state detectors. It is a fact that high-energy radiation induces changes in the mechanical, electrical, and optical properties of polymers. And although any one of these changes might be used to measure radiation dosage, the the optical changes, particularly in the visible region, are generally employed because they are relatively readily measured. Indeed such optical changes as the turning yellow of polymethylmethacrylate (PMMA), known commercially as Plexiglas, Lucite, or Perspex, on irradiation persist for a time after radiation and thus lend themselves conveniently to total (or integrated) dose measurements.

On the whole, solid-state detectors are not yet as capable of high-precision measurements as is the ionization chamber, which is based on the ionization of a gas as the result of interaction with radiation. No doubt these solid-state detection methods will be coupled with an improved technology such that the precision of solid-state detectors will become increasingly better. The obvious advantages of solid-state detectors— small size, ruggedness, and ultimately low cost—will then probably result in their replacing devices of the ionization-chamber type in many areas of radiation dosimetry.

The Solid-State Ionization Process

In recent years there has been considerable development in the field of semiconductor junction devices, consisting essentially of a p-n junction (Section 6.5) such as, for example, a silicon diode. When one electron is freed from a valence bond by radiation, we have, of course, an electron-hole pair. This situation is somewhat analogous to the electron-ion pairs which appear in a gas as the result of radiation interacting with the gas. For this reason, these p-n junction devices are sometimes called *solid-state ionization chambers*.

The Thermal Effect

Probably the most direct and possibly most difficult method of detecting and measuring the absorbed dose of radiation is to observe the temperature of the absorber rise as energy is absorbed. This is the method of *calorimetry*. It is difficult because, as we have indicated earlier, large doses of radiation, that is, large from the point of view of potential hazard, result nevertheless in exceedingly small temperature increases. The whole premise of this method of radiation detection is, of course, that essentially all radiation energy transferred to, that is, absorbed in, a material is ultimately degraded to heat.

Biological Effects

The destruction of living tissue, such as bacteria, phage, or drosophila (fruit fly) eggs, is presently still being used as a relatively crude radiation measurement technique in some contexts. However, this physiological effect, this damaging of living tissue, on the part of ionizing radiation, was frequently used for measurement in the early days of radiography and radiotherapy. It was observed, for example, how much radiation was required to produce reddening of the skin, that is, to produce a mild erythema. This unit of radiation was known as an *erythema dose.*

On the whole, it would seem that unless particular biological indicators, such as the destruction of phage, are required for certain experimentation, the biological method of detecting radiation is hardly convenient or desirable, and moreover, from the standpoint of measurement neither precise nor accurate. For example, estimates of erythema exposures vary as widely as from 400 R to 1000 R, depending on the particular circumstances of the irradiation. On the other hand, one must admit that the death by irradiation of drosophila eggs is a much more reliable indicator. Almost invariably the same percentage of a large number of eggs is destroyed by a certain exposure, say 90% by 500 R.

11.4 RADIATION MEASUREMENT DEVICES

The measurement of radiation, as we implied earlier, is known as *dosimetry.* The instruments involved are variously known as *dosemeters, dosimeters,* and *dose-rate meters.* As a general rule, the "dose" these meters measure is what we have previously defined as "exposure." Hence these meters are calibrated in terms of roentgens.

Modern dosimetry may be considered to have begun in 1928 when the roentgen was internationally accepted as the unit of exposure. Since the R is defined in terms of the ionization produced in air, it is not surprising that the standard instrument for measuring exposure, in R, is the so-called free-air ionization chamber, which we shall describe shortly.

Dosemeters and Dose-Rate Meters

In the measurement of radiation exposures, two different types of information may be sought: the total exposure, in R, or the time rate of exposure, in R/min. If we restrict ourselves for the moment to radiation measurements made via the ionizing effect of radiation on a gas such as is involved in Fig. 11.3, then this distinction between exposure and exposure rate can be clarified in terms of our knowledge of electric charge and electric current.

The dosemeter, which measures exposure, ultimately gives a reading on the basis of the electric charge which transfers during the time of the exposure. However, since charge per unit time is current, we see that a dose-rate meter would be one in which the reading is based on electrical current.

The above distinction is shown in Fig. 11.4. In the case of both the devices shown, radiation produces ionization, which provides the vehicle for charge transfer. In the case of the dosemeter, one first charges the capacitor C by closing switch S. Then switch S is opened. The capacitor will remain charged until ionizing radiation permits charge to transfer through the ionization chamber, thus discharging the capacitor. The more

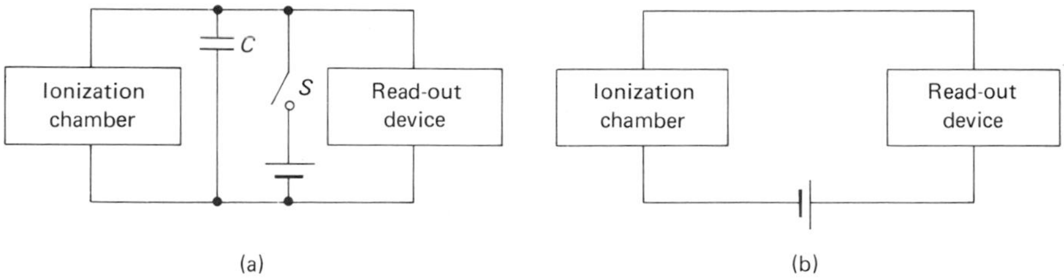

FIG. 11.4. The essential difference between a dosemeter (a), and a dose-rate meter (b).

intense the radiation and the longer it is in effect, the more the ionization in the chamber and hence the more charge leaves one side of the capacitor to neutralize the charge on the other. From Eq. (2.6), we see that as the capacitor's charge decreases so does the voltage across the capacitor plates. This means the readout device could be a voltmeter, which in turn could be calibrated directly in roentgens.

The ratemeter, on the other hand, supplies a continuous constant voltage across the ionization chamber. This means that as long as ionization is taking place there will be a current through the readout device. This readout device is therefore an ammeter. The size of the current through the ammeter will vary as the intensity of the ionizing radiation varies and will, of course, be zero when the ionizing radiation stops. The instrument must consequently be read while the irradiation is taking place. Since, as we said before, the current gets larger as the ionizing rate increases with increased radiation intensity, it is possible to calibrate this readout device directly in R/min.

Because the importance to the patient of weighing the risks of examination against its merits cannot be overemphasized, it is fair to say that diagnostic x-ray departments should have both dosemeters and dose-rate meters available.

From the standpoint of x-ray personnel monitoring, of course, it has become standard practice to wear a dosemeter, based on the photographic effect of radiation, that is, a film badge.

The Standard Ionization Chamber

To satisfy the definition of the roentgen, that is, to provide a primary standard for the calibration of other radiation meters, a so-called standard free-air ionization chamber is required. Such a chamber is shown in Fig. 11.5. In actual practice this chamber may look considerably more complicated, as may be seen in Fig. 11.6, which shows a modern standard free-air chamber employed by the National Research Council of Canada for the calibration of radiation-measuring instruments in use in therapy and diagnosis.

Let us look at the essential features of operation of the free-air chamber. The same basic principles will suffice to clarify the operation of the condenser-R chamber which we shall describe later.

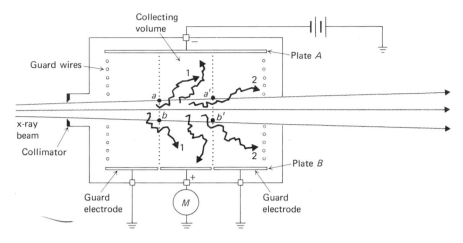

FIG. 11.5. Schematic of a standard free-air ionization chamber. *M* is the measurement device, such as an electrometer. Note that the grounded side is the high-potential side in this case. The guard wires are maintained at a series of intermediate potentials between the low potential of plate *A* and the ground potential of plate *B*. Along with the guard plates these guard wires help to keep the electric field perpendicular to plates *A* and *B* throughout the collecting volume.

A relatively narrow beam of x-rays passes through the collimator and enters the region between the two parallel plates *A* and *B*. These plates are connected to a source of EMF such that there is a potential gradient of the order of 200 volts/cm between them. In essence, then, the ionization chamber is a capacitor.

Because of the potential difference between the plates, the freed electrons and negative ions produced as the result of the x-rays will go one

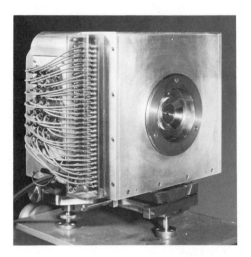

FIG. 11.6. Standard free-air ionization chamber, designed and built at the National Research Council of Canada (Photograph courtesy NRC)

way, while the positive ions will go the other. In Fig. 11.5 this means that the positive ions will be collected by plate A.

So that the ion pairs may be collected from a specified volume of air, as is required if the definition of the roentgen is to be fulfilled, two important factors must be considered in the design of the free-air chamber. First of all, a uniform electric field must be achieved in the critical volume of air. This volume is indicated by the letters a, a', b', b. Only if the electric field is uniform in this region can one be assured that only the charged particles originating in this region are collected. So that this end may be achieved, the actual collecting part of plate B is in the center (shaded part), while insulated from it on either side are what are known as *guard electrodes*. These electrodes prevent the fringing of the electric field at the outer edges of the collecting plate and thus help to accurately define the active, or critical, air volume $aa'b'b$.

The second consideration involves the fact that some of the ions collected will undoubtedly have been produced by electrons originating outside the critical volume represented by $aa'b'b$. An example is a charged particle of track 1. However, if the geometry of the chamber is properly designed, for every such track-1 outsider collected, there is a track-2 charged particle due to electron action within the critical volume, but not collected. So things can be arranged so that the net effect is that the charge collected at the plates is equivalent to that of all ions arising from the action of the photo and Compton electrons produced by the x-rays in the region of $aa'b'b$. As we have already learned, this situation is referred to as *electronic equilibrium*.

But what if the plates of the ionization chamber are closer to the critical volume $aa'b'b$ than the maximum range of the primary and secondary electrons originated by the x-ray beam? This would mean that some electrons would be collected before they had expended all their energies in the production of ions; then the electrometer, the device which measures the charge collected, would give a false indication. In terms of roentgens, the electrometer would indicate a lower exposure value than the true one. Fortunately, this problem is obviated relatively easily, if the x- or γ-ray energy is not too high: Plates A and B are arranged far enough away from the critical volume so as to be beyond the range of electrons liberated by the x-ray beam. Similar considerations apply with respect to the distance of the collimator from the active volume $aa'b'b$. In short, $aa'b'b$ must be surrounded by a thickness of air greater than the range of the most energetic of the liberated electrons. For x-rays produced at 200 kV this means that plates A and B must be some 40 cm apart, while the active region has dimensions something like $\overline{aa'} = 10$ cm, and $\overline{ab} = 2$ cm. Obviously the plate separation must increase as higher-energy x-rays are employed. In the case of 500-keV x-rays, the plates would have to be almost 1 meter apart. Such an increase in dimension demanded by higher-energy radiation soon places the free-air chamber outside the realm of practicality. For this reason, among others, the standard air chamber is not employed for energies in excess of 3 MeV. As a consequence, the roentgen is not defined for photon energies above 3 MeV.

As we have described it, the standard air chamber is a dosemeter. That is, it has an electrometer that measures collected electric charge. It is also possible to have a current-detecting meter, which means that the chamber is turned into a dose-rate meter.

Because of their size and complexity, standard air chambers are not generally employed except as primary standards in standardization laboratories. In actual practice the x-ray technician will, however, find various modifications of this device, such as a condenser R-meter, which we shall describe next.

The Condenser R-Meter

We have just mentioned that, because of the requirement of achieving electronic equilibrium, the free-air chamber becomes impractical for general-purpose use. However, if the air could be compressed, then in principle, at least, a chamber of smaller dimensions could be devised, since the range of the ionizing particles decreases as the density of the medium being ionized increases. Therein lies a practical solution to the problem of size.

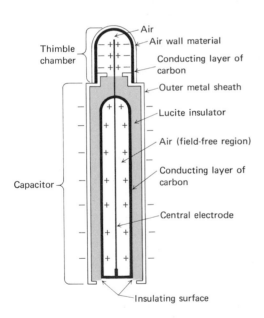

FIG. 11.7. Schematic of a Victoreen condenser chamber, showing the thimble ionization chamber affixed to a cylindrical condenser.

What is done, in effect, is not to compress air but something simpler: to construct the chamber of an air-equivalent material. By that we mean a material which is much denser than air but has about the same atomic number as air ($Z \approx 7.6$). Such an air-equivalent chamber is shown in the top part of Fig. 11.7. It is called a *thimble chamber*. It may be made of bakelite coated on the inside wall with carbon to act as one electrode, with the other, an axial electrode, made of aluminum.

The *condenser chamber* itself consists of the thimble chamber, in which the important ionization processes take place, connected to a cylindrical capacitor. (Capacitors used to be, and still are, called condensers by some people; hence the name condenser chamber.) Condenser chambers may be made in a variety of shapes, depending on their particular use. One of the commonly employed chambers is the Victoreen R-chamber. A cross section of an R-chamber is shown in Fig. 11.7. The overall dimensions of this device are about 6 in. by $\frac{3}{4}$ in. in diameter. The thimble chamber itself may be about 1 in. long.

The purpose of connecting the thimble chamber, which itself is like a capacitor, to the larger cylindrical capacitor is simply to increase the capacitance. This arrangement permits the measurement of reasonably large exposures without completely discharging the capacitor when ionization takes place in the thimble chamber. In other words, one avoids placing a low upper limit on the measurable exposure by this means. In this connection it can be shown, as is indeed plausible, that if we want to measure large exposures we need only a small thimble chamber but a large overall capacitance, while for very low exposures for which extreme sensitivity is required we need a large thimble chamber but a relatively small capacitance.

Looking carefully at Fig. 11.7 might raise at least one interesting question. For example, does not ionization of the air within the main capacitor chamber take place and thus upset the whole intent of simulating the air chamber? After all, the capacitor sheath is not air-wall material. We can find the answer if we recall our discussion in Section 2.2, in which we said that the electric field inside a hollow conductor is zero. In the absence of an electric field in the region (marked field-free region in Fig. 11.7), whatever ions are formed rapidly recombine.

Incidentally, note that the region between the carbon layer and the outer sheath is, of course, not a field-free region. But there is no significant charge transfer in this region because it is filled by a good solid insulator in which there is little electron migration and at the surface of which few electrons are emitted.

If we now provide this condenser R-chamber with some device to charge its capacitor and a device for reading how much it has discharged upon exposure to ionizing radiation, we have what is called a *condenser R-meter*. The device used to indicate the loss of charge on the capacitor and thus the exposure in R or mR is called an *electrometer*. Let us discuss electrometers next.

Electrometers

Electrometers are basically devices for indicating potential differences. In that sense the electroscopes mentioned in Section 2.1 are electrometers. In fact, a clever modification of the gold-leaf electroscope is the so-called *string electrometer*, of which there are several versions.

One version of a string electrometer is shown in Fig. 11.8. The "string" is actually a platinum-coated quartz fiber, which is charged oppositely to the deflection electrode. The deflection electrode is a long screw which

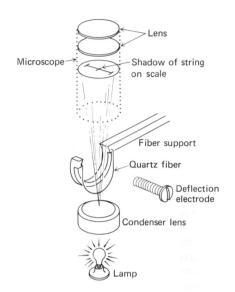

Lens

Microscope

Shadow of string on scale

Fiber support

Quartz fiber

Deflection electrode

Condenser lens

Lamp

FIG. 11.8. Quartz-fiber or "string" electrometer, as employed in the Victoreen Model 570 R-meter. (Courtesy Victoreen Instrument Co.)

is adjustable and which projects from the side of the electrometer casing. By properly adjusting the screw, one can arrange it so that the Coulomb attractive force of the screw on the fiber is such that the shadow of the quartz fiber moves across the scale in an approximately linear fashion with changes in voltage between the fiber and the deflection electrode.

So what happens? We charge the condenser chamber and the electrometer together by some means. This can be done several ways: for example, with the appropriate charging circuitry supplied by energy from the mains. That is, one can plug the cord of the charging device into a wall socket. The Coulomb force of the fixed-deflection electrode on the oppositely charged quartz fiber now causes the quartz fiber to move toward the deflection electrode against the restoring force, that is, spring action, of the quartz fiber as it becomes twisted from its normal equilibrium position. At some predesignated maximum charging voltage, say 400 volts, the quartz fiber has its maximum deflection. The shadow of the fiber rests at zero R on the viewing scale.

Next the condenser chamber is removed from the charging device and the charging device becomes disconnected from the electrometer. We have now, separately, a fully charged condenser chamber and a fully charged electrometer.

The chamber is then exposed to ionizing radiation. Charge in the condenser chamber "leaks off," that is, recombines. We now reconnect the condenser chamber to the electrometer and some charge will flow from the electrometer to the partially discharged condenser chamber, thereby lowering the potential difference between the quartz fiber and the deflection electrode. We can note the deflection of the quartz fiber to a new position by looking at its shadow on the scale calibrated in roentgens. The greater the exposure, the greater the charge loss in the condenser

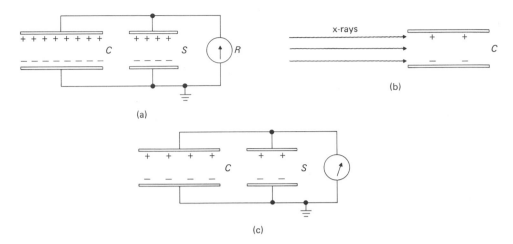

(a)

(b)

(c)

FIG. 11.9. The steps in using a condenser R-meter. *C* is the condenser chamber, *S* the capacitor part of the electrometer, and *R* the electrometer read-out device, a voltmeter calibrated in roentgens. (a) Charging the chamber *C* and electrometer *S*. (The voltage source for charging is not shown.) (b) X-rays partially discharge the chamber *C*. (c) Reading is taken. Charge drifts from *S* to *C* until the voltage across both *S* and *C* is the same. (The number of charged particles shown in each case must not, of course, be taken literally.)

chamber, the greater the charge migration from the electrometer to the condenser chamber. But the lower the charge on the electrometer, the less the Coulomb force and the more the quartz fiber moves back toward its uncharged equilibrium position. This sequence of events is summarized in Fig. 11.9.

So-called electronic or valve electrometers are also employed. Figure 11.10 shows, in simplified form, how such a device might work. Note that both one electrode and one side of the electrometer circuit are grounded. If the central electrode of the electrometer is now negative with respect to ground, the grid of the triode (see Section 7.7) is negative with respect to the cathode and thereby impedes the current in the measuring circuit, as we note by looking at the meter *M*. As the condenser chamber becomes

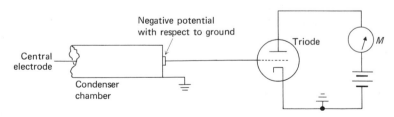

Fig. 11.10. Electronic or valve electrometer.

partially discharged through exposure to ionizing radiation, the central electrode of the chamber becomes less negative with respect to ground, the potential difference between it and ground becomes less. Hence also the grid of the triode becomes less negative with respect to the cathode, thus offering less opposition to current, and the meter reading in terms of current goes up. In this particular simplified version, then, the larger the exposure of the condenser chamber the larger the current reading of the meter M. This meter could be calibrated in roentgens.

The Pocket Dosimeter

The pocket dosimeter, shown in Fig. 11.11, is about the size of a fountain pen. This instrument is essentially one of the condenser R-meter type discussed earlier; in other words, it is an integrating-type ionization chamber. In its simplest form it consists of a cylindrical ionization chamber with a central wire electrode.

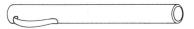

FIG. 11.11. A pocket dosimeter.

As well as the actual ionization chamber, pocket dosimeters frequently also include their own built-in electrometers, of the quartz-fiber type shown in Fig. 11.8. In this case all that is required in addition to the dosimeter itself is a charging device; dosimeters that even include their own chargers have recently become available.

What goes on in a self-reading dosimeter? When the central axial electrode of the dosimeter is charged, the stirrup fiber (of the type shown in Fig. 11.8) which is connected to the central electrode is displaced by Coulomb repulsion. After the device is exposed and there is resulting ionization in the chamber, the charge on the axial electrode is reduced, the Coulomb force is reduced, and the fiber moves toward the position it would occupy when no net electrical charge were on the electrode. One may read the various positions of the fiber by looking lengthwise through the chamber at a light and thus viewing it through a small optical magnifying system, including a scale calibrated in roentgens or milliroentgens. If the pocket dosimeter is employed for routine personnel monitoring, perhaps as an adjunct to the film badge, it is usually calibrated in mR.

The advantages of the pocket dosimeter are its convenient size, fairly high sensitivity and, unlike the film badge, its capability of being instantaneously read. On the other hand, because of electrical leakage, this dosimeter is not generally employed for measuring accumulated exposure over a protracted period of time. Frequently the procedure is to read and record the result daily. Another disadvantage of the pocket dosimeter is that when it gets a mechanical shock, such as happens when someone drops it, the position of the electrometer's fiber may change enough to give a spurious reading.

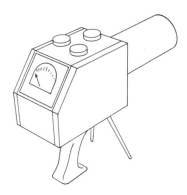

FIG. 11.12. The Cutie Pie, an ionization-chamber type ratemeter which yields immediate readings of x- and γ-radiation levels.

The Cutie Pie

The Cutie Pie, originated at the U. S. National Laboratory at Oak Ridge, is a small device for measuring β- and γ- rays; it has a pistol-grip handle, as shown in Fig. 11.12. It is an ionization-chamber type ratemeter which can detect radiation as low as a fraction of 1 mR/hr. Such meters offer various sensitivity ranges; for example, 0–5, 0–50, 0–500, and 0–5000 mR/hr.

The Cutie Pie is a very useful survey meter in that, although it is not as sensitive as the Geiger counter (which we shall discuss shortly), it has a flatter response to variations in x-ray energies than does the Geiger counter. What this means is that the exposure reading does not fluctuate significantly with changes in the quality of the x-ray beam. The reader will appreciate that it is possible to produce an exposure of a certain number of roentgens with one setting of kV and mA, and reproduce the exposure with a variety of different settings such as, say, reducing the kV and appropriately increasing the mA. If a meter does not have a flat response it will not show the same reading in the second case as in the first. It is said to be responsive to the photon energy. From the practical standpoint in the x-ray department, this means that a meter with a relatively flat response need have only one scale. A meter that is responsive to x-ray photon energies, on the other hand, would need to be calibrated on various scales for the various values of kV.

The Geiger Counter

The Geiger counter, more properly known as the Geiger-Müller or G-M counter, evolved from the work that Rutherford and Geiger did in connection with the counting of alpha particles in the early 1900's. The first counter of the type to be discussed here was constructed by Geiger and Müller in 1928. Since that time the G-M counter has become perhaps the mostly widely used of all radiation-measurement devices which can detect individual particles or photons.

Like the Cutie Pie, the Geiger counter is a ratemeter. It is a highly sensitive device which will detect radiation at levels as low as 0.1 mR/hr. On the other hand, as we mentioned in the discussion of the Cutie Pie, the Geiger counter is responsive to photon energies. If it has been calibrated with a radium source, it may be out by as much as a factor of 4 in the monitoring of x-rays produced at 100 kV.

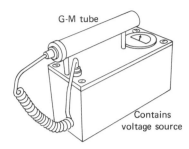

FIG. 11.13. Portable Geiger counter.

Figure 11.13 shows what a portable Geiger counter looks like. We shall investigate its operation by reviewing first of all what might happen in a device such as that represented schematically in Fig. 11.14 as the voltage across the electrodes is varied. One electrode consists of an axial conductor inserted through an insulating plug into a metallic gas-filled chamber which itself forms the second electrode.

Let us now suppose that a constant voltage of about 100 volts is applied between the central axial electrode, the anode, and the chamber, the cylindrical cathode. What happens when x-rays enter the chamber? Most of the x-ray photons pass right through it, but some are absorbed, and transfer energy to the gas via the ejection of photo and Compton electrons from the atoms of the gas. Ionization is achieved. At voltages from about 100 to 200 volts these electrons and ions are sufficiently affected by the electric field to prevent their recombining. The electrons move toward the axial anode under the influence of the applied electric field, and the positive gas ions migrate toward the chamber walls. Thus, as long as the x-ray intensity remains constant there will be a small constant current indicated by the meter, M. This current will increase if more ions are produced, and more ions can be produced by increasing the x-ray intensity. In other words, the current is a measure of x-ray intensity. When operated in this manner (with, incidentally, measuring circuitry that is slightly more complex than shown), this instrument is obviously of the same sort as the standard free-air chamber and the Cutie Pie. It is not surprising, therefore, that it is called an *ionization chamber*. Such a device was used in the original Bragg spectrometer (Fig. 9.14).

Now let us suppose that the voltage across the electrodes is raised to 500 volts, or perhaps somewhat higher. The electric field is now suffi-

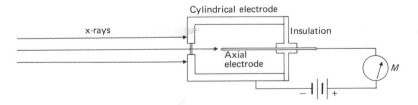

FIG. 11.14. A chamber for measuring x-ray intensity via the ionization process.

ciently large that the primary electrons produced by the interaction of the x-rays with gas gain considerable energy in being accelerated toward the axial electrode. These electrons knock electrons out of other gas atoms, and the secondary electrons themselves repeat the process. An avalanching process takes place, which greatly increases the amount of ionization produced by a single photon, over what such a photon would have produced at the ionization-chamber voltage of, say, 100–200 volts. The effect of a single photon can now readily be detected because it will result in perhaps 10^4 more ions than it would have at the ionization-chamber voltage.

We note one more point regarding this avalanching process. The greater the x-ray photon energy, the more the energy of the primary electron, the more secondary electrons produced, the larger the current pulse due to the photon. In other words, the size of the current pulse is proportional to photon energy. Therefore a chamber operated in this voltage region is called a *proportional counter*. The proportional counter is a very fast counter, capable of distinguishing between separate current pulses triggered at a rate of some 10^6 per sec. This rapid response rate is due to the fact that the ionization avalanche is confined to a very short part of the axial electrode. The avalanche does not spread along the length of the counter chamber.

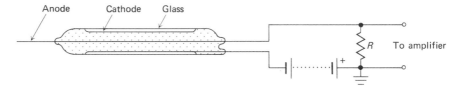

FIG. 11.15. Geiger-Müller counter tube.

If we next increase the potential difference across the electrodes still further, say to around 1000 volts, a new development takes place. We have a Geiger-Müller counter which works as follows. Because of the extremely large electric field in the chamber now, any ionization avalanche triggered by an x-ray photon, no matter what its energy (within limits, of course) will spread through the entire length of the counter chamber. This means two things: First, the G-M counter is even more sensitive than the proportional counter in that it provides greater amplification of any single ionizing event. And second, the counter's current pulses are less dependent on the energy of the x-ray photons.

In Fig. 11.15 we show a schematic of a G-M tube with part of its detection and amplification circuitry. The complete device of G-M tube and associated circuitry is what is generally called a Geiger counter. The G-M tube is essentially like the ionization chamber of Fig. 11.14. Specifically, the G-M tube consists of a cylindrical glass tube inside of which there is a metallic cylinder or metallic coating, and an axial electrode of thin wire. The tube is filled with a special mixture of gases (special for reasons we do not intend to pursue in this text) at a pressure of about 10 cm of Hg.

When an ionizing event takes place in the tube, an avalanche occurs along the entire length of the tube; a large current pulse appears. The current pulse causes a corresponding voltage drop across R. This voltage pulse is then amplified by electronic circuitry, employing either vacuum tubes such as the triode (Section 7.7) or transistors. If this amplified pulse is fed to a speaker, one hears the generally familiar "clicks" of the Geiger counter. Usually the circuitry also includes a meter which indicates the number of ionizing events per unit time, usually in counts/sec. If the Geiger counter is designed for radiological use, it may also be calibrated in R/min as well as counts/sec.

To sum up: a portable Geiger counter is a ratemeter which may be employed as a radiation survey monitor, particularly where very low radiation intensity is found. Perhaps one of the most useful applications of this device in the medical field is as a monitor to check possible contamination in radioisotope laboratories and to locate small lost radioactive sources. This is so because a Geiger counter is sensitive enough to detect the disintegration of a single nucleus.

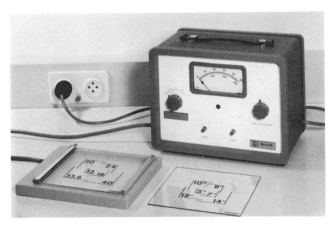

FIG. 11.16. Diagnostic x-ray monitor with transparent ionization chamber for various field sizes. (Courtesy N.V. Philips' Gloeilampenfabrieken, Eindhoven, Nederland.)

A Diagnostic X-Ray Monitor

Let us close our discussion of instruments based on ionization by considering a practical diagnostic x-ray monitor of considerable sophistication. This monitor employs a flat ionization chamber which has been calibrated by referral to some standard ionization chamber. Such a monitor chamber is essentially the same as the flat ionization chamber employed in an ionization chamber timer. A device of this type, including the associated electrometer, is shown in Fig. 11.16.

This particular device has an interesting advantage over a number of other radiation meters in that it takes account not only of the exposure at a point but also of the field size undergoing irradiation. It has a flat chamber to cover the different possible fields the technician may wish to employ. With circuitry which integrates, that is, adds, the exposure over the entire area of the x-ray beam, a reading in R-cm² is given. This is an obvious advantage since, as we shall indicate in Fig. 11.19, the deleterious effect of radiation increases roughly in proportion to the surface area exposed.

Another aspect of considerable significance of the instrument shown in Fig. 11.16 is that it has been devised to take account of the quality of the x-ray beam, thus allowing for the specific behavior of the beam with respect to the tissue being irradiated. In that sense, such an instrument approaches the measurement of what the medical practitioner is most interested in, namely the locally absorbed dose. Actually, this instrument doesn't go quite that far. But it does measure the total energy imparted to the patient. Hence it could be calibrated in foot-pounds, calories, joules, or watt-seconds. Actually some such meters are calibrated in milliwatt-seconds. However, although the measurement quoted in milliwatt-seconds or milli-joules is correct in that this expresses the actual energy imparted to the patient, the current practice is to calibrate such meters in R-cm², since the roentgen has found more ready acceptance in the medical field.

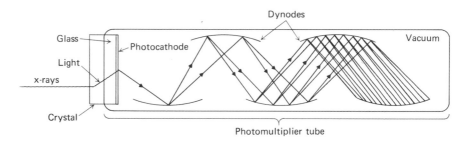

FIG. 11.17. Schematic of a scintillation counter. The electrical connections are not shown.

The Scintillation Counter

The scintillation counter is, in essence, a fluorescent phosphor (see Section 10.6) coupled to a photomultiplier tube (see Section 7.8).

The phosphor generally used to detect x-rays is a sodium iodide crystal activated with a small amount of thallium. This phosphor emits blue light when subjected to x-rays. The phosphor crystal is cemented to the end of a photomultiplier tube, as shown in Fig. 11.17. Every x-ray photon interacting with the phosphor produces a flash of light which passes into the photomultiplier tube and there causes the emission of electrons from the photocathode. Then by the process of secondary emission, as discussed in Section 7.8, ultimately a very large number of electrons is collected at the final dynode. The result is a relatively large signal for as little as one x-ray photon. Furthermore, this whole fluorescent and multiplying process requires less than a microsecond, so that a scintillation counter can operate at an exceedingly high count rate, thus permitting wide latitude in the x-ray intensity which can be measured.

Scintillation counters can, of course, be used for α- and β-radiations as well as for x- or γ-rays. In fact, in the days before the photomultiplier tube, the scintillation method of measurement was largely restricted to α-rays, since the fluorescent effect is much less effective with β- and γ-rays than with α-particles.

At present scintillation counters are finding wide use in medicine. An example is the use of a scintillation counter in thyroid scanning, as was shown in Fig. 1.18. Scintillation counters have also recently been used in the determination of diagnostic x-ray spectra, such as was shown in Fig. 9.20.

One outcome of the development of large organic phosphor crystals, as well as liquid scintillators, is of prime interest to the health physicist. We are referring to whole-body counters, employed for the direct evaluation of the radioactivity in humans. In the case of the liquid whole-body counter, the subject lies on a pallet inside a cylindrical housing and is surrounded by an annular tank of liquid scintillator. Such a counter also lends itself to the determination of the effects of radioactive fallout materials lodged in the body.

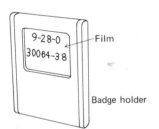

FIG. 11.18. A film badge.

The Film Badge

Undoubtedly the most widely used device for radiation monitoring of personnel is the film badge (Fig. 11.18). The film badge is particularly suitable for measuring the cumulative exposure resulting from low-level exposures over a period of time. In x-ray departments, for example, it is common practice for personnel to wear the same badge for a two-week period. At the end of this time the film is removed from the badge holder and the exposure is evaluated, generally by some outside agency. Usually the permissible amount of exposure is specified in protective regulations set forth by the government.

The film badge, as the name implies, is based on the photographic effect of x-rays, as is the whole science and art of radiography. Although nowadays special films are available for film badges, it would be quite possible to establish such a monitoring system by using small dental x-ray films. The exposure is evaluated by measurements of the density of the film as compared to the density of a control film. Thus density may be correlated directly to exposure in roentgens, which—on the basis of the relationship between exposure and absorbed dose, Eq. (11.2), and of the relationship between dose equivalent and absorbed dose, Eq. (11.3)—can then be translated into rems. Consequently, as a rule, the evaluation of the radiation dosage is presented to the badge wearer in terms of millirem.

The badge holder is commonly fitted with several different filters and a "window." The purpose of the filters is to aid in the approximation of the quality of the radiation. The "window" permits the detection of low-energy beta-rays which could be stopped by the badge-holder material.

Film badges have a number of advantages as personnel-monitoring devices. They are relatively cheap; they are extremely rugged; they are not subject to gross errors as is delicate electronic equipment; and they provide a permanent record.

On the other hand, film badges have a distinct *dis*advantage in that the wearer does not become aware of any unusually high exposure to radiation until the film is developed. When the person does receive a report of a high reading, he may no longer be able to track down the cause of the high exposure.

11.5   RADIATION HAZARDS AND PROTECTIVE MEASURES

Biological Effects of Radiation

As we have said, all absorbed x-radiation, no matter how small the dose, has deleterious biological effects. We would like to comment on the fact that all medical radiography is harmful. The fact that it nevertheless continues to be used is due to the undoubted benefits it also brings. But if some harmless method of diagnosis could be invented to take the place of the x-ray method, we could dispense with the decision which has to be made each time radiography is contemplated; that is, which will do the patient more harm, the exposure to radiation or the failure to utilize this diagnostic procedure?

As implied earlier, the harmful consequences result from the ionizing effects of the radiation within the body. For example, electron bonds between different parts of large molecules in the human organism may be disrupted. The broken molecules may then react with other molecules and so form substances which are detrimental to life. Or, by changing some molecules from their original form, the radiation may deprive some vital cells of materials they require to continue living. Little is known of the exact mechanism by which damage is produced.

Radiation hazards may be classified as either somatic or genetic. Somatic hazards are those which concern the cells which constitute the body as a whole. Genetic hazards are those which concern the reproductive cells, although, of course, somatic cells are involved in genetics (when such cells divide to produce new cells). By "genetics" in the present context we mean the genetics of new people rather than the genetics of new tissue in the same person.

The somatic effects of medical radiography form a much smaller hazard today than was the case in the past. Patients undergoing radiography no longer receive burns, or suffer from epilation (hair falling out). As time goes on and films, screens, and image intensifiers become more efficient, such happenings will become even less likely than today. But still so little is known about such things as the carcinogenic effects of radiation that every care must continue to be taken to keep all irradiation to an absolute minimum. Research into this and other aspects of radiation hazards is hampered by the long latent period which may occur between exposure and clinical manifestation. At least one well-documented case exists in which the latent period was known to be nearly 50 years.

Table 11.4 lists some exposures and their somatic effects on humans.

Table 11.4

SOME EXPOSURES AND THEIR EFFECTS ON HUMANS

Exposure, roentgens	Effect
25–50 R whole body	Possible blood changes (e.g., blood-cell destruction)
~ 100 R whole body	Possible radiation sickness
~ 250 R to gonads	Temporary sterility (~ 1 year)
~ 300 R localized	Loss of hair, reddening of skin
~ 400 R whole body	Death to 50% of exposed human population, or 50% chance of death in average individual
600 R or more, whole body	Death

Genetic damage due to radiation is manifested in the uniting of a sperm and an ovum, one or both of which have suffered radiation damage, and the subsequent production of an abnormality in an offspring. Such a change is called a *mutation*. Some mutations may confer an advantage on the child; nevertheless, many are harmful. Genetic hazards are even harder to pinpoint than somatic hazards so far as individuals are concerned. Although many people are alarmed by the population explosion, the radiation geneticist regrets that humans produce further generations so slowly. He has so little opportunity for seeing what happens to a person's great-great-grandchildren.

Also, genetics and radiobiology deal so much with averages and total populations that, when one is talking about hazards to the individual, one can comment only in terms of probabilities. We can discuss the increase of mutation rates in populations following a rise in radiation doses to those populations, but we cannot predict the future for an individual. What we do know is that there seems to be no threshold to the genetic effects; any increase of the dose to a population, no matter how small, appears to increase the mutation rate.

It must be made clear at this point that in a discussion of the biological effects of any absorbed radiation, the body region irradiated is of considerable consequence.   For example, the three x-ray exposures shown
in Fig. 11.19 are by no means biologically equivalent, even if the exposure
specified in roentgens is the same for each case.   The whole-body radiation
of case C is considerably more harmful than the specific-area exposure of
case A because of the larger number of cells irradiated and the consequently relatively more limited opportunity for cellular repair.   Case B,
which represents gonadal radiation, is of special significance with regard
to genetic defects.   Changes to genes are cumulative and irreversible.

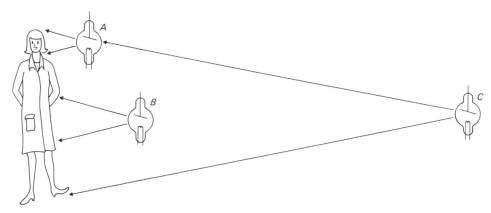

FIG. 11.19. The amount of radiation injury depends not only on the exposure in roentgens,
but also on the area exposed. Hence R-cm² and the body part irradiated give a better indication of possible deleterious effects than just the exposure in R.

From the standpoint of possible genetic hazards, the contribution of
diagnostic radiation is not entirely insignificant. Averaged out over whole
populations, this contribution appears to be of the order of the contribution
by natural background radiation (100 mR/yr), although available estimates
vary widely from 14 mR/yr* to 136 mR/yr.†

Radiation Guides

Radiation guides are dealt with by the International Commission on
Radiological Protection (ICRP). This commission consists of internationally recognized experts in the various disciplines necessary to formulate
acceptable radiation protection standards.   The commission specifies
maximum permissible absorbed doses (MPD) for different groups of per-

---

* British Medical Research Council, *The Hazards to Man of Nuclear and Allied Radiations*.
London: Her Majesty's Stationery Office, 1960.

† Laughlin, J. S., and I. Pullman, *Gonadal Dose Received in the Medical Use of X-rays*. Prepared for the Genetics Panel of the National Academy of Sciences, Washington, D.C., 1956.

sons. Such a dose is defined as that dose which, in the light of present knowledge, is not expected to cause detectable bodily injury to a person at any time during his lifetime. Although these maximum permissible doses are recommended as upper limits, the overriding consideration must be in all cases to keep irradiation to an absolute minimum. We should also note that current radiation guides may be changed in future ICRP publications. In general, in the past, each time the ICRP has come out with a new publication, it has stated values of maximum permissible dosage that are lower than the MPD's suggested as guides in the previous publications. You are urged, now as a student and later as an x-ray technician, to refer to the latest publications of the International Commission on Radiological Protection.

Table 11.5

RECOMMENDED LIMITS ON ABSORBED DOSE DUE TO EXTERNAL RADIATION*

Occupational Critical organs (includes the whole body, head and trunk, active blood-forming organs, gonads)	*Nonoccupational* Individuals in vicinity of controlled areas	*General population* Average exposure, exclusive of background radiation
3 rems/13 weeks Cumulative for life: [5 (Age − 18)] rems	1.5 rem/yr (adult workers occasionally entering radiation areas) 0.5 rem/yr (general public, including children, living in the neighborhood of controlled areas)	5 rems by age 30

* ICRP (latest recommendations)

Some radiation guides, in the form of maximum permissible doses as recommended by the ICRP, are shown in Table 11.5 for three groups of persons: (a) those occupationally exposed, (b) those living in the vicinity of a controlled area (that is, an area in which a radiation hazard exists), and (c) the general population. On the whole, these ICRP recommendations are supported in Canada (Atomic Energy Control Act), the U.K. (British Medical Research Council), the U.S., (National Committee on Radiation Protection and Measurements), and in many other countries.

The implication of these recommendations is that the chief concern is a problem of genetics. Occupationally exposed persons are permitted higher maximum doses because they form such a small minority of the general population.

It should be pointed out that the recommendations of Table 11.5 are by no means comprehensive. They represent basic recommendations only. Other considerations, such as minimum ages, maximum dose rates,

Table 11.6

DOSE TO THE GONADS PER YEAR RESULTING FROM BACKGROUND RADIATION*

External radiation	
Cosmic rays	24
Local gamma rays (strongly dependent on locale)	50
Radon in the air (3×10^{-13} curies/liter)	1
Internal radiation	
Potassium 40	21
Carbon 14, radon, and its decay products	4
Total gonadal dose per year	100

* Approximate values in mrads/year per person in the U.K. (Varies considerably with locale.) Based on data in *The Hazards to Man of Nuclear and Allied Radiations*, London: 1956 and 1960. Report to the Medical Research Council. Crown copyright.

and dose rates to individual parts of the body are given in detail in the reports of the ICRP.

For the radiographer, perhaps the most important figures of Table 11.5 are 3 rems/13 weeks, and the total MPD for a given age, calculated by the formula, [5 (Age − 18)] rems, which really just means 5 rems/year after age 18. This is not to suggest that x-ray technicians should strive for 3 rems/13 weeks. Far from it. As a matter of fact, perusal of the formula [5 (Age − 18)] rems shows that one would exceed the limit implied by the formula if one experienced doses of 3 rems in each and every 13-week interval. (On the other hand, an emergency radiation guide in case of nuclear fallout sets the maximum dose at 100 rem in 6 weeks.)

In other words, 3 rems/13 weeks is the upper limit, the MPD. As we shall suggest again later, with reference to film-badge monitoring, the technician should become seriously concerned if he averages half this MPD in any 13-week period. Competent radiography can be done with considerably less than 0.5 rem/13 weeks to the operator. And remember: Don't wear your film badge when having your own x-ray taken! The MPD's quoted for radiation workers are exclusive of radiation received for medical purposes.

Some Significant Doses

So far in this chapter we have dealt with dosage and dosimetry and have supplied occasional examples of exposure, particularly from the x-ray department. It will now be instructive to note a number of typical absorbed doses. These measured and estimated doses are presented in Tables 11.6 and 11.7. Of course, the actual doses vary from place to place, but one can get some idea of the orders of magnitude of doses from the figures given. The reason why a gonadal dose is specified is, of course, the concern with regard to genetic hazard.

Radiation Protection

Although this text is not intended to serve as a basis for a radiation protection program, in the present section we shall, however, outline the

Table 11.7

GONADAL DOSE ESTIMATIONS, MILLIRAD*

Sweden				
Some typical examinations	Gonad dose per examination		Gonad dose per person per year without regard to age and fertility	
	Male	Female	Male	Female
Pelvis and hips	1080	200	7.7	1.0
Barium enema	255	2065	0.9	7.4
Lumbar spine and sacrum	375	680	2.7	3.9
Hysterosalpingography		2650		2.5
Urethrocystography	2500		2.1	
Pelvimetry		1500		0.7
Stomach	8.5	32	0.1	0.4
Lung	1.6	4.6	small	0.1

United States				
Some typical examinations	Gonad dose per examination, ages 12–30 yr		Probable significant gonad dose per person per year	
	Male	Female	Male	Female
Skeleton, pelvic region	2000	1000	20.5	9.2
Abdomen and colon	200	500	4.8	4.9
Lower GI (fluoroscopy)	750	1500	6.4	9.7
Stomach and upper GI	200	300	1.6	2.1
Urinary tract	300	1000	0.5	1.4
Obstetric examination, mother		260–2500		9.5
Pyelography	2000	1200	4.9	2.6
Salpingography		1000		1.6
Chest	1.2	0.3	2.3	1.1

Probable significant gonad dose $= 135 \pm 100$ mrad per person per year

* Based on findings of the ICRP and the ICRU, as published in *Physics in Medicine and Biology* 2, 2, 107 (1957).

methodology of protection, indicate relevant sources of information, and bring to a focus some points which have arisen elsewhere in the book and which are pertinent here. We include a discussion of protection measures to bring home to the student the importance of recognizing the ever-present hazards associated with his work.

A program of protection against radiation hazards in medical radiography must concern itself with patients, radiation workers, and others likely to be exposed to hazard. Such a program should consist of foresight in the design of the x-ray installation, careful control of working methods, and the taking of radiation surveys.

Fundamental to any such program are the three basic principles of radiation protection, which may be summarized in three words: *time, distance,* and *shielding.*

By "time" is meant keeping the time of exposure to radiation at a minimum.

"Distance" means that if exposure is necessary, then, within the limits of practicality, one should keep as far away from the radiation source as possible. Recall that radiation intensity in air falls off approximately as the square of the distance from the source.

"Shielding" means availing yourself of as much shielding from the radiation as the job permits. For x-ray technicians this implies such procedures as making radiographic exposures only when behind the lead shielding of the control booth, and wearing a lead apron when assisting the radiologist in fluoroscopy. At this point we should recall again that, as discussed in Chapter 10, both atomic number and thickness of the shielding material have a bearing on the attenuation of the radiation. In general, the higher the atomic number and thickness of the shielding material, the better the protection from x-rays.

With these ideas in mind, the design of x-ray installations from a protection point of view consists basically of limiting the primary beam at the tube to that part of the patient being examined; of protecting staff and others from the primary beam by means of suitable primary barriers; and of the protection of staff and others from secondary radiation. To these ends, design recommendations deal with such things as maximum permissible rates of leakage of tube housings and also with the computation of the thicknesses of lead or concrete primary and secondary barriers. Such computations take into account radiation guides (maximum permissible doses), the distance of the protected area from the source, the type of machine, how the machine is to be used, and the occupancy rate of the areas to be protected.

Filtration of the primary beam and limitation of dose rates received by the patient are also taken into account in the design of the installation. This latter point will come up in Chapter 12 when we discuss the shortcomings of conventional fluoroscopy.

All these matters and recommendations for working methods, surveys, and inspections are referred to in Handbook 76, *Medical X-ray Protection up to Three Million Volts,* listed at the end of this chapter. In Handbook 76 specific installations are discussed separately. Each discussion is arranged in three sections: "operating procedures," "equipment," and "structural shielding."

Proper working methods have two objectives: (1) keeping the dose to the patient at a minimum consistent with obtaining good radiographs, and (2) suitable protection of x-ray personnel.

Besides methods used to keep radiation to the patient to a minimum, operating procedures are greatly concerned with the protection of staff. Protection of operators can be achieved if the operators keep out of, and away from, the primary beam and avoid irradiation by scatter (see Section 10.5), and by means of adequate shielding and regular personnel monitoring.

Protection surveys and inspections (also dealt with in Handbook 76) are carried out, before the use of new equipment, to determine the suitability of the installation design. Thereafter regular checks are carried out to see that there has been no deterioration of conditions. Additional surveys are required whenever any changes are made in the type of equipment or in the manner of its use. If any survey should show that improvements in protection are necessary, a further survey is made to confirm that the alterations to the installation are satisfactory.

As stated above, all radiation workers should maintain a continuing program of personnel monitoring, such as mentioned in Section 11.4. Let us underscore the importance of personal responsibility, that is, the importance of the technician's serious consideration of all protective measures. Strict adherence to safety rules and control measures, such as wearing film badges, is to be highly recommended.

If it is common practice (as it should be) that film-badge readings are regularly evaluated, say at two-week intervals, then the radiographer should make it his business to be aware of his own badge reading. Although the most desirable reading would be above background by only a negligible amount a reading of 20 millirems per two-week interval is presently considered quite reasonable. Even readings of 40 millirems per two weeks are perhaps not unusual. On the other hand, if readings such as 200 millirems per two weeks, or higher, turn up more than occasionally, the procedures followed and the equipment used should be carefully scrutinized.

QUESTIONS

1. Define the roentgen.

2. The exposure due to an x-ray beam at a given point in space can be altered by five factors over which the radiographer has control. What are those five factors?

3. If an x-ray tube delivers 20 R/min in air at 50 cm from the target when operating at 10 mA and 200 kV, estimate the exposure at a distance of 100 cm, given that the tube operates for 30 sec at 20 mA and 400 kV. [*Hint:* See Sections 9.2 and 11.1.] Why is your answer only an approximate one?

4. Will an ionization chamber placed at the position occupied by the skin surface read the same for the same technique whether or not the patient is in position? If there is a difference in reading, indicate the nature of the difference (that is, larger or smaller reading) and explain.

5. Assume that a chest PA is taken with a technique which results in an exposure of 300 mR in air. If the back-scatter factor is 1.4, what would be the actual skin or surface exposure of the patient?

6. As a rule, in which case is more radiation exposure involved for both patient and operator: radiography or fluoroscopy? Suggest why there is a difference.

7. Distinguish between exposure and absorbed dose, giving the units in which each is usually measured.

8. Would you expect the ratio of rads to roentgens to be larger for low-energy photons or for high-energy photons in the case of the exposure of a given absorber? Explain.

9. The quantitative relation between absorbed dose D in rads and exposure R in roentgens is given by $D = fR$. Suppose that one wanted to decrease the tube voltage in the interests of contrast but keep f approximately constant. What changes would one have to apply in filtration?

10. Perform the calculation which shows that an absorbed dose of 300 rads will raise the temperature of 1 gm of soft tissue about $7 \times 10^{-4} C°$.

11. State any six specifically different effects of x-rays which could be exploited for purposes of detection and measurement of exposure and/or absorbed dose.

12. What is the most direct method of measuring absorbed dose?

13. a) What is meant by solid-state detectors?
    b) Give an example of a radiation effect involved in one such detector.

14. Many radiation-detection devices depend on ionization.
    a) Name such a device.
    b) Describe fully the actual processes of primary and secondary ionization by x-rays.
    c) With the aid of a diagram, explain the basic operation of an ionization chamber.

15. a) Describe how photographic film is commonly used to monitor x-ray dosage.
    b) What is the purpose of the different metal strips often found in film-badge holders?

16. a) Explain the difference between a dose meter and a dose-rate meter.
    b) Indicate in what units each might be calibrated.

17. a) Describe the essential features of a condenser R-meter.
    b) List the steps involved in the actual use of such a meter.
    c) What is the major difference between a condenser R-meter and a standard free-air ionization chamber?

18. Would you employ a dose-rate meter to monitor a radiographic exposure of $\frac{1}{10}$ sec? Comment.

19. a) Describe the construction and the working principle of a Geiger-Müller tube.
    b) In what way is the Geiger-Müller counter different from an ionization chamber?

20. About what fraction of whole-population exposure to radiation may be attributed to diagnostic x-rays?

21. Assuming that you were to set up a diagnostic x-ray department, what features would you incorporate to ensure adequate protection of the staff and how would you test to see to what extent your measures were effective?

22. Explain how it is possible to employ an exposure of as much as 1000 R in radiotherapy, and yet 500 R is considered a lethal exposure.

23. a) Give, in roentgens, the approximate localized exposure which causes epilation and erythema.
    b) Which of the above two biological effects found use in the past as an indicator of radiation dosage?

24. Suggest a maximum weekly whole-body exposure permissible for radiation workers, based on the ICRP recommendations.

25. Describe measures you might employ to keep the x-ray exposure at a minimum for (a) the patient, and (b) the operator.

SUGGESTED READING

BRAESTRUP, C. B., and H. O. WYCKOFF, *Radiation Protection.* Springfield, Ill.: Charles C. Thomas, 1958. This book, by authors closely connected with the ICRP, and the NCRP of the U.S., presents a careful and fairly detailed summary of present knowledge of the application of radiation physics to the field of radiation protection, including the relevant instrumentation. It is written in a manner such as to be comprehensible to the interested professional who is not a specialist in this field.

CHESNEY, D. N. and M. O., *Radiographic Photography.* Oxford, England: Blackwell Scientific Publications, 1965. This is a text written especially for student radiographers, and contains most of the material given in the syllabuses of instruction (under the subject heading Radiographic Photography) of the Canadian, American, and British x-ray societies. The authors have considerable experience and authority in medical radiography. This book is highly recommended to the x-ray student, as part of his/her professional library.

DUGGAN, H. E., "Radiation Protection in Canada," *Canadian Medical Association Journal*, 91, 1964. "Radiation Protection in Canada" consists of several papers on the topic, written by a radiologist, and published in serial form. Part IV, the paper on "Factors of Importance in Minimizing Radiation Exposure of Patients, Operators and Others Involved in Diagnostic and Therapeutic Radiology" is particularly recommended to any x-ray technician. The paper deals in specifics, giving much useful information in the form of actual operating procedures, dosages, and practical recommendations.

ETTER, L. E., *The Science of Ionizing Radiation.* Springfield, Ill.: Charles C. Thomas, 1965. This book has an excellent chapter on protection from ionizing radiation, including a discussion of doses received in diagnostic radiology.

GURNEY, R. W., and N. F. MOTT, "The Theory of the Photolysis of Silver Bromide and the Photographic Latent Image," *Proc. Roy. Soc. 1938*, 164A: 151. This 17-page paper is well worth an investigation by the more ambitious student who wishes to enquire into sources. Again, as with some of the suggested reading in Chapter 7, this paper makes easier reading than many subsequent "explanations" of it.

THE INTERNATIONAL COMMISSION ON RADIOLOGICAL PROTECTION, *Recommendations of the ICRP* (ICRP Publication 6). Oxford: Pergamon Press, 1962. Publications of the ICRP deserve careful scrutiny by the x-ray technician, in that these reports represent the considered opinions of outstanding world authorities on radiation protection.

JOHNS, H. E., *The Physics of Radiology,* second edition. Springfield, Ill.: Charles C. Thomas, 1964. Chapter VII gives some details on radiation measurement devices, including certain circuits and some numerical examples. In Chapter XVI there is an excellent summary of steps which might be taken to reduce the patient-absorbed dose in diagnostic x-ray work.

NATIONAL COMMITTEE ON RADIATION PROTECTION AND MEASUREMENTS, *Medical X-Ray Protection up to Three Million Volts* (National Bureau of Standards Handbook 76). Washington, D.C.: U.S. Department of Commerce, 1961. This 52-page handbook contains much that is pertinent for the medical radiographer so far as protection is concerned. Every student and qualified radiographer would do well to be familiar with the contents of this booklet. Handbook 76 also contains a useful list of references for those who would pursue the subject further.

NEBLETTE, C. B., *Photography: Its Materials and Processes* (sixth edition). Toronto: D. Van Nostrand (Canada) Ltd., 1964. This text is more advanced than that of the Chesneys, and is concerned with the theory of photographic materials and processes. However, the senior student radiographer who wishes to read further will probably be pleasantly surprised to find how much of it he can understand. Much of the physics of medical radiography covered in the earlier chapters of our text will be found useful in the study of the book by Neblette.

RADIOACTIVE SUBSTANCES STANDING ADVISORY COMMITTEE, *Code of Practice for the Protection of Persons Against Ionizing Radiations from Medical and Dental Use.* London: Her Majesty's Stationery Office, 1964. This is the British equivalent of the American Handbook 76.

THOMPSON, J. T., and R. L. STRAUBE, *Radiation Biology and Medicine.* Reading, Mass.: Addison-Wesley, 1958. Interesting reading across the entire spectrum of the use of x-rays and radioisotopes in medicine.

YOUNG, M. E. J., *Radiological Physics,* second edition. London: H. K. Lewis and Co., 1967. Chapter 10 makes interesting reading for those students wishing to discover a little more about some of the chemical and biological effects of ionizing radiations. Since this text is written at a higher level than ours (and oriented toward therapy), it could serve well as supplementary reading to our chapters 7–11, for those students with a sound understanding of basic physics.

CHAPTER 12

Physics and Recent Advances in Medical Radiography

The objective of this chapter is twofold: first, to provide you with a survey of most of the recent advances in medical radiography and so to give you a map of this large and ever-growing territory; and second, to demonstrate the extent to which a knowledge of basic physics provides the vehicle for understanding many of the changing aspects of your profession. But, as we said before, the text is not intended to supplant an apparatus text, rather we intend to indicate briefly some of the underlying physics of the various pieces of equipment. Consequently particular use is made of cross references to the basic physics of the earlier chapters. We hope that, with the aid of this survey, you will be able to comprehend the scope of the entire diagnostic x-ray field, and also be able to fit in new pieces of information as they appear. You will then, in some measure, be better prepared for the future in the world of medical radiography.

Although it is of great practical importance for the x-ray technician to understand the application of new x-ray equipment, the understanding of its principles is, in the long run, even more important. For instance, many x-ray machines appear at first to be widely different from one another, even though they may all have the same function and principles of operation. Obviously, the technician who wishes to become versatile needs a familiarity with basic principles. The details of application readily follow with experience. Moreover, changes in x-ray equipment are likely to occur even more quickly in the future than they have in the past; hence an understanding of physics will make it much easier to understand the new equipment, and even to understand new physics. Note particularly how much use is made, even in the relatively brief excursion into newer equipment and ideas in this chapter, of the basic vocabulary of physics we established earlier. Much of this vocabulary—that is, words like voltage, potential, electric field, resistor, semiconductor, intensity, photoemission, frequency, luminescence, and many others—finds extensive use in the literature of medical radiography, from manufacturers' advertising to equipment instruction manuals to research papers.

12.1 FLUOROSCOPY

The Fluoroscopy Table

Many recent advances in medical radiography stem from the production of a fluoroscopic image. For this reason, it will be well for us to examine the fluoroscopy table or unit in some detail before we go further.

Figure 10.20 illustrates a conventional fluoroscopy apparatus, with the table in the upright position. The fluoroscopy x-ray tube is suspended below the table top. High-tension cables from the transformer are connected to this tube. Above the tube is a collimator with adjustable shutters which can be operated from controls close to the fluoroscope screen. The shutters are usually independent; that is to say, the vertical dimension of the field may be varied independently of the horizontal dimension. It is possible to move the tube along the length of the table or across it.

Above the table top, which is usually made of some relatively radioparent plastic material, is the fluoroscope screen. This is connected with the tube underneath. Any movement of the screen moves the tube as well. In this way the useful beam is always confined to the area of the screen and so cuts down the radiation hazard to people in the room. For further radiation protection, the screen is provided with a lead glass front and suitable hanging lead rubber aprons. One movement of the screen is made independent of the tube, that is, it may be pushed closer to the tube or pulled farther away. So as to provide full utilization of its area, the screen sometimes has an electrical connection to the shutters of the collimator. These shutters then automatically open as the screen is moved closer to the tube, and close again as the screen is moved away. The design of this control is such that the shutters when open at their fullest extent in any position of the screen never permit primary radiation to fall outside the screen area.

Alongside the fluoroscope screen there is usually a *spot film* device. This is a cassette holder which throughout the fluoroscopic examination holds a loaded cassette behind a suitable metal screen to protect it from radiation. As the radiologist wishes, the cassette may be slid across between the patient and the screen for a radiographic exposure by the undercouch tube. This spot film device usually includes some mechanism whereby a sequence of exposures may be made on one film, commonly two or four. The mechanism is set by the radiologist and the films taken in rapid succession, if necessary.

The tube current for fluoroscopy is usually controlled from the control panel elsewhere in the room and is most often of the order of 3–5 mA.

The kV may be controlled from both the fluoroscopic screen and the control panel, and may vary from 60 kV up to 140 kV.

Further controls mounted next to the fluoroscopic screen may include a density control for phototiming of the radiographic exposure for spot films, an exposure button for fluoroscopy and radiography which is in addition to the normal foot switch, and a five-minute-interval timer which will terminate fluoroscopic exposure after five minutes of viewing time have elapsed. This timer can then be reset at the requirement of the radiologist but has, in the meantime, warned him of the growing dose to the patient.

The standard fluoroscopy table is equipped with a motor-driven tilting mechanism. By means of this, one can tilt the table from a horizontal to an upright position and stop it at any point between these two extremes. Often the degree of tilt is extended into a 20° or 25° head-down or *Trendelenburg* position. Other tables again may tilt further, into the head-down vertical position. Some tables are equipped with a variable-speed motor and switch. These tables may be tilted at any speed, up to some maximum, merely by depressing the switch to a greater or lesser extent.

Because of the fact that the distribution of weight changes when the tilt of the table changes from one position to another, the screen and its appurtenances may require counterbalancing through cables and weights or springs.

So that they may be used for routine radiography, many fluoroscopy tables have an over-table tube, either floor or ceiling mounted, and an under-table Potter-Bucky tray.

In addition to these features, conventional fluoroscopy equipment may have many more pieces of accessory apparatus installed, but from what we have said you can see that this type of equipment represents a considerable engineering problem.

The Uses of Fluoroscopy

The greatest value of the fluoroscope is that it offers a method of studying the dynamics of the body, such as the movement of joints, or the swallowing process. The fluoroscope is much used in the examination of the gastrointestinal tract, after the patient has first ingested a barium sulfate solution or had a barium enema. (We referred to this contrast medium in Section 10.4.) The fluoroscope may also be used in bronchography to control the placing of a catheter in the bronchus, in myelography, in the investigation of the thoracic contents, and in the x-ray examination of the circulatory system, especially with regard to the positioning of catheters in the heart or great blood vessels. The fluoroscope is also used, although to a lesser extent, in the examination of other parts of the body such as the renal tract and the biliary tract.

The Shortcomings of Conventional Fluoroscopy

The use of the conventional fluoroscope which we have described suffers from many disadvantages. The level of intensity of the image is very low. The screen must be viewed in complete darkness after a considerable time of dark adaptation (20 or 30 minutes at least). When one views the image, only the rods of the retina are used. For this reason, much small detail on the screen cannot be seen at all.

Because the room has to be darkened for viewing, the inconvenience to the staff is considerable. Also, the cooperation of elderly or infirm patients is frequently more difficult to obtain under these conditions.

For routine fluoroscopy the exposure rate measured at the table top should be as low as possible and must not exceed 10 R per minute (ICRP recommendation). Even within these limits the patient dose may reach quite high levels in an extended x-ray investigation.

Conventional fluoroscopy also poses a radiation hazard to the operator and other staff, even though this may be kept within certain limits by proper protection devices and suitable personnel monitoring. The size of this hazard depends to a great extent on the tube current and voltage and the time for which the fluoroscope is operating.

The radiologist and his technical staff are restricted by cumbersome radiation protection devices such as lead rubber aprons and gloves. These, together with the darkness, certainly add nothing to the efficiency of the team.

The image on the screen is rather like the fish that got away. The radiologist may report on it but, in order to substantiate his diagnosis, he must have some sort of permanent record. This is obtained by means of the spot film radiographic device, which is consequently of considerable value. However, spot films can provide a permanent record only of arrested movements, so that in any examination of body dynamics their usefulness is restricted.

By reason of the shortcomings that have been mentioned here, the conventional fluoroscope has only a very limited value in consultation and teaching, both of which activities are necessary in radiology as in any other branch of medicine.

Because of the radiation hazard to the patient, this method of x-ray examination should be used only where clearly indicated. In particular, fluoroscopic examinations should be kept to an absolute minimum in the case of pregnant women, children, and adults within the child-producing age range.

A Digression on Alternatives to Medical Radiography

Although fluoroscopy, because of the prolonged time of exposure, usually produces a greater radiation hazard to the patient than radiography, any use of radiation is accompanied by hazard. For this reason, diagnostic methods are being constantly sought and developed in an effort to (ideally) replace radiography in medicine. At the time of writing, total replacement seems unlikely, but two fields of research seem particularly encouraging. These are *thermography* and *ultrasonics*. Both these techniques are stimulating interest in some areas of medicine.

In thermography, a heat-sensitive camera records a picture of the patient in which different densities in the image indicate regions of different temperatures at the skin surface. As mentioned before, differentiation of areas with temperature differences of 0.5 C° or less can be made by this method. Or the skin may be photographed after being treated with a phosphor which, upon irradiation with ultraviolet light, emits visible light at different intensities depending on temperature. In either case, the value of thermography, in addition to its freedom from unavoidable hazard, lies in the fact that many pathological conditions, such as certain tumors, produce local changes of temperature.

Ultrasonics, as implied in Section 9.1, is defined as the science of mechanical vibrations of frequencies greater than those normally audible to the human ear. In medical diagnostic procedures, known as *ultrasonography,* such sound waves are reflected from internal structures of the body. Both a source and a detector are required for the examination, the detector being used to record the intensity of the reflected waves from region to region of the area scanned. This intensity varies depending on the density of the structure from which the waves are reflected. By means of the resulting "map," it is possible to detect abnormalities of position, shape, or size of internal structures and so form a diagnosis.

12.2 PHOTOFLUOROGRAPHY

Photofluorography is the photographic recording of fluoroscopic images on small films. It may be taken to mean photography of the fluorescent screen during a single radiographic exposure by a single photographic exposure. It is therefore of no use for the study of body dynamics.

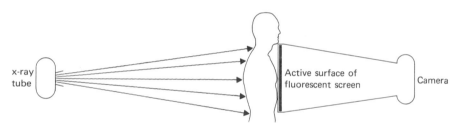

FIG. 12.1. The photofluorographic unit. The camera photographs the fluorescent-screen image of the patient's chest.

Mass Miniature Radiography

Photofluorography is very useful in mass surveys because of the economy of film. Its greatest use is to be found in x-ray examination of the chest, as this is the site of many common diseases and the chest lends itself to convenient radiographic examination.

Figure 12.1 is a diagram of a photofluorographic unit that might be used in mass miniature radiography of the chest. The camera on the right is enclosed in a light-tight tunnel at the wider end of which is the fluorescent surface of the screen. During the radiographic exposure a light image is produced on the screen and is recorded by the camera. In this figure, only the essentials of the method are shown. The actual equipment may include many refinements, such as automatic advance of the film so as to avoid double exposure, automatic marking of the film with the patient's name or other particulars, phototiming of the exposure, and a motor-driven platform for automatic height adjustment of either the tube and screen or the patient.

The film used in photofluorography has a photographic rather than a radiographic type of emulsion with a sensitivity designed to match the color of the fluorescence of the screen. This fluorescence is usually either green or blue. Since it is a light image arriving from one direction which is to be recorded, the film is coated on one side only. The film size is much smaller than the screen because the image produced by visible light in the camera is greatly diminished. The most common sizes of film in use are 35 mm, 70 mm, 100 mm, and 4 by 5 inches.

This convenient reduction in image size is, of course, dependent on first producing a visible image on the fluoroscopic screen. X-rays themselves could not be directly employed for producing reduced images because x-rays are not readily refracted. Hence conventional radiographs obviously require a film of the same size as the part being examined.

The Lens Camera

We now digress for a moment into a realm of physics known as *geometrical optics* or *ray optics*. A simple device amenable to explanation by means of elementary ray optics, as shown in Fig. 12.2, is the pinhole camera.

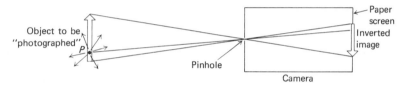

FIG. 12.2. The pinhole camera. If the object is illuminated, light is reflected from all points of it and, as shown at *P*, is reflected in all directions. Only one "ray" from each point, however, can reach the screen through the pinhole (providing the pinhole is very small). Since light travels in straight lines, the resulting image will be inverted and reversed from left to right.

Only if the pinhole in the camera is very small will the image be sharply defined. If the hole is made large (Fig. 12.3), more than one ray of light from a single point on the object will gain admission to the camera. As these rays diverge they will be some distance apart. Because this can happen from every point on the object, the resulting image is composed of many such overlapping areas. The result is a generalized blur which will be more severe the larger the hole. Hence it seems advisable to keep the hole small. But if the hole is kept very small, there is obviously a severe limitation on the total quantity of light which enters the camera. Therefore, the image is not very bright. For this reason, long exposures will be required if the screen is to be replaced by a photographic film of some sort. In other words, we may either have a sharp, dim image or a bright, blurred image in the pinhole camera. This dilemma may be resolved by employing a lens.

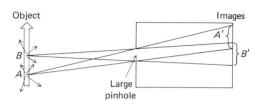

FIG. 12.3. The effect of a large hole in a pinhole camera. Rays of light from any point *A* enter the camera and produce an image *A'*, which is larger than a point. Rays from any other point *B* on the object produce another region of image, *B'*. Two adjacent points on the object are shown as overlapping regions of image. Since this happens for all points on the object, the resulting image is blurred.

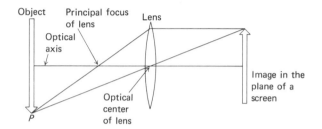

FIG. 12.4. The lens camera. All rays of light which enter the lens from any point *P* on the object reach the screen at a point. The image is therefore sharply defined. The image may always be easily located by drawing two rays: one through the optical center of the lens, which ray is not appreciably refracted, and one through the principal focus of the lens, which ray is refracted to emerge parallel to the optical axis.

Figure 12.4 shows a camera in which the pinhole has been replaced by a lens. The lens admits much more light to the camera, as it has a much greater diameter. At the same time it is a property of the glass of the lens to bend or refract rays of light. This phenomenon derives from the fact that the velocity of light in glass is different—that is, less—than the velocity of light in air. Note that, as may be construed from Fig. 12.4, the rays which strike the lens farthest from its optical center are refracted most. The end result is that any given point on the object is shown again on the image as a point, even though many rays from the point on the object enter the camera. The lens is said to *focus* the light. We now have an image that is both sharp and bright. Such an arrangement forms the basis of a lens camera which may be used in photofluorography. We should add that the simple ray diagram of Fig. 12.4 refers to relatively thin lenses. For thick lenses the situation becomes somewhat more complex.

The Mirror Camera

Another type of camera which is frequently used in photofluorography is the concave-mirror camera. Figure 12.5 illustrates the principles of this device. The unit shown is one which uses 100-mm cut film.

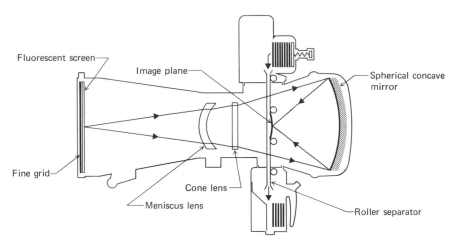

FIG. 12.5. The mirror camera. (From a diagram supplied by courtesy of N. V. Optische Industrie, De Oude Delft, Delft, Holland.)

The mirror camera, like the lens camera, employs a fluorescent screen and a light-tight tunnel, but the photographic recording system uses a front-silvered concave mirror instead of a lens. In the diagram, two rays of light originating from the center of the image on the fluorescent screen are shown entering the optical system. The meniscus lens and cone lens are included to improve resolution, but the essential point of concern for us is that the light rays fall onto the surface of the mirror and are reflected back to the center line, or optical axis of the system. Here the rays form an image in the curved plane where the film is held during an exposure. Any light ray from the fluorescent screen not absorbed by the blackened walls of the interior of the apparatus will enter the optical system and be reflected by the mirror to the film. A more detailed ray analysis shows that an image, smaller than the object, will be formed on the film. The object in this case is, of course, the image on the fluorescent screen. Note that during the actual exposure the film is curved to match the curvature of the mirror. The reason for this is that the plane of the image in this optical system is a curved plane. Note also that the sensitive emulsion of the single-sided film faces away from the fluorescent screen, that is, toward the mirror. As we can see in Fig. 12.5, the film and its pressure plate obstruct some of the light rays from the fluorescent screen which might otherwise have reached the mirror. Although this obstruction will cut down the number of light rays reaching the mirror from the fluorescent screen, it will not produce a sharp shadow on the mirror. Some rays from anywhere on the fluorescent screen pass around the film and its pressure plate, reach the mirror, and take part in image formation. Therefore there is no part of the fluorescent screen that is not "seen" by the film.

In this particular type of camera, the cut sheets of film are moved forward by a spring-and-hook device into a film-guide system. Here they are moved by rollers onto the face of the film pressure plate. This plate then presses the film into its curved exposure position. After the film has been exposed, rollers move it into the exposed-film container while the next sheet is brought into the exposure position. Roll film is often used in an alternative arrangement.

12.3 CINEFLUOROGRAPHY

Cinefluorography consists of the production of x-ray motion pictures by photographically recording fluorescent screen images on 16-mm, 35-mm, or 70-mm film.

Motion pictures, we should recall, are of course no more than a series of still pictures taken in quick succession. Now therefore by means of cinefluorographic apparatus, people can record the dynamics of the body. And, moreover, make these dynamics available for viewing at some later time, since the processed cine film can be run through a movie projector and shown on a screen.

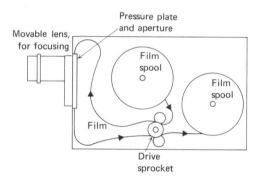

FIG. 12.6. The cine camera. Loops of film are required above and below the region of the aperture (which includes the pressure plate, shutter, and pull-down mechanism) to permit transition of the film from continuous movement to intermittent movement.

The Cine Camera

The cine camera is basically the same as the lens-type camera already described, except that the film is moved intermittently at variable speeds. Figure 12.6 is a diagram of the basic components of a cine camera. The lens of the camera focuses an image onto the film which is held by a pressure plate against the aperture during an exposure. The duration of the exposure is controlled by the shutter which rotates between the lens and the aperture. Details of the shutter are shown in Fig. 12.7. As the shutter rotates, it alternately covers and uncovers the aperture. When the aperture is uncovered by the shutter blade, the film is held firmly by the pressure plate and kept stationary. But as soon as the shutter blade covers the aperture, the film is released by the pressure plate and moved on to the next frame by means of a pull-down mechanism which engages perforations on the film edge. The cycle is then repeated. Because of this mechanism, the movement of the film past the aperture is an intermittent movement, even though the film drive sprocket moves the two film spools continuously. Because of these differences of film travel in the camera, it is necessary to have a loop of film on either side of the aperture in which the change of movement from continuous to intermittent may take place without damage to the film.

Camera speeds in cinefluorography may vary from 15 frames (or fewer) per second up to as high as 270 frames per second. Speeds of fewer than 15 frames per second may be necessary in cases in which the x-ray machine output is not sufficient to supply an adequate exposure during the brief shutter opening of the camera at the faster camera speeds.

Other limitations, such as motion of the part being examined, the size of the patient, and patient dose may have to be taken into account and may restrict camera speeds to fifteen frames per second, or fewer. Otherwise, camera speeds in this radiographic specialty are frequently the same as those of ordinary movie cameras, which for silent films usually run at 16 frames per second. The standard camera speed for sound films is somewhat faster, 24 frames per second.

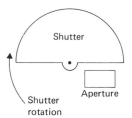

FIG. 12.7. The cine-camera shutter. As the shutter rotates, it alternately covers and uncovers the aperture of the camera. While the aperture is closed, film is moved to the next frame. During exposure the film is held stationary.

Cinefluorography

Although, as we have said, cinefluorography involves photography of a fluorescent screen, in practice this screen is rarely photographed directly. The intensity of the fluoroscopic image is too low. Without some method of intensification, either the image is too dim to provide adequate cine pictures or the dose to the patient becomes impractically large. Consequently, today the image is intensified or brightened by some means or other (see Section 12.5), and the cine-film record is made of the intensified image.

Aside from image intensification, other avenues are employed to reduce patient dosage. Let us review what is happening in cinefluorography. While the cine camera is operating and exposing the film intermittently, the x-ray tube may be making a continuous fluoroscopy-type exposure. In this case, the patient will receive radiation not only during the shutter-open position but also during the shutter-closed position when no film exposure is being made. One way of resolving this problem of

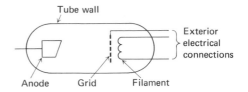

FIG. 12.8. The grid-controlled x-ray tube. Shown in diagram form, a negatively charged grid will repel electrons produced by the filament and prevent their reaching the anode. A grid of zero bias will permit electrons to reach the anode and x-rays will be produced.

unnecessary exposure is a method meeting with increasing use today. It is to produce the x-rays in pulses synchronized with the shutter openings of the cine camera. This may be achieved by controlling the exposure from the x-ray tube by means of a grid within the tube, as shown in Fig. 12.8. The x-ray tube shown in this figure operates in the same way as a conventional x-ray tube but the third electrode, the grid, is maintained at a substantial negative potential with respect to the filament during the intervals for which no x-rays are desired. The difference in potential between the grid and the filament may be something like 2 or 3 kV, which is sufficient to prevent the thermionically emitted electrons from the filament from striking the target. When an exposure is required, the grid voltage relative to the filament is momentarily reduced to near zero. We referred to this triode electronic control mechanism in Section 7.7. In summary then: By suitable control of the grid voltage, one can produce x-ray exposures of very short duration and start and stop them almost instantaneously in whatever synchronization desired.

A further refinement of this method is to omit the shutter from the camera altogether and to make exposures from the grid-controlled x-ray tube during those periods when the film in the cine camera is stationary in the aperture. When the film is moving from one frame to the next, no x-rays are produced. This procedure, of course, requires a phosphor of very rapid response. Image afterglow cannot be tolerated.

X-ray Cinematography

Whereas cinefluorography is widely used, it is by no means the only approach to viewing body dynamics. There are many different methods by which these dynamics may be studied by means of x-rays. As a student radiographer, you may have come across some of these methods and may have perhaps been puzzled as to where each fits in the general scheme of things. Let us look at the various methods under the common heading of x-ray cinematography.

By x-*ray cinematography* is meant the making of movie films by means of x-rays. The terminology we are using has not been universally adopted, but until such time as standardization has been effected, it is convenient to use the most common terms for the various relevant methods.

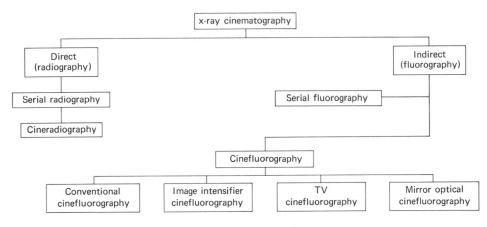

FIG. 12.9. The various branches of x-ray cinematography.

Perhaps we can use Fig. 12.9 to reduce the most common methods to an orderly presentation. This figure shows that x-ray cinematography may be divided into two large areas: direct and indirect.

We use the word "direct" in the sense that no fluoroscopy screen is involved. The films produced are the result of direct x-radiation, or perhaps x-rays with intensifying screens, as in conventional radiography. The first type of direct x-ray cinematography is serial radiography. This means the taking of a number of radiographs of a part of the body in a sequence, with certain time intervals between films. Probably the most common example of this type of work is to be found in the intravenous pylogram, or I.V.P., although this is seldom referred to as serial radiography *per se*. When the four or five films of the I.V.P. have been processed, they form a continuing record of the dynamics of the urinary system. However, in this example, although it illustrates serial radiography very clearly, there are large time gaps between the successive films.

Serial radiography may be undertaken either by changing the cassettes between exposures, perhaps in a cassette changer, or changing the film between intensifying screens in a film changer (see Section 12.4). Some serial radiography is performed by methods such as these at a rate of as many as 12 exposures per second. The apparatus may vary from the hand-operated cassette tunnel to very sophisticated automatic machinery.

A further step which may be taken is to photograph the radiographs produced during serial radiography and reproduce them on a cine film, a procedure called *cineradiography*. When these films are projected on a screen, an impression of movement will be produced. However, this further step entails added expense and at the present time is rarely undertaken.

The other major division of x-ray cinematography, the indirect methods, may all be called fluorography, in that they entail the photography of a fluoroscopic screen. These methods may be divided into two groups, *serial fluorography* and *cinefluorography*.

Serial fluorography is the direct photography of a fluoroescent-screen image on a small film. This process is as illustrated in Fig. 12.1, except that in serial fluorography a series of exposures is made. Because of the low level of intensity of the fluoroscopy screen this method, as suggested earlier, does not lend itself to cine photography, which requires a greater screen intensity because of the very short exposure times necessary. The limitation of direct photography of the fluorescent screen, that is, serial fluorography, is obvious. The resulting films produce a record of the dynamics of body processes, but usually with gaps between consecutive projections. One important exception to this is the mirror-camera unit, described in Section 12.2. Because of the optical properties of the mirror camera, such as a large aperture, it is possible to make as many as 6 exposures per second of the nonintensified fluoroscopic screen, thereby obviating the limitation expressed above. Mirror-camera serial fluorography is therefore of great value.

As we pointed out in the previous section, cinefluorography is the continuous recording on cine film of the fluoroscopic image. Although it is not spelled out in the literal definition of the word cinefluorography, in order to be practical this group of procedures includes some sort of brightening or intensification of the fluoroscopic image to be photographed.

In Fig. 12.9 we have subdivided this category of x-ray cinematography into only four different procedures, because these are probably the most common types you are likely to meet. However, there are other types of procedures not mentioned here. They are presently in less common use, but during the coming years may well achieve greater prominence. As further discoveries are made in the future and new equipment is produced, you should have no real difficulty in fitting the new procedures into place in a diagram such as the one we are discussing. Note that, of the four types of cinefluorography mentioned, each includes a word or phrase which explains the method by which the fluoroscopic image is intensified before being photographed; for example, image-intensifier cinefluorography and TV cinefluorography.

Conventional cinefluorography holds some promise, especially as research is carried out into the production of brighter fluoroscopic screens, faster films, and faster lenses.

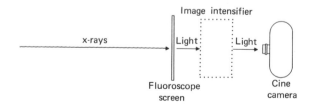

FIG. 12.10. Image-intensifier cinefluorography. The visible-light image leaving the image intensifier may be as much as 3000 times brighter than the visible-light image received by the intensifier.

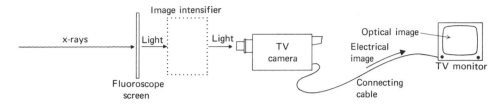

FIG. 12.11. Television cinefluorography. The fluoroscope screen image is viewed by the TV camera and relayed by coaxial cable to a monitor. Although not necessary in an explanation of the principles of TV cinefluorography, the image intensifier is included in the chain to show the combination of units often used.

Image-intensifier cinefluorography is the recording of the fluoroscopic image on cine film as a continuous process after the image has been intensified. This sequence of events is shown in Fig. 12.10 by means of a block diagram. We shall deal with the principles of operation of an image intensifier in Section 12.5.

Television cinefluorography is the recording of a TV image on cine film. In this method, the television image has been obtained by means of a TV camera from a fluoroscopic screen. This process is demonstrated in Fig. 12.11, which shows the components involved. The method is discussed more fully in Section 12.6, which deals with television and cinefluorography.

The fourth method of cinefluorography, that which utilizes a mirror optical system, is yet another way in which a gain in brightness is obtained between the fluoroscopic screen and the cine camera. We shall discuss an example of this in Section 12.5.

12.4 CINERADIOGRAPHY

Cineradiography is included in the general field of recent advances in medical radiography. As such, it will certainly appear to you to be closely connected with such matters as cinefluorography. Although cineradiography has, of course, already been briefly discussed in connection with the chart of Fig. 12.9, it warrants some further elucidation.

The production of direct radiographs as a sequential record of body function, either rapid or otherwise, may be obtained by one of two pieces of equipment: cassette changers or film changers.

Cassette Changers

The name given to these pieces of equipment is self-explanatory. Whatever form the changer takes, it consists of a device for moving a cassette from a radiation-proof magazine into place beneath the part to be x-rayed, holding the cassette still during the exposure, and then moving it into another magazine. The removed cassette will then be replaced beneath the patient by the next cassette in the series. Figure 12.12 shows, in

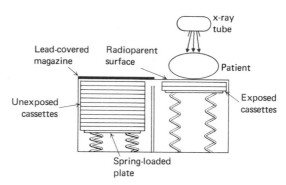

FIG. 12.12. Principles of a cassette changer. Between exposures cassettes move from left to right. The mechanism which moves them is not shown. During exposure a fresh cassette is held by springs against the radioparent magazine cover. Those cassettes below the one being exposed are protected from fogging by thin sheets of lead which are included in the backs of all the cassettes.

diagrammatic form, the principles of operation of a typical cassette changer. Such a mechanism provides up to 12 exposures per second.

Film Changers

Because of the limitations of weight and numbers inherent in moving cassettes in a cassette changer, another method for obtaining a series of radiographs is to use a film changer. In a film changer, only the film is moved between exposures. During the exposure the film is held at rest between a pair of intensifying screens. Figure 12.13 shows two types of film changer: (a), the cut-sheet changer, and (b), the roll-film changer. Apparatus of the roll-film type can presently be used to obtain 12 exposures per second for 70 to 80 exposures. The cut-sheet changer produces up to 6 exposures per second, for 30 exposures.

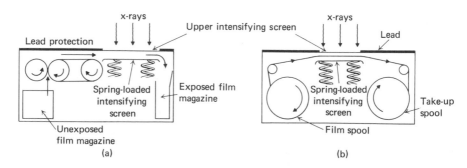

FIG. 12.13. Film changers. (a) Cut sheet changer. Each sheet is flipped up by a lever from the unexposed magazine. It later falls by gravity into the exposed magazine. (b) Roll film changer. The roll film passes between the intensifying screens as shown. In both types film is transported between the parted screens while no exposure is being made. During exposure film is held stationary between the closed intensifying screens.

To complete this subsection on film changers, we must also mention the 70-mm and 100-mm cut-film and roll-film mirror-camera systems already discussed in Sections 12.2 and 12.3.

12.5 IMAGE INTENSIFICATION

In the search for a means of making the fluoroscopic image brighter, people have discovered one method which has become widely used. It depends, like the x-ray tube, on the acceleration of electrons. The device involved is known as an *image intensifier*. The process involved is known as image intensification, or image amplification.

The Image Intensifier

The most common type of image intensifier is a vacuum tube which converts the light image from a fluoroscopic type of screen into an electron image. The electrons so produced are then accelerated, focused, and made to form a smaller and much brighter light image. Figure 12.14 illustrates this device.

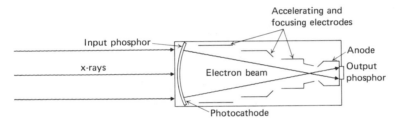

FIG. 12.14. The image intensifier. An x-ray image is converted to an electron image. The electrons are focused and accelerated, to produce a much smaller and brighter light image on the output screen.

Let us look at it in some detail. This type of image intensifier consists of a large evacuated glass tube, the actual diameter of which may be anything from about 6 in. to about 11 in., while its length may be of the order of 18 in. An x-ray beam, after traversing the patient, arrives at the input phosphor screen, where it produces a light image. This phosphor, zinc sulfide or a similar substance, coated on the convex side of the curved glass input end of the tube, fluoresces, as we discussed in Section 10.6. At this stage the light image is very similar to that on a fluoroscopic screen. But now, instead of being viewed directly, the image is transmitted through the glass of the tube to a photocathode. The photocathode is coated on the concave side of the glass, with a photoemissive material such as cesium antimony. (What is involved here was discussed in Section 7.8.) By means of this photocathode the light image is converted into an equivalent electron image because the number of electrons emitted per unit area per unit time is proportional to the intensity of light received.

At the smaller end of the tube is a metal anode shaped somewhat as shown. Located in this anode is the output phosphor, a small circular screen of zinc sulfide or other fluorescent material. Between the input assembly, or cathode, and the anode a potential difference of some 25 kV is applied to accelerate the electrons toward the output phosphor. The output phosphor, coated on the inside of the small glass end of the tube, then fluoresces with an intensity proportional to the intensity of the incident electron beam.

In their passage through the tube, the accelerating electrons are focused on the output phosphor, as shown, by means of circular electrodes positioned down the length of the tube. These charged focusing rings, or electron lenses, going from the largest to the smallest, are at potentials of something like $+300$, $+2000$ and $+5000$ volts, respectively, relative to the cathode. The focusing effect on the electrons is, of course, due to the electric field which is shaped by these circular electrodes. Although these electrodes are positively charged with respect to the cathode, they do not capture many of the electrons in the beam. The reason is that, as they follow the electric field lines at their approach to the next electrode and so are made to converge, the electrons are also greatly accelerated, and acquire great speeds. Thus, by the time they are abreast of an electrode they are too energetic for the local field of any one electrode to have sufficient effect to divert them from their general direction toward the output phosphor.

The visible image on the output phosphor is many times brighter than the visible image at the input phosphor, for two reasons. The electrons originating at the photocathode are accelerated in the tube and therefore gain energy. This energy is surrendered at the output phosphor and manifests itself as a gain in brightness. Also, a gain in brightness is produced because of the diminution of the image size brought about by focusing of the electron beam; that is, the intensity increases because the energy per unit area is increased if the area is decreased. Altogether the brightness gain may be something in the order of 3000 times.

The metal casing of the image intensifier tube, in addition to supplying mountings for its attachment to the x-ray equipment, has two other important functions. It provides magnetic shielding (see Section 4.2) so that any magnetic fields produced by electric brakes, used for tube immobilization, for example, or by any other electromagnetic components of the x-ray machine, are prevented from affecting the electron beam through the tube. (We saw in Section 4.3 that there is a force on a charge moving in a magnetic field.)

The other function of the housing is to attenuate any x-rays produced by the electrons striking the output phosphor, and x-rays transmitted and scattered by the input phosphor. From one point of view, the image intensifier tube appears to be somewhat like an inefficient x-ray tube, with a voltage of 25 kV and a tube current of something like 0.5 μA.

Typical sizes for input phosphor diameters in image-intensifier tubes are 6 inches, 9 inches, and 11 inches. Output phosphor diameters, on the other hand, are much smaller: $\frac{3}{4}$ in. to 1 in.

What about viewing the output from the image intensifier? The simplest method is to connect it to a system of lenses and an eyepiece. Or the image from a lens system may be received in a large mirror system, after suitable enlargement, so that two viewers may see the image. It is also possible to connect a TV camera to the image intensifier and hence have the image displayed on a TV screen (see Section 12.6). Various types of cine cameras may be used to record the intensified image on 16-mm or 35-mm film (see Section 12.3). A mirror camera may also be used to produce 70 mm- or 100-mm spot films either singly or in rapid sequence (see Section 12.2).

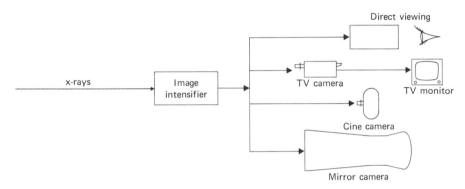

FIG. 12.15. Viewing and recording the intensified image.

Figure 12.15 illustrates these various viewing and recording possibilities, which may be used singly or in any combination. Reference to this figure may aid you in determining which method or combination has been adopted in your x-ray department for any particular machine.

The advantages of the image intensifier may be briefly summarized. During fluoroscopy, if there is an image intensifier as part of the equipment, the x-ray tube current, instead of being 3 to 5 mA as in the case of conventional fluoroscopy, may be reduced to 1 mA or less. The dose rate to the patient is obviously similarly reduced. At the same time, the greatly increased brightness of the image means that it is no longer necessary to carry out viewing in complete darkness. The gain in brightness also means that the radiologist is able to see more with less uncertainty: a desirable diagnostic feature which in itself leads again to smaller patient dosage. Finally, there is the advantage that with the brighter image the various recording media mentioned may be used to better advantage to record body dynamics; again this helps to make a diagnosis more certain.

An Electro-Optical Image Intensifier

Before we go on to the next section, which concerns television in medical radiography, let us talk about two more fairly recent developments. The first, the *electro-optical image intensifier,* we include in order to show you one of the ways in which image intensification may be put to use. The

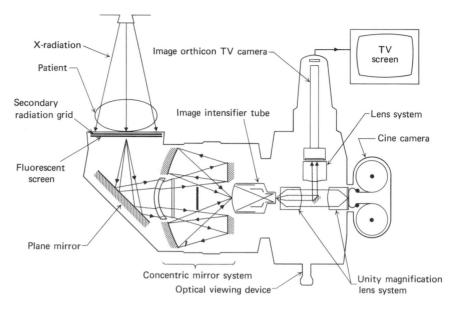

FIG. 12.16. An electro-optical image intensifier. The large (approximately 12 in.) fluoro-scopic screen image is transferred (and diminished) by the mirror optical system to the input phosphor of the image-intensifier tube. Another optical system transfers the output phosphor image of the intensifier tube, without a change in size, to a 35-mm cine camera. (Courtesy N. V. Optische Industrie, De Oude Delft, Delft, Holland.)

approach to brightness gain is somewhat different from the approach we have described for the image-intensifier tube alone. We feel that discus-sion of at least one other method of intensifying the fluoroscopic image should enable you to regard the image-intensifier tube as a building block or component in a chain of devices. The variety of available components allows considerable flexibility of design. Once you are aware of these possibilities, any new developments in the future along these or similar lines will, we hope, present fewer problems to you.

The particular electro-optical image intensifier in question requires only a small image-intensifier tube; its replacement is made simple by suitable design. Such replacement might be necessary in the event of failure or the development of better tubes. Figure 12.16 illustrates the principles of this type of intensifier.

The optical part of the system depends on the principles of the mirror camera, which we discussed in Section 12.2. But in the intensifier the light optical system receives the light from a circular fluoroscopic screen of approximately 12 in. diameter. The light image is brought to a focus at the input phosphor of the image-intensifier tube, which is about 3 in. in diameter. The two plane mirrors, one of which is at 45° to the fluoroscopic screen, reflect the light beam as shown. The output of the image-intensifier tube is approximately 0.5 in. in diameter. The output image, unchanged in size, is transmitted through a second smaller optical system to a 35-mm cine camera. However, there are other final recording medium possibilities. The overall brightness gain in the equipment shown is something in the order of 1000 times.

Solid-State Amplification

The last subject we shall consider under the general heading of "image intensification" is *solid-state amplification.* The indisputable advantage of having quantities of solid materials to perform tasks by means of electronics make development in this direction almost certain. When the technology has become sufficiently advanced, it seems likely that the vacuum tube in image intensification will be superseded by solid-state devices, as it has been already in radio and many other applications. Even though for practical purposes solid-state image intensification is in its infancy, if you gain an understanding of the principles now, it will certainly pay you dividends later.

Photoconductors are materials, such as cadmium sulfide, which act as current carriers when radiant energy, such as light or x-rays, is applied to them. Photoconductors belong to the group of materials known as semiconductors; recall that we discussed the theory of semiconductors in Section 3.1.

Electroluminescent phosphors are materials, such as zinc sulfoselenide, which emit light when electric fields are applied to them directly.

The use of photoconductors and electroluminescent phosphors in solid form has made it possible to convert x-ray images into intensified light images. A thin sandwich of these materials between suitable electrodes is arranged as shown in Fig. 12.17. An alternating voltage is applied between the two outermost electrodes.

While the photoconductor is not irradiated no current flows through it, and much of the voltage appears across this layer. The remainder of the voltage, appearing across the electroluminescent layer, is not sufficient to cause the emission of light.

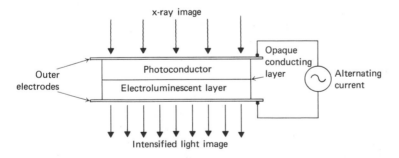

FIG. 12.17. Solid-state image intensification. An alternating voltage is applied between the two outer electrodes. Due to this alternating voltage, emission of light from the electroluminescent layer will increase when the photoconductor is irradiated. The central opaque conducting layer prevents feedback of light from the electroluminescent layer to the photoconductor.

When an x-ray image is permitted to fall on the photoconductor, current is produced and the voltage drop across the layer decreases. A greater proportion of the applied voltage therefore appears across the electroluminescent layer, which then emits light. The current in the photoconductor and therefore the emission of light from the electroluminescent layer depends on the local intensities in the x-ray image beam. Where the x-ray intensity is greatest, the final light emission will be brightest.

A thin, opaque, but conducting layer is placed between the two active layers. This is done so that only the x-rays and not the light emitted by the electroluminescent layer trigger the photoconductor into the conducting state.

In a practical unit, which looks something like a conventional fluoroscopic screen, the layers, each a few thousandths of an inch thick, are supported by a sheet of glass. The alternating voltage may be applied between a front electrode of silver paint and another, transparent, electrode of an oxide of tin. Typical operation might be at 500 volts and 400 cycles per second. The intensity of the emitted light increases with increasing frequency and size of the applied voltage.

The active layers are composed of small crystals, in the order of microns in diameter, embedded in a plastic, nonconducting bonding material. Alternating voltages are used, since direct current cannot flow from crystal to crystal through the plastic binder. Electrically, the layer may be regarded somewhat as a capacitor.

Electroluminescence is a combination of semiconductor charge movement and luminescence. Somewhat simplified, it may be described as follows. Within each crystal of the electroluminescent phosphor is a crons in diameter, embedded in a plastic, nonconducting bonding material. of the host crystal and impurity atoms diffused in from the surface. The application of an electric field to the crystal produces a field across the junction. Electrons are raised to conductor band energy, migrate across the junction under the influence of this field, and create electron-hole pairs. As the applied field falls to zero, the electron-hole pairs recombine, the electrons fall back into the valence band, and emit photons of energy in the visible-light region. This sequence of events is repeated for the next half cycle of input voltage. The duration of the light flash produced at each half cycle is 10^{-3} to 10^{-2} sec, depending on the phosphor.

At the present stage of development of solid-state amplifying screens for medical radiography, several problems remain to be overcome. The brightness per x-ray exposure rate is presently only about 100 times that of a conventional fluoroscopic screen, but this will no doubt be improved. Also, the most sensitive phosphors are those which exhibit the longest decay periods. This means that the light image may persist for 30 sec or more after x-irradiation has ended. This is generally a disadvantage. Graininess and nonuniformity of the amplified image are also undesirable characteristics. But despite these difficulties, it seems safe to predict at this time that devices of this nature will find very wide application in radiography in the years to come.

12.6 TELEVISION AND CINEFLUOROGRAPHY

In Fig. 12.9, which summarizes much of the field of cinefluorography, one of the methods noted is *television cinefluorography*. The intensified fluoroscopic image is viewed on a television monitor after being picked up from the output phosphor of the image intensifier by a television camera. The advantage of television is that several people may view the image at the time it is produced. This is not the case with other cinefluorographic methods. For consultation and teaching purposes, the image may be relayed to other TV monitors either in the same room or elsewhere. The television image may, of course, also be photographed to provide a permanent record, although more recently video tape is being increasingly used for television recording purposes in diagnostic radiology. We shall discuss this aspect later in this section.

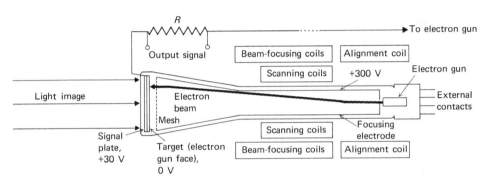

FIG. 12.18. The vidicon camera tube. Wherever light reaches the target, current will flow through the target to the signal plate and so through the resistor, *R*. The varying voltage drop across *R* constitutes the output signal. Scanning coils on the reader's side of the tube and beyond the tube are not shown. All voltages shown are with respect to the electron gun emitter.

The Television Camera

Although the television camera in practice contains a number of electrical and electronic circuits which will not be discussed here, at the heart of it is the television camera tube. This is an electronic vacuum tube, the operation of which depends on physical principles we have to some extent already discussed in previous chapters. Figure 12.18 shows the main components of the television camera tube. The type we have chosen to illustrate is the tube referred to as a *vidicon*. This is the simplest and least expensive of a variety of available tubes. Other television camera tubes—such as the image orthicon, the plumbicon, and the x-ray-sensitive vidicon —are more or less variations of the vidicon tube.

The vidicon camera tube consists of an evacuated glass cylindrical envelope about an inch in diameter and about six inches long. Metal pins pass through the glass wall of the tube at one end to provide a means of making electrical contact with the elements inside the tube. The other end of the tube contains a light-sensitive material on which a light image from the output of an image-intensifier tube is focused. This focusing may be achieved by means of a suitable lens system. The camera tube contains a source of electrons, called an electron gun, consisting of an oxide of thorium or some other metal with suitable thermionic emission characteristics. This electron gun is indirectly heated by an adjacent but separate filament. Note here that so far there are many similarities between this television tube, other electron tubes, and J. J. Thomson's *e/m* apparatus of Fig. 1.8.

Now then, at operating temperature the oxide emits electrons which are focused into a tiny beam by means of electrically charged cylinders which surround the electron source, and suitably shape the electric field in this region. Focusing is also aided by focusing coils outside the tube. The electron beam is accelerated away from the electron gun, by an electrode within the gun, toward the anode, which is at the opposite end of the tube. This anode consists of a double layer of materials supported as a thin disk at the end of the tube. The layer onto which the electron beam falls is called the *target*. The target is at 0 volts relative to the electron source. It consists of a very thin coating of photoconductive material, such as antimony trisulfide. The other layer of the sandwich, called the *signal plate*, receives the light image from the image-intensifier tube. This signal plate, as pointed out earlier, is composed of a transparent conductive material, such as an oxide of tin, and is at a potential of, perhaps, + 30 volts with respect to the gun side of the target, and also with respect to the cathode of the electron gun.

Between the electron gun and the target there is a cylindrical accelerating electrode which supports a fine wire mesh a few millimeters from the surface of the target. The cylinder and mesh are at + 300 volts with respect to the gun.

Outside the tube two pairs of electromagnetic coils are positioned above and below it and to either side of it. These coils, with their varying magnetic fields, are so energized as to produce a scanning of the target by the electron beam, in accordance with Eq. (4.3). Other electromagnetic coils which surround the tube for most of its length provide a magnetic field whose lines of force lie parallel to the long axis of the tube. This field focuses the electrons into a narrow beam.

During operation the signal-plate side of the target is at a potential difference of, for example, + 30 volts with respect to the target. When an image from the output phosphor of the image-intensifier tube falls on the end of the vidicon tube, it passes through the transparent signal plate and reaches the target. At whatever point sufficient light reaches the target, the photoconductor material will emit electrons which will be attracted toward the signal plate, leaving a positive charge on the target at that particular point. As the electron beam of the camera tube is made to scan the face of the target, by means of its deflecting coils, regions of the target with positive charge will permit electrons from the beam to pass through the semiconductor to the signal plate.

As the scanning electron beam is made to pass across the inner surface of the target, it therefore gives rise to a current through the resistor, R. This current varies in magnitude and depends on the brightness of the light image falling on the target at the spot in question. By this means, and with a very rapid scanning of the electron beam, the image is converted to an electric current which varies very rapidly with respect to time. This varying current, in passing through the resistor R, results in a voltage across the resistor. It is this voltage which is used as the output signal from the camera tube.

The scanning pattern followed by the electron beam across the face of the target is known as a *raster*. In the television camera, the electron beam scans the whole frame of the target face 30 times per second. The beam follows a pattern somewhat as shown in Fig. 12.19. The total frame is composed of 525 lines so the tiny electron beam scans 15,750 lines in each second. If it could be seen, the target plate would appear to be uniformly covered at any given moment.

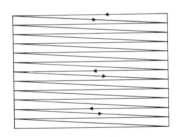

FIG. 12.19. A raster: the type of pattern traced on the camera (and picture tube) screen by the electron beam.

The size of the current through the resistor R may vary many times during the period for which the electron beam scans one line of the raster; as much as 7 million times per second. Your acquaintance with Ohm's law will thus lead you to note that the voltage across R will change with a similar frequency.

A fairly recent experimental development in electronics is a tubeless television camera about the size of a man's hand. The image-sensing element occupies a one-inch-square glass slide and consists of 32,400 dots of photoconductive material. Each photoconductive dot is deposited at the intersection of thin metal conductors which have been evaporated onto the glass slide to form a grid pattern.

A light image is focused onto this grid array, where the photoconductive dots lower their electrical resistance in proportion to the intensity of the light falling on them. The grid array is continuously "scanned" by arranging a tiny pulse of voltage to be applied to each dot in turn by a direct connection with supporting circuitry. Each dot then passes on a pulse of current which is proportional to the intensity of the incident light at that point. These pulses of current represent the output signal of the camera.

The use of the solid-state television camera in medical radiology has yet to be demonstrated, but, from the brief description we have given, the student who has understood the basic physics discussed in the present text should have no great difficulty in understanding this and other future developments.

The Television Receiver

The television picture tube consists basically of a cathode-ray tube in which a tiny beam of electrons strikes a fluorescent screen, the phosphor of which forms a layer on the inner surface of the expanded end of the glass tube. We made a brief reference to this matter in Section 4.3, in which the principles of the television picture tube were related to Eq. (4.3), which deals with the force on a charge moving through a magnetic field. (Refer again to Fig. 4.21.) In the picture tube the source of electrons is an electron gun similar to that in the television camera tube (vidicon). For uniform illumination of the viewing surface of the tube, the electron beam is made to produce a raster pattern similar to the pattern in the camera tube. The direction of the electron beam is controlled by means of electromagnets positioned as shown outside the tube close to the source of the beam. These magnets are composed of vertical and horizontal elements. The current in the pairs of magnets above and below and from side to side is made to alternate, as in the camera tube. These fields then produce a rapid side-to-side movement of the beam and a slower up-and-down movement, thus producing the raster. The television picture is formed by applying the output voltage from the television camera tube between the source of electrons in the picture tube gun and a small electrode immediately in front of the source. This changing voltage thereby changes the intensity of the electron beam. As the beam scans the phosphor it therefore varies in intensity from point to point, and when it does this very rapidly, it produces an image made up of various degrees of brightness.

In the television image intensifier the camera and picture tube are joined together by electric cables. Such a system is called closed-circuit television, as opposed to broadcast. The cable, besides transmitting the output voltage from the camera tube to the picture tube, also provides a connection to other auxiliary circuits which control the raster on each tube face and also synchronize the electron scanning of camera and picture tubes.

As in the case of the camera tube, the picture tube unit also contains other circuitry to supply currents and voltages for the operation of the tube.

Videotape Recording

As implied earlier, in television cinefluorography it is becoming more common to record the final intensified image on a magnetic videotape rather than on photographic film. Videotape is a thin, plastic material, usually 1 or 2 inches wide in the case of the x-ray videotape recorder. Videotape recording equipment used in conjunction with present-day television image-intensification equipment utilizes a tape speed of from 3.7 in./sec to 120 in./sec. This tape is available in rolls of 1800 ft, for example. The tape is coated on one side with a layer of magnetizable material, such as perhaps an iron oxide. So that the image will be transferred to the tape, the varying output voltage from the television camera is used to produce a varying magnetic field which magnetizes the tape by different amounts along its length. When the visible television picture is required, this tape is used to induce a varying current within a coil, the voltage from which is then used to control the intensity of the electron beam in the picture tube. In this fashion we have access to a picture stored on tape.

The basic principle of operation, as we have seen, is relatively simple. In practice, a little more is involved, such as some arrangement whereby the signal to be recorded may be packed tightly on the tape instead of being spread out in a linear fashion along its length. Consequently, it is arranged that the recording head moves from side to side across the tape as well as along it. To obtain fairly high fidelity of picture reproduction, it is necessary to run the tape at high speed relative to the recording head, but a zigzag pattern can accomplish this even though the linear movement of the tape is much slower.

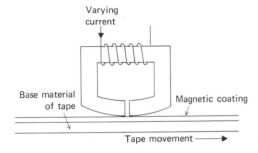

FIG. 12.20. The videotape recording and playback head. The current in the electromagnet coil is varied by the camera tube output signal. The changing field strength at the head gap magnetizes the tape coating to various degrees. A permanent record of the camera tube signal is the result.

The basic arrangement for recording is shown in Fig. 12.20. The output signal from the camera tube is made to produce a varying current in the small electromagnet of the recording head in the figure. The recording-head electromagnet has a very narrow gap between its poles and across this gap the magnetizable tape passes. The intensity of the magnetic field in the gap varies with the varying current in the coil and magnetizes each small portion of the tape as it passes through. Each tiny area of the tape is therefore more or less magnetized, depending on the field strength at the time of its movement across the gap. The tape is then wound onto a storage reel and forms a permanent record of the output signal from the camera tube.

When the picture is to be viewed by the radiologist or others, the tape is simply passed through the recording head again, but now the electromagnet functions as a playback device. As the different regions of the magnetized tape pass across the gap of the electromagnet, they induce EMF's in the electromagnet coil which vary in proportion to the degree of magnetization of the tape in that area. The resulting varying current may then be employed to furnish a correspondingly varying voltage across some resistor. This voltage is then applied to the electron gun in the picture tube in order to vary the electron beam intensity. Thus we obtain a television picture on the screen.

What are some advantages of videotape recording? By means of videotape, one can play back a record of the x-ray examination any number of times at some later period for reporting, consultation, or teaching. Playback can also be made immediately following recording, for a confirmation of a finding, thus avoiding a repeat fluoroscopic x-ray exposure to a patient. Or the image may be held at one point on a screen for more prolonged study or even run in reverse in the case of the study of certain dynamics.

Color Television

The use of color television is beginning to be increasingly considered in medical radiography. The color-television camera consists of three camera tubes. Each tube sees a scene, through a colored filter, in terms of one of the additive primary colors only: red, green, or blue. The three "colored" signals are then transmitted to a receiver or picture tube. This tube has screen phosphors which produce these three colors. The signal from the red camera tube is made to excite the red emission phosphor, the green signal produces a green image, and the blue signal produces a blue image. The individual phosphor elements are so small, and arranged in trios of the three colors, that the viewer is unable to resolve the separate elements. One simply sees an overall colored image which is very nearly the same as the original colored scene, since the colors are mixed by the picture tube in the same proportions and intensities as in the original scene.

Color television finds application in medical radiography, for example, in subtraction techniques. A certain radiographic image is recorded on videotape by the television system. Perhaps the part to be examined is a skull. Shortly afterward a series of exposures is made following the injection of contrast material into the carotid artery. Both the arterial and the venous phases of the cerebral circulation are recorded and stored. The television system can then superimpose a negative image of the first exposure onto positive images of the series. The net effect in the new image is zero in all areas of the skull except the contrast-filled vascular system. The skull image becomes nearly invisible and the blood-vessel images stand out clearly on the screen. In addition to this, the venous part of the system can be shown in one color, blue for example, and the arterial part in red.

Color television may also be used to increase contrast in an image. Although in a conventional radiographic television image, contrast consists of differences in brightness within the image, it is now possible to view these differences in terms of color as well. The television system can arrange to make brighter parts of the image more blue, for example, and darker parts more red. In this way the density differences between one region of the body and another, say between the kidneys and the surrounding perirenal fat, are further highlighted.

12.7 FIELD EMISSION RADIOGRAPHY

Field emission is the emission of electrons from a metal under the influence of a strong electric field. A high voltage is applied between the metal in question, which is made negative, and a suitable anode. Unlike the case of thermionic emission, no heat is applied to the cathode.

As an aside we might just note that field emission is the fourth type of electron emission we have encountered. Let us review: First there is *thermionic* emission, as in the x-ray tube; then there is *photo* emission, as in the photo-timer; third, there is *secondary* emission, as employed in the photo-multiplier tube; and finally, the process of concern at this point, *field* emission.

In field emission, if the electric field E at the emitter surface has a sufficiently high value, say 10,000 kV/cm or more, then the current, that is, the number of electrons emitted per unit time, increases exponentially with the applied electric field. A 1% change in field causes a change of approximately 10% in current. It is thus possible, by means of suitable design, to obtain currents as high as 100 million amperes per square centimeter of emitter.

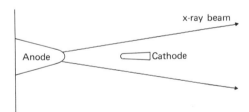

FIG. 12.21. The field-emission x-ray tube. A high voltage is applied between the electrodes. Because of the small area of the cathode (perhaps 10^{-6} cm), the current density is large. The focal spot of such a tube might be about 1 mm in diameter.

Figure 12.21 represents an x-ray tube which uses the field-emission principle. At the application of a high voltage between the two electrodes, electrons will be emitted, bombard the anode, and produce x-rays.

From the foregoing information you can see that the exposure times required for medical radiography employing field emission are extremely short; something in the order of 0.05 microsecond.

The conventional x-ray generator is, of course, inadequate to supply the high tension for field-emission radiography. Instead a pulsed supply is used. Figure 12.22 shows the wave form of such a pulsed high-tension

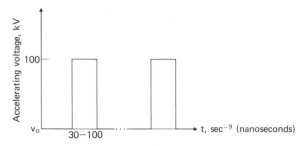

FIG. 12.22. A pulsed voltage supply. The squareness of the pulses is somewhat idealized. The pulse rate in field-emission radiography is typically 10 to 25 pulses/sec. The accelerating voltage is the voltage above the minimum very high voltage, V_0, required for field emission; that is, the accelerating voltage is that part of the total applied voltage which corresponds to the tube voltage in the case of a Coolidge tube.

supply. During exposures of a field-emission x-ray tube, the exposure rate at the tube face may be as high as 10^9 R/sec.

A practical x-ray machine utilizing the field-emission principle may consist of two units, the tube and its housing and the pulse generator. These are connected by a single coaxial cable. The tube unit is a cylinder of approximately 2 ft in length and 3 in. in diameter. The high tension supply is a small case approximately 10 in. by 10 in. by 20 in., and weighs approximately 60 pounds. The machine operates from a standard power outlet of 110 to 125 volts AC.

Although still undergoing further intensive research, this type of apparatus is already in use in industry, especially in the radiographic investigation of rapidly moving objects such as bullets and exploding charges. In medical radiography at present, its chief use is in portable x-ray machines.

12.8   COMPUTERS AND MEDICAL RADIOGRAPHY

You may well understand from your general reading that a computer is often a complex electronic device which can make calculations, store information, and produce answers, all at great speed. Computers, as you are no doubt fully aware, are becoming more and more common in every branch of human activity.

In the x-ray department, the computer can be used to calculate and produce all timetables, work schedules, salary and tax scales, accounts, records of film stocks, maintenance costs, and other routine business management figures. It can also, with far greater efficiency than humans, record and make rapidly available all patient records, reports, notes, and index systems, providing that a suitable computer input format for all this information can be devised. The computer is also beginning to be used as part of the direct chain between the x-ray image and the final diagnosis, but before we discuss the way this can be done, let us enquire into the methods of operation of these machines.

First, what is a computer? The dictionary describes it as an apparatus for carrying out mathematical operations by mechanical or electrical means, or both. In other words, a computer does not necessarily mean a large electronic device. In this section we shall discuss the two main types, digital and analog. No attempt will be made to give a comprehensive account of the operation of a computer. What we shall do is explain the principle at the heart of each type and then point out the feasibility of using this principle to produce the final machine. For further study, we would refer you to the section on suggested reading at the end of this chapter. One other point might be made at this time: contrary to many popularized comments, the computer is not "smart." It supplies no intelligence, as yet at least! In fact, the computer does nothing except what it is told to do by some intelligent being, A "thinking" computer, if there should ever be one, would probably first require a better understanding of the brain than we have today, and also some significant development in computer technology.

Digital Computers

The digital computer is a machine which receives numbers and performs mathematical operations with them. It can only add (and subtract by complementary addition). But by being able to do this much it is, of course, also capable of multiplication and division.

Any computer is made up of the functional parts shown in Fig. 12.23. Let us look first at the memory.

Suppose that we have a giant perforated board with holes regularly spaced, but in groups of three, as shown in Fig. 12.24. Each right-hand hole of the three represents the number 1, the center hole represents 2, and the left-hand hole 4.

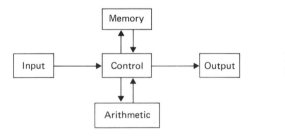

FIG. 12.23. The functional components of a computer.

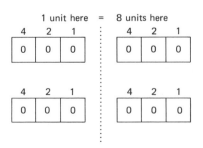

FIG. 12.24. The pegboard memory. Numbers are recorded by putting pegs in the appropriate holes.

To record a number in this memory, we place pegs in the appropriate holes. For example, to store and record the number 5 we would put pegs in holes 4 and 1. Each trio of holes will record as high as 7. To record higher numbers we merely begin a new trio, shown to the left in the figure. Each unit in this new trio represents the number 8. Here we have a system which counts in 8's instead of 10's. More importantly, it is a *binary system*. That is, the numbers are recorded on the board by having a peg in the hole, or leaving the hole empty. Each indicator (hole) is either filled or empty.

Suppose now that on our giant board each trio of holes has an address. That is, each hole group may be uniquely referred to by a number. For instance, on our board suppose that we have 10,000 such groups in rows. Then we may address the groups by means of the numbers 00,000 through 9,999. Whenever we wish to refer to a memory location we have only to give its numerical address.

The arithmetic unit of the computer has a structure similar to the memory unit, but is used to add (and subtract) numbers taken from the memory. We have separated the two units because the memory may be nearly full with numbers, but the arithmetic unit will contain only a transient number population. This arrangement allows more arithmetic flexibility.

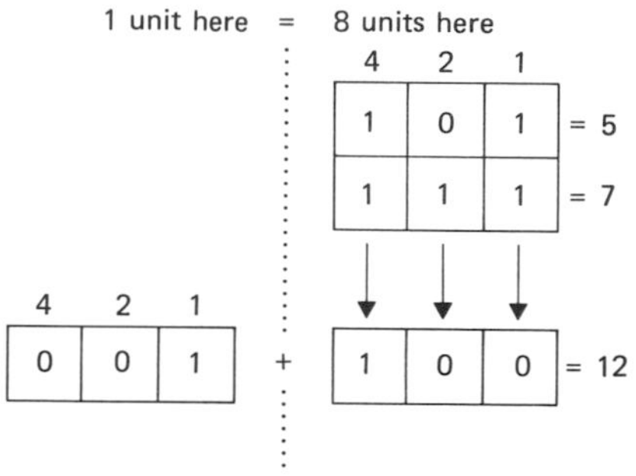

FIG. 12.25. The arithmetic unit. Here 5 has been added to 7 to give 12, indicated by 8 + 4.

Let us take two numbers from the memory, say 5 and 7, place them in the arithmetic unit and add them. They will appear as in Fig. 12.25. The number 1 represents a peg in the hole, 0 represents an empty hole. We need four simple rules for this operation. You can test their validity for yourself. Here we shall merely state them. Adding two 0's results in 0; adding 0 and 1, or 1 and 0, gives a sum of 1; and adding two 1's results in 0, with a 1 to carry. Follow the operation in the figure and see if you agree.

When this new number has been obtained, it may either be stored in the memory to be combined in some way with another, or may be read out as an output.

Referring again to Fig. 12.23, we can see the function of the other units. The input might be a sheet of paper with a problem on it carried by yourself. The output unit could be another piece of paper, or your voice announcing the results. The control unit would be made up of yourself jumping about between two giant pegboards, moving pegs in the correct order. And there we have a computer of the digital type; using binary digits (called *bits* for short) for its operation.

Now you may ask what use is it? We could have performed these computations more easily in our heads, or with pencil and paper. But suppose the computer to be an electronic device with a memory of many millions of bits. Furthermore, suppose the time required to store or obtain information from the memory to be in the order of millionths of a second. Then, of course, such a machine would be very useful. The digital computer's vast information capacity and almost incomprehensible speed of operation, together with its accuracy, indicate some of the possibilities for its use.

The units of transfer, storage, and computation, which we have represented by trios of holes, with or without pegs, may in practice consist of any one of many electronic or other devices. They all have in common the fact that they are either ON or OFF. One material used is a magnetic tape. Each tiny spot on the tape may be magnetized either in one direction or the other. Or a punched card may be used; each space on the card is either punched out or not. There are many possibilities.

We can get some idea of the capabilities of the modern electronic computer by considering its very high speed of operation. Such machines are often called "electronic brains" which, as we pointed out earlier, they are not. In fact, we can readily understand the dependence of the machine on human beings and the enormous labor involved in putting a computer to work by making a study of computer programming.

Essentially, programming consists of arranging for the control unit to operate the other units of the computer in a given order. This includes every single movement of numbers from one address to another throughout whatever complex operation is required to attain the desired output. Devising the program may occupy several people for many months. But once the program is completed, and once the machine is told what to do, it is able to perform computations in a few seconds or minutes. These computations might well have required the people who devised the program to spend many years or even lifetimes, if they had tried to do the computations themselves.

The format of the input is naturally very important. It has to be in some form, such as numbers, which the machine can digest. Also it has to be free of errors and ambiguities.

How may computers be used to store radiographic images? A television picture or an x-ray film may be recorded, by means of a scanning device, as a variable brightness with respect to scanning time. In the computer this variation may produce a series of numbers, for example. These numbers, in their proper sequences, have then only to be recalled from the computer and applied to a suitable display apparatus, such as a television picture tube, in order to make the image available. You may think of the numbers from the computer as being voltage variations at the picture tube input.

While the x-ray images are in the storage facility, or memory, of the computer, certain of their characteristics may be enhanced. Their contrast may be increased, or fog due to scattered radiation may be removed; that is, in the language of electronics, the signal-to-noise ratio may be increased. Or subtraction techniques such as those mentioned in Section 12.6 may be carried out.

Finally, of course, diagnostic processes may be performed. The computer may be supplied with a normal radiograph, perhaps of a chest, and instructed to compare all subsequent chest radiographs with it. In this way a preliminary division of normal and abnormal radiographs is made. The selected radiographs are then further processed by the computer or a radiologist. The ultimate diagnosis, of course, will still have to be performed by a radiologist who supplies the necessary subjective intelligence for each individual case.

The first steps of these processes involving computers have already been carried out in some medical schools, although many problems remain and a great deal of further research is still to be done. However, you can see that we live in exciting times. Elsewhere in radiology and medicine one of the most challenging problems yet to be fully overcome is that of the human-machine interface. The ultimate answer would permit human speech to be used as an input medium to the computer.

Analog Computers

To perform computations, an analog computer, instead of using separate digits, uses continuous quantities such as electric currents. By so doing, it constructs analogies which represent input and output information. In other respects its methods of operation are quite similar to those of the digital computer. For instance, if a certain current is flowing in a given circuit, then, by adding another current to it, we get the algebraic sum of the two. By virtue of the laws of electric circuits, some of which you already know, it is possible to perform other mathematical processes. Ohm's law expresses a linear relationship; other circuit elements such as diodes can be used to produce nonlinear relationships.

One common and simple analog computer is the slide rule. Here length is the analogous quantity: Length is made to represent the logarithms of numbers, so that when one length is added to another we may say that two numbers have been multiplied. The result is the product of the two.

In general, analog computers are not as widely used as digital computers. An example of the use of analog computers in a field of medicine allied to radiology is the study of the dynamics of blood flow in blood vessels. If an analog computer is given sufficient information from a normal patient regarding blood flow rates, as obtained from angiographic studies, vessel diameters, flow patterns, viscosity, and other factors, the computer can construct a model of these circumstances in its memory. Then various other factors may be added. A stoppage, that is, zero flow, may be arranged at a certain point to represent a blood clot. This factor changes the previous model and we are able to see exactly in what way it changes it. Consequently, by this means we may conduct research without endangering the well-being of a patient. This fact alone indicates that analog computers are very likely to find increasing uses in research and teaching hospitals.

SUGGESTED READING

BLUEMLE, A. (editor), *Saturday Science.* New York: E. P. Dutton, 1960. Written by scientists of the Westinghouse Research Laboratories for high school students and informed laymen, and requiring little mathematics, this book includes information about electroluminescence.

CHESNEY, D. N. and M. O., *Radiographic Photography.* Oxford: Blackwell Scientific Publications, 1965. The last four chapters of this book deal with optics, cameras, fluorographic equipment, and the photographic aspects of fluorography. The book is written for the student radiographer, and deals in greater detail with matters discussed in our Section 12.2. Some photographs of mirror camera equipment are included.

DE FRANCE, J. J., *Electron Tubes and Semiconductors.* Englewood Cliffs, N.J.: Prentice-Hall, 1958, fourth reprint 1964. This is a book for students of technical institutes and for electronic technicians. For senior x-ray students who are interested in electronics, and who have a background of basic physics as covered in our text, this book will make absorbing reading. It includes chapters on such topics as cathode ray tubes, semiconductor rectifiers, basic transistors, phototubes, and photoelectric cells.

DYKE, W. P., "Advances in Field Emission," *Scientific American,* January 1964. This short article by a leading scientist is presented at a level suitable for the senior student radiographer, and includes a bibliography.

ETTER, L. E. (editor), *The Science of Ionizing Radiation.* Springfield, Ill.: Charles C. Thomas, 1965. For all student radiographers we recommend Chapter 5, "Equipment of All Types." Many excellent photographs are included.

FINK, D. G., and D. M. LUTYENS, *The Physics of Television.* New York: Anchor Books, Doubleday, 1960. This 160-page paperback belongs to the Science Study Series and is intended for high school students and laymen. Although not oriented toward the uses of TV in medical radiography, this book nevertheless is a valuable addition to the bookshelf of a radiographer.

JACOBOWITZ, H., *Electronic Computers Made Simple.* New York: Doubleday, 1963. We suggest this book for the advanced student. A knowledge of elementary calculus is helpful.

NEBLETTE, C. B., *Photography, Its Materials and Processes.* Princeton, N.J.: D. Van Nostrand, 1962 (sixth edition). For those students who would know more about photographic optics, photographic lenses, shutters, and cameras, we recommend Chapters 4 through 7. The text is very detailed, but should be easily understood by student radiographers.

RAMSEY, G. H. S., T. A. TRISTAN, J. S. WATSON, S. WEINBERG, and W. S. CORNWELL (editors), *Cinefluorography*.   Springfield, Ill.: Charles C. Thomas, 1960; also published by Blackwell Scientific Publications in Oxford, England, and by the Ryerson Press, Toronto, Canada.   The book is a very informative report of the proceedings of a symposium on cinefluorography held in New York.   In 18 chapters, this book presents in an orderly fashion a wealth of information and comment on topics we have touched on in our Sections 12.3 through 12.6. References are included at the end of each chapter and a lengthy bibliography follows the text.   Recommended for the senior student and new graduate.

YOUNG, F. H., *Digital Computers and Related Mathematics*.   Boston, Mass.: Ginn and Co., 1961.   We recommend this 40-page pamphlet as further reading for the x-ray student with a certain degree of maturity in mathematics.   (However, despite this qualification, only elementary algebra and the use of exponents is assumed as a prerequisite.)

Mathematical Review

In writing this book we have assumed that the reader has a knowledge of elementary algebra, geometry, and trigonometry. For the benefit of those readers whose mathematics needs a little refreshing, a brief review of some relevant mathematics is given here.

We wish especially to draw the attention of all readers to the list of Suggested Reading at the end of this appendix. The book by Kemp, referred to there, can be highly recommended to all.

A.1 EXPONENTS

Calculating with Exponents

It is often necessary to multiply a quantity by itself a number of times. This process is indicated by a superscript number called the *exponent*, according to the following scheme:

$$A = A^1,$$
$$A \times A = A^2,$$
$$A \times A \times A = A^3,$$
$$A \times A \times A \times A = A^4,$$
$$A \times A \times A \times A \times A = A^5.$$

We read A^2 as "A squared" because it is, or may be conceived as, the area of a square of length A on a side; similarly, A^3 is called "A cubed" because it may be the volume of a cube each of whose sides is A long. More generally we speak of A^n as "A to the nth power." Thus A^5 is read as "A to the fifth power."

When we multiply a quantity raised to some particular power (say A^n) by the same quantity raised to another power (say A^m), the result is that quantity raised to a power equal to the sum of the original exponents. That is,

$$A^n A^m = A^{n+m}.$$

For example,

$$A^2 A^5 = A^7,$$

which we can verify directly by writing out the terms:

$$\underbrace{(A \times A)}_{A^2} \times \underbrace{(A \times A \times A \times A \times A)}_{A^5} = \underbrace{(A \times A \times A \times A \times A \times A \times A)}_{A^7}.$$

From the above result we see that when a quantity raised to a particular power (say A^n) is to be multiplied by itself a total of m times, we have

$$(A^n)^m = A^{nm}.$$

For example,

$$(A^2)^3 = A^6,$$

since

$$(A^2)^3 = A^2 \times A^2 \times A^2 = A^{2+2+2} = A^6.$$

Reciprocal quantities are expressed in a similar way with the addition of a minus sign in the exponent, as follows:

$$\frac{1}{A} = A^{-1}, \qquad \frac{1}{A^3} = A^{-3}.$$

Exactly the same rules as before are used in combining quantities raised to negative powers with one another and with some quantity raised to a positive power. Thus

$$A^5 A^{-2} = A^{5-2} = A^3, \qquad (A^{-1})^{-2} = A^{-1(-2)} = A^2, \qquad (A^3)^{-4} = A^{-4 \times 3} = A^{-12},$$

It is important to remember that *any* quantity raised to the zeroth power, say A^0, is equal to 1. Hence

$$A^2 A^{-2} = A^{2-2} = A^0 = 1.$$

We can see this more easily if we write A^{-2} as $1/A^2$:

$$A^2 A^{-2} = A^2 \times \frac{1}{A^2} = \frac{A^2}{A^2} = 1.$$

Fractional exponents are frequently useful. The simplest case is that of the square root of a quantity A, commonly written $\sqrt{A}$, which when multiplied by itself equals the quantity:

$$\sqrt{A} \times \sqrt{A} = A.$$

Using exponentials, we see that, because

$$(A^{1/2})^2 = A^{2 \times (1/2)} = A^1 = A,$$

we can express square roots by the exponent $\frac{1}{2}$:

$$\sqrt{A} = A^{1/2}.$$

In general, the nth root of a quantity, $\sqrt[n]{A}$, may be written $A^{1/n}$, which is a more convenient form for most purposes. Some examples may be helpful:

$$(A^4)^{1/2} = A^{(1/2) \times 4} = A^2, \qquad (A^3)^{-1/3} = A^{-(1/3) \times 3} = A^{-1}.$$

Fractional exponents may also be expressed as decimals:

$$A^{1/2} = A^{0.5}, \qquad A^{1/3} = A^{0.333}, \qquad A^{7/4} = A^{1.75}.$$

Quantities raised to decimal exponents are manipulated in the same manner we have become accustomed to:

$$(A^{1.8})^{-4} = A^{-4 \times 1.8} = A^{-7.2},$$
$$(A^{0.6})^{0.5} = A^{0.5 \times 0.6} = A^{0.3}.$$

Exponents and Units

All this dealing with exponents is as true in the case of units (for example, centimeters) as it is in the case of some number A. For example, we say that the linear attenuation coefficient of lead, μ, is 0.12 per cm, and we can write this in either one of the two equivalent ways:

$$\mu = 0.12/\text{cm} = 0.12 \text{ cm}^{-1}.$$

Or we might consider the frequency f of alternation of an alternating current which may be 60 cycles per second (or hertz), and write:

$$f = 60/\text{sec} = 60 \text{ sec}^{-1}.$$

As a final example, we consider a fluoroscopy screen 12.0 in. long and 12.0 in. wide. We write its area A as

$$A = (12.0 \text{ in.}) (12.0 \text{ in.})$$
$$= (144) (\text{in.} \times \text{in.})$$
$$= 144 \text{ in}^2.$$

Exponential Notation

Now that we have recalled the essential principles of dealing with exponents, we note that exponential notation is a convenient and widely used method for abbreviating large and small numbers. The method is based on the fact that all numbers (in decimal form) may be expressed as a number between 1 and 10 multiplied by a power of 10. To see this, we must first construct a table of powers of 10, such as Table A.1.

Table A.1

Powers of 10 from 10^{-10} to 10^{10}	
$10^{-10} = 0.000,000,000,1$	$10^0 = 1$
$10^{-9}\ = 0.000,000,001$	$10^1 = 10$
$10^{-8}\ = 0.000,000,01$	$10^2 = 100$
$10^{-7}\ = 0.000,000,1$	$10^3 = 1000$
$10^{-6}\ = 0.000,001$	$10^4 = 10,000$
$10^{-5}\ = 0.000,01$	$10^5 = 100,000$
$10^{-4}\ = 0.000,1$	$10^6 = 1,000,000$
$10^{-3}\ = 0.001$	$10^7 = 10,000,000$
$10^{-2}\ = 0.01$	$10^8 = 100,000,000$
$10^{-1}\ = 0.1$	$10^9 = 1,000,000,000$
$10^0\ \ \ = 1$	$10^{10} = 10,000,000,000$

Now let us look at a few examples:

$$600 = 6 \times 100 = 6 \times 10^2,$$
$$7940 = 7.94 \times 1000 = 7.94 \times 10^3,$$
$$0.023 = 2.3 \times 0.01 = 2.3 \times 10^{-2},$$
$$93,000,000 = 9.3 \times 10,000,000 = 9.3 \times 10^7.$$

This method of writing very large and very small numbers has a great advantage in that it makes numerical calculations less cumbersome and therefore less prone to errors in many cases. An example that obviously supports this contention is the calculation suggested in Question 18 of Chapter 9, in which both Planck's constant and the speed of light become involved. Imagine calculating with Planck's constant as

0.0000000000000000000000000000000000663 joule-sec,

instead of simply 6.63×10^{-34} joule-sec.

A.2   SIGNIFICANT FIGURES

Significant Figures and Precision

As this term implies, significant figures are figures which are meaningful. For example, if one were to guess the diameter of a coin to be 1.0396 inches, the .0396 is obviously not significant. These figures have no real meaning because they indicate a degree of precision far beyond that which can be achieved by guessing. Now if one were to measure this diameter using a ruler marked off in 0.1 inch, the diameter could be quoted as 0.95 inch (see Fig. A.1). Note that although the 5 was guessed, it is still a significant figure. One figure beyond the smallest graduation may be used as significant, since one can make a reasonable guess to that extent. However, since the figure is doubtful, it would be meaningless to quote another

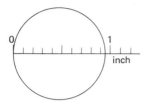

FIG. A.1. Measuring the diameter of a coin: 0.95 inch.

figure after the one in doubt. If you are not quite sure how many hundredths there are, you surely cannot suggest how many thousandths. To quote the diameter of the coin in this case as 0.953 in. would be nonsense.

However, if one were to use a more precise instrument, say with 0.01 inch as the smallest division, the diameter could be quoted, for example, as 0.953 inch. Note that in this case the 5 is definite and the 3 is guessed.

So we see that when one writes the value found from a measurement one must be careful to indicate the precision of the instrument by writing only the appropriate number of significant figures. Zeros being used to indicate the position of the decimal point are not significant figures. Writing numbers using exponential notation is a convenient way of indicating significant figures. For example, if one reads the voltage indicated by a panel meter on an x-ray unit as 35,000 volts, not all the zeros are likely to be significant figures. If the meter were graduated in kV (see Fig. A.2), the first zero after the five would be doubtful, and hence it would be the last significant figure. The voltage would properly be quoted as 3.50×10^4 volts, or 35.0 kV.

Note that when we write a number that employs exponential notation, it is a simple matter to retain only the significant figures, and yet indicate the proper order of magnitude, that is, the proper position of the decimal point.

Now consider the tube current reading shown in Fig. A.3. The meter reads 23.5 milliamperes or 0.0235 ampere. The first zero after the decimal is not a significant figure. In exponential notation we would properly write the current as 2.35×10^{-2} ampere, or 23.5 mA.

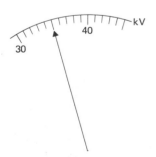

FIG. A.2. Reading a kV meter: 35.0 kV.

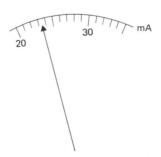

FIG. A.3. Reading an mA meter: 23.5 mA.

Calculating with Significant Figures

Care must be taken when adding and multiplying numbers to maintain the correct number of significant figures. For example, let us add:

$$
\begin{array}{r}
390.1 \ \ \text{ft} \\
6.44 \ \ \text{ft} \\
\underline{8.553 \ \text{ft}} \\
405.093 \ \text{ft}
\end{array}
$$

What is the meaning of this result? In any number obtained by measurement, all the digits following the last significant figure are unknown. For example, the digits to follow the .1 in the first measurement, 390.1, are unknown. Clearly if one adds an unknown quantity to a known quantity, one gets an unknown answer. Consequently the last two figures, 93, in the sum above have no real meaning. The answer is therefore reported simply as 405.1 ft.

Since 0.1 ft. was the smallest unit known for the least precise measurement, the answer was rounded off to the appropriate number of tenths (0.1) of a foot. Since 0.093 is greater than 0.05, it was changed to 0.1. Generally if the first figure to be dropped is equal to or greater than 5, the last significant figure is raised by one; if the figure to be dropped is less than 5, it is simply dropped.

In addition and subtraction the number of significant figures after the decimal in an answer should be equal to the least number of significant figures found after the decimal in the addends. Obviously all the addends must be written to the same power of ten. One could not directly add 3.90×10^2 and 6.7.

For multiplication and division, it is the total number of significant figures in the least precise value that is important. For example, if we were to calculate the power being used by an x-ray machine (Power = voltage × amperage) that was operating with 203.4 mA at 35.0 kV, then we would write:

$$
\begin{aligned}
\text{Power} &= (3.50 \times 10^4 \text{ volts}) (2.034 \times 10^{-1} \text{ amperes}) \\
&= [(3.50) (2.034) \, 10^{4-1}] \text{ watts} \\
&= 7.119 \times 10^3 \text{ watts},
\end{aligned}
$$

which is properly reported as 7.12×10^3 watts.

The answer is written to only three significant figures because the least-precise value (3.50) has three significant figures. If the product were 7.114×10^3, the final answer would be rounded off to 7.11×10^3.

A.3 ALGEBRA

Symbolism

Algebra may be thought of as a generalized arithmetic in which symbols are used in place of specified numbers. The advantage of algebra is that with its help we can perform calculations without knowing in advance the numerical values of all the quantities involved. Sometimes algebra is no more than a help, perhaps because it shows us how to simplify complex calculations, and sometimes it is the only way in which we can solve a problem.

The symbols of algebra are normally letters of the alphabet. If we have two quantities, a and b, and add them to give the sum c, we would write

$$a + b = c.$$

If we subtract b from a to give the difference d, we would write

$$a - b = d.$$

Multiplying a and b to give e may be written $a \times b = e$, or $a \cdot b = e$, or more simply, as just

$$ab = e.$$

Whenever two algebraic quantities are written together with nothing between them, it is understood that they are to be multiplied.

Dividing a by b to give the quotient f is usually written

$$\frac{a}{b} = f,$$

but it may sometimes be more convenient to write

$$a/b = f,$$

which has the same meaning.

Parentheses and brackets are used to show the order in which various operations are to be performed. Thus

$$\frac{(a + b)c}{d} - e = f$$

means that we are first to add a and b, multiply their sum by c, then divide by d, and finally subtract e.

Equations

An equation is simply a statement that a certain quantity is equal to another one. Thus

$$7 + 2 = 9,$$

which contains only numbers, is an arithmetical equation, and

$$3x + 12 = 27,$$

which contains a symbol as well, is an algebraic equation. The symbols in an algebraic equation usually cannot have any arbitrary values if the equality is to hold. Finding the possible values of these symbols is called *solving the equation.* The solution of the latter equation above is

$$x = 5,$$

since only when x is 5 is it true that $3x + 12 = 27$.

In order to solve an equation, one must keep a basic principle in mind.

Any operation performed on one side of an equation must be performed on the other.

An equation therefore remains valid when the same quantity, numerical or otherwise, is added to or subtracted from both sides, or when the same quantity is used to multiply or divide both sides. Other operations, for instance squaring or taking the square root, also do not alter the equality if the same thing is done to both sides. As a simple example, to solve $3x + 12 = 27$, we first subtract 12 from both sides:

$$3x + 12 - 12 = 27 - 12,$$
$$3x = 15.$$

To complete the solution we divide both sides by 3:

$$\frac{3x}{3} = \frac{15}{3}, \qquad x = 5.$$

To verify the correctness of a solution, we substitute it back into the original equation and see whether the equality is still true. Thus we can check that $x = 5$ by reducing the original algebraic equation to an arithmetical one:

$$3x + 12 = 27, \qquad 3 \cdot 5 + 12 = 27,$$
$$15 + 12 = 27, \qquad 27 = 27.$$

Two simple rules follow directly from the principle stated above. The first is,

One can transpose any term on one side of an equation to the other side by changing its sign.

To verify this rule, we subtract b from each side of the equation $a + b = c$ to obtain

$$a + b - b = c - b,$$
$$a = c - b.$$

We see that b has disappeared from the left-hand side and $-b$ is now on the right-hand side.

The second rule is

A quantity which multiplies one side of an equation may be transposed so as to divide the other side, and vice versa.

To verify this rule, we divide both sides of the equation $ab = c$ by b. The result is

$$\frac{ab}{b} = \frac{c}{b}, \qquad a = \frac{c}{b}.$$

We see that b, a multiplier on the left-hand side, is now a divisor on the right-hand side.

Examples

1. Given that $V = IR$ (Ohm's law), $V = 12$ volts, and $R = 6$ ohms, determine I.

    $V = IR$ is the same as $IR = V$.

    Now, dividing both sides by R, we get

    $$I = \frac{V}{R} = \frac{12 \text{ volts}}{6 \text{ ohms}} = 2 \frac{\text{volts}}{\text{ohms}}.$$

    (The unit volt/ohm is called an ampere.)

2. The relation between equivalent temperatures on the Celsius and Fahrenheit temperature scales is given by $C = \frac{5}{9}(F - 32°)$. What is the Fahrenheit reading for a Celsius temperature of 25°?

    $$\tfrac{5}{9}(F - 32°) = C = 25°, \qquad F - 32° = 25° \times \tfrac{9}{5} = 45°.$$

    Therefore the Fahrenheit reading F is given by

    $$F = 45° + 32° = 77°.$$

Proportionality

The notion of proportionality is frequently encountered in physics. This is natural, because physics has its roots in experiment and a common result of an experiment is a proportional relationship. Let us look into just what is implied in relationships of this kind.

When the value of a quantity A depends on the value of another quantity B in such a way that doubling B causes A to double, tripling B causes A to triple, and so on, A is said to be *directly proportional* to B. If A is directly proportional to B, then we may have, for example,

$$A = 0 \text{ when } B = 0,$$
$$A = 1 \text{ when } B = \tfrac{1}{2},$$
$$A = 2 \text{ when } B = 1,$$
$$A = 4 \text{ when } B = 2,$$
$$A = 6 \text{ when } B = 3,$$

and so on. No matter what the value of B, the ratio between A and B remains constant:

$$\frac{A}{B} = 2 = \text{constant} = c.$$

Hence we may express the fact that A is proportional to B by the equation

$$A = cB,$$

where c is called the *constant of proportionality*. In our particular case, the proportionality constant is 2.

A practical example of such a proportionality is Ohm's law: $V = RI$. Here the two variables analogous to A and B in our example are V, the voltage, and I, the current. The proportionality constant is R, the resistance.

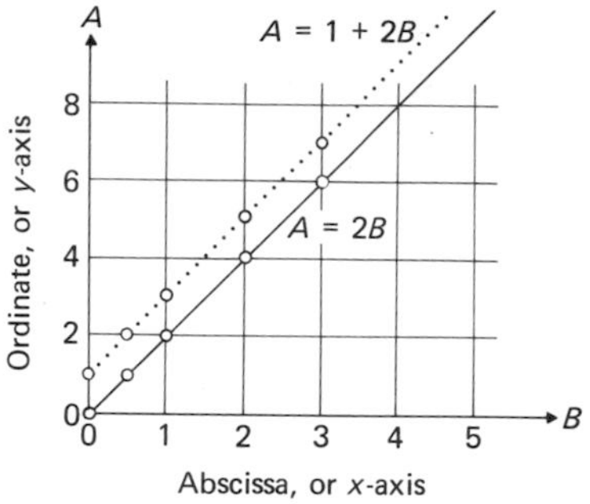

FIG. A.4. Graphing linear equations.

If we were to graph such a proportionality, we would get a straight line, as shown in Fig. A.4, in which we have plotted the values of A of our example along the ordinate (or y-axis) and the values of B along the abscissa (or x-axis).

In the parlance of mathematics, we say that we have plotted A *as a function of B*. Moreover, since we obtain a straight line, we say that:

a) A is a linear function of B, or
b) $A = 2B$ is a linear equation, or
c) A is *directly* proportional to B (written simply as $A \propto B$).

All these statements infer the same relationship.

Now suppose that instead of the values for A and B, as given earlier, we had the following:

$$A = 1 \text{ when } B = 0,$$
$$A = 2 \text{ when } B = \tfrac{1}{2},$$
$$A = 3 \text{ when } B = 1,$$
$$A = 5 \text{ when } B = 2,$$
$$A = 7 \text{ when } B = 3.$$

In this case we note that $A \neq 2B$, but rather

$$A = 1 + 2B.$$

If we plot this (dotted line on Fig. A.4), we still get a straight line. This is still a linear relationship. In analytic geometry, in which it is common practice to use y as the dependent variable and x as the independent variable, such an equation is frequently written in the quite general standard form

$$y = mx + b,$$

where in our specific case $y = A$, $x = B$, $m = $ slope of line $= $ proportionality constant $= 2$, and $b = y$-axis intercept $= 1$.

Proportionalities other than direct proportionalities are, of course, also found in physics. We might find, for example,

$$A = 0 = 0 \times 3 \text{ when } B = 0,$$
$$A = 12 = 4 \times 3 \text{ when } B = 2,$$
$$A = 27 = 9 \times 3 \text{ when } B = 3,$$
$$A = 48 = 16 \times 3 \text{ when } B = 4.$$

In this case, $A = 3B^2$. We say that A is directly proportional to B^2. An example is in the heating of the x-ray tube target, the heating effect of an electric current being given by

$$P = I^2 R,$$

where P is the power, or the rate that heat energy is developed.

We say that P varies as I^2 (written $P \propto I^2$). (With reference to our A and B example: P is analogous to A, I to B, and $R = 3$.)

Another possibility is an *inverse proportionality*; that is,

$$A = c\,\frac{1}{B} \qquad \text{or} \qquad AB = c.$$

Such a situation exists in the case of gases. In a given mass of a gas at a constant temperature, the volume varies inversely as the pressure, that is,

$$PV = \text{constant.}$$

Inverse-Square Law

Of course, the inverse proportion, like the direct proportion, could be to higher powers. That is, we could have

$$A = c\,\frac{1}{B^2} \qquad \text{or} \qquad AB^2 = c.$$

Omitting the proportionality constant and therefore writing the relationship as a proportionality instead of an equation, we would have

$$A \propto \frac{1}{B^2}.$$

Either way of writing, this is the familiar case of an inverse-square law, of which Coulomb's law is one. Coulomb's law states that the force F of one electrical charge on another varies inversely as the square of the distance s between them; that is

$$F \propto \frac{1}{s^2}.$$

Another example is in the field of radiation intensity. The x-ray intensity I, due to a point source, varies inversely as the square of the

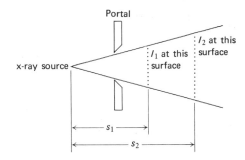

FIG. A.5. The inverse-square law:
$I \propto 1/s^2$.

distance s from the anode of the x-ray tube; that is,

$$I \propto \frac{1}{s^2}.$$

Let us try this relationship in a practical case. We refer to Fig. A.5. For distance s, we write

$$I_1 \propto \frac{1}{s_1{}^2} \quad \text{or} \quad I_1 = k\frac{1}{s_1{}^2},$$

where k is some constant of proportionality. Similarly for s_2 we have

$$I_2 = k\frac{1}{s_2{}^2}.$$

Dividing these latter two equations, we have

$$\frac{I_1}{I_2} = \frac{k/s_1{}^2}{k/s_2{}^2},$$

which is in effect

$$\frac{I_1}{I_2} = \frac{s_2{}^2}{s_1{}^2}.$$

This format of the inverse-square law is probably the most useful one for radiographic physics.

Now with some numbers: What happens to the intensity of irradiation from a small x-ray source (point source) if the surface originally to be x-rayed at 30 in. is moved 10 in. farther away?

$$\frac{I_2 \,(\text{at 40 in.})}{I_1 \,(\text{at 30 in.})} = \frac{30^2 \text{ in}^2}{40^2 \text{ in}^2};$$

hence

$$I_2 = I_1 \left(\frac{30}{40}\right)^2 = \frac{9}{16}\,I_1.$$

A.4 LOGARITHMS

The logarithm of a number to a given base is the power (or exponent) to which the base must be raised in order that the result yield the given number. For example, given that $y = 10^2$, then the logarithm of y to the base ten is 2. We could thus write

$$\log_{10} y = 2.$$

Other examples are

$$\log_{10} 10 = 1, \text{ since } 10^1 = 10,$$
$$\log_{10} 1 = 0, \text{ since } 10^0 = 1,$$
$$\log_2 16 = 4, \text{ since } 2^4 = 16,$$
$$\log_e 0.5 = -0.693, \text{ since } e^{-0.693} = 0.5.$$

Let us look at some of the essentials of common logs. Logarithms have two parts: a decimal fraction which is always positive (called the *mantissa*), and an integer which may be positive or negative (called the *characteristic*). For example, in the case of log $256 = 2.408$, the 408 is the mantissa and the 2 is the characteristic (see Fig. A.6).

Note that the common logarithms of all numbers expressed by the same figures in the same order but with different positions of the decimal point all have the same mantissa but a different characteristic, determined by the position of the decimal point in the particular number. If the number is greater than 1, the characteristic is positive, and its value is 1 less then the number of digits to the left of the decimal point. This may be seen by the previous example of the logarithm of 256, which yielded a characteristic of 2. Had the number been 25.6, the characteristic would have been 1: that is,

$$\log 25.6 = 1.408.$$

If the number is less than 1, say 0.0256, then the characteristic is negative, and has a numerical value 1 greater than the number of zeros between the decimal point and the first integer to the right of the decimal point. A negative characteristic is shown with a bar over the top of it to indicate that it alone, and not the mantissa, is negative. Example:

$$\log 0.0256 = \bar{2}.408,$$

which means $0.408 - 2$.

L-scale (mantissa of logarithm of number)

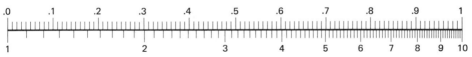

D-scale (number)

FIG. A.6. Scales for finding the logarithms of numbers.

The mantissa, on the other hand, is independent of the position of the decimal point in the number in question. The mantissa is generally found to 5 or more digits in a table of logarithms. Slide rules may also be employed for this purpose, but with a lesser degree of precision. Figure A.6 shows two scales on a slide rule (D- and L- scale) which may be used to find the logarithm of a number. We used this to find that the mantissa for log 256 was 408.

Let us look at a few further examples:

$$\log 150 = 2.176,$$
$$\log 15 = 1.176,$$
$$\log 1.5 = 0.176,$$
$$\log 0.15 = \bar{1}.176,$$
$$\log 0.015 = \bar{2}.176.$$

The essential point to note about logarithms is that a logarithm is no more than an exponent, and hence the rules for calculations with logarithms are the same as the rules employed for exponents. Hence, for example, if we want to multiply two numbers, we may achieve this by adding the logarithms of those two numbers and then finding the number which has a log equal to this sum.

Logarithms are generally employed either to base 10, in which case one simply writes log, the subscript 10 being understood, or to base e ($e = 2.71828 \ldots$), in which case one writes simply ln, where ln means $\log_e$.

To get from base 10 to base e, or vice versa, we have the relationships:

$$\ln x = (2.3026) \log x, \qquad \log x = (0.4343) \ln x.$$

For further details, we refer the reader to the book by Kemp listed at the end of this appendix.

A.5 GRAPHS

Linear Graph Paper

It is often instructive to exhibit the relationship between two quantities in the form of a graph. Frequently the information is more useful in this form than in the form of an equation because it immediately shows what value the one quantity has if the other quantity has some given value, and it also immediately displays a general trend. Anode cooling curves, such as are posted in many x-ray control booths, are an example of the way graphs provide ready information in an easily accessible manner.

In our previous discussion of proportionality, we have already shown the graph of a linear relationship (Fig. A.4). Linear graph paper—that is, paper which has all equal spacings along the axes—is the one most commonly employed. It can be used, of course, to plot nonlinear relationships.

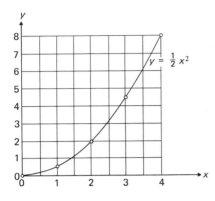

FIG. A.7. A nonlinear relation plotted on linear graph paper. (Data from Table A.1.)

An example is seen in Fig. A.7, in which is plotted the equation

$$y = \tfrac{1}{2}x^2,$$

for which some values are tabulated in Table A.1.

Table A.1

x	x^2	y
0.0	0.0	0.0
1.0	1.0	0.5
2.0	4.0	2.0
3.0	9.0	4.5
4.0	16.0	8.0

Logarithmic Graph Paper

When a large range of quantities is to be displayed, it is often practical to employ logarithmic, for example, log-log, graph paper. Instead of plotting, say, A as a function of B, one plots $\log A$ as a function of $\log B$.

Figure A.8 shows such a case. Note that in the same space taken up for ten units in the first cycle, or series of divisions, we are able to go from

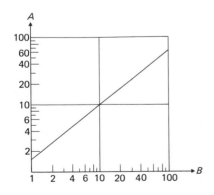

FIG. A.8. Log-log graph paper. Log A is plotted as a function of log B.

10 to 100. If a third cycle were added, we could go, in the same space again, from 100 to 1000.

Another advantage of log-log paper is that a relationship such as an inverse-square law can be plotted as a straight line, which is easier to draw than a curve, and yields more precise values in the regions between actually calculated points. In using log-log paper for plotting an inverse-square relationship such as

$$A = \frac{1}{B^2} = B^{-2},$$

we are in fact taking the logs of both sides of the equation, i.e.,

$$\log A = -2 \log B,$$

which has the linear form $y = mx$, where $m = -2$. Hence plotting values of A and B on log-log paper indeed yields a straight line.

Semilogarithmic Paper

Of more concern in the present text is the case of semilog paper, which is discussed in connection with the linear attenuation coefficient.

This type of graph paper is shown in Fig. A.9. Note that one axis is scaled logarithmically and the other linearly.

The advantage of this type of graph paper comes to the fore when we have an exponential relation like the following (A and B are the variable quantities, c is a constant):

$$A = 10^{cB}.$$

This may be written $\log A = cB$, which is linear, of the form $y = mx$, where $y = \log A$, $m = c$, and $x = B$.

Note the example of a semilog graph from the x-ray room (Fig. A.9b).

More frequently in physics one encounters relationships in which e, the base of natural logarithms, appears. For example:

$$N = N_0 e^{-\lambda t},$$

which is the radioactive decay law. Here the variables are N and t, while N_0 and λ are constants. In logarithmic form this expression is

$$\ln N = -\lambda t + \ln N_0,$$

which is of the linear form

$$y = mx + b,$$

with

$$\ln N = y, \ -\lambda = m, \ t = x, \text{ and } \ln N_0 = b.$$

Since it is more usual to find log paper to base 10 rather than to base e, one therefore changes this expression to base 10, according to the relationship between base 10 and base e logs given in Section A.4.

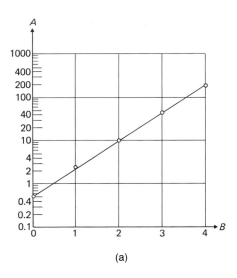

(a)

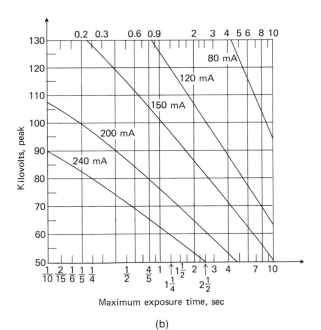

(b)

FIG. A.9. Semilog paper. (a) Log *A* is plotted as a function of *B*. (b) *X*-ray tube rating chart in which kV is plotted as a function of the logarithm of the maximum exposure time. The numbers across the top indicate the decimal divisions of two logarithmic cycles. The numbers across the bottom are as they are likely to be found on an actual chart in the x-ray room.

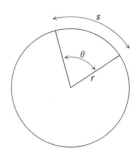

FIG. A.10. Radian measure: θ (in radians) = s/r.

A.6 GEOMETRY

Radian Measure

We now recall some elements of plane geometry.

First, something about angles. A right angle has 90°; in a circle there are 360°; and the sum of the interior angles of any triangle is 180°.

Another way of measuring angles is in terms of radian measure. An angle in radians is given by dividing the arc, s, which subtends the angle, θ, at the center of a circle by the circle's radius r (see Fig. A.10); that is

$$\theta = s/r.$$

From this definition we can see that for a full circle we get

$$\text{Angle in radians} = \frac{2\pi r}{r} = 2\pi.$$

In other words, 360° are equivalent to 2π radians, 180° = π radians, and 90° = $\pi/2$ radians. Also, since $\pi \approx 3.14159$, 1 degree is about equivalent to 0.01745 radian.

Similar Triangles

The other useful point to recall relates to similar triangles. Stating it very loosely, one might say that similar triangles have the same shape but not necessarily the same size. Figure A.11 shows two similar triangles. It can

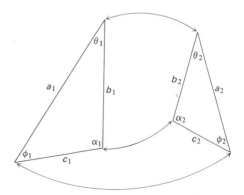

FIG. A.11. Similar triangles.

be shown that for these triangles the ratio of the corresponding sides is a constant; that is,

$$\frac{a_1}{a_2} = \frac{b_1}{b_2} = \frac{c_1}{c_2},$$

and, of course, from the definition of similar triangles,

$$\theta_1 = \theta_2, \qquad \phi_1 = \phi_2, \qquad \text{and } \alpha_1 = \alpha_2.$$

A.7 TRIGONOMETRY

Trigonometric Functions

It is often necessary to know the relationships among the various sides and angles of a right triangle, which is a triangle two of whose sides are perpendicular. The three basic trigonometric functions are defined in terms of the triangle shown in Fig. A.12 as follows:

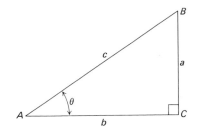

$\sin \theta = \frac{a}{c}$

$\cos \theta = \frac{b}{c}$

$\tan \theta = \frac{a}{b}$

FIG. A.12. A right, or right-angled, triangle, with trigonometric functions defined.

We shall label θ the angle at A included between the side b of the triangle and its hypotenuse c. The sine of this angle, which is abbreviated $\sin \theta$, is the ratio between the side a of the triangle opposite to θ and the hypotenuse c. Hence

$$\sin \theta = \frac{a}{c} = \frac{\text{opposite side}}{\text{hypotenuse}}$$

The cosine of the angle θ, abbreviated $\cos \theta$, is the ratio between the side b of the triangle adjacent to θ and the hypotenuse c. Hence

$$\cos \theta = \frac{b}{c} = \frac{\text{adjacent side}}{\text{hypotenuse}}.$$

The tangent of the angle θ, abbreviated $\tan \theta$, is the ratio between the side a opposite to θ and the side b adjacent to θ. Hence

$$\tan \theta = \frac{a}{b} = \frac{\text{opposite side}}{\text{adjacent side}}.$$

From these definitions we can obtain a useful result:

$$\frac{\sin \theta}{\cos \theta} = \frac{\text{opposite side/hypotenuse}}{\text{adjacent side/hypotenuse}}$$

$$= \frac{\text{opposite side}}{\text{adjacent side}} = \tan \theta.$$

The tangent of an angle is equal to its sine divided by its cosine.

Numerical tables of $\sin \theta$, $\cos \theta$, and $\tan \theta$, for angles from $0°$ to $90°$, can be found in many mathematics books (see Suggested Reading at the end of this appendix). These tables may be used for angles from $90°$ to $180°$ with the help of the following formulas:

$$\sin (90° + \theta) = \cos \theta,$$
$$\cos (90° + \theta) = -\sin \theta,$$
$$\tan (90° + \theta) = -\frac{1}{\tan \theta}.$$

Trigonometric functions can be treated algebraically, just as any other quantity. Suppose that we know the length of the side b and the angle θ in the right triangle of Fig. A.12, and wish to find the lengths of the sides a and c. From the definitions of sine and tangent, we see that

$$\tan \theta = \frac{a}{b}, \qquad \sin \theta = \frac{a}{c},$$

and so

$$a = b \tan \theta, \qquad c = \frac{a}{\sin \theta}.$$

The Pythagorean Theorem

Another useful relationship in a right triangle is the Pythagorean theorem, which states that the sum of the squares of the sides of such a triangle adjacent to the right angle is equal to the square of its hypotenuse. For the triangle of Fig. A.12,

$$a^2 + b^2 = c^2.$$

Hence we can always express the length of any of the sides of a right triangle in terms of the other sides:

$$a = \sqrt{c^2 - b^2}, \qquad b = \sqrt{c^2 - a^2}, \qquad c = \sqrt{a^2 + b^2}.$$

Graphing a Trigonometric Function

Recalling the concept of plotting a mathematical expression on linear graph paper, we now present the equation $y = \sin \theta$ so graphed (see Fig. A.13).

Note that the maximum value for $\sin \theta$ is $+1$ and the minimum value is -1, and that these extreme values are for values of $\theta = 90° = (\pi/2)$ rad or whole-number multiples thereof. A look back at Fig. A.12 suggests that indeed these extreme values make sense, for as θ approaches $90°$ in Fig. A.12 we can mentally visualize side "a" closing up on "c" and becoming

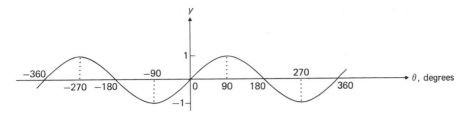

FIG. A.13. Graphical representation of the sine function: $y = \sin \theta$.

closer to "c" in length. At $\theta = 90°$, of course, $a = c$, hence

$$\sin 90° = a/c = c/c = 1.$$

Also to be noted on the graph is that $\sin \theta = 0$, for $\theta = 0$, $180°$, and $360°$. The zero value is also readily apparent from the triangle of Fig. A.12. Imagine θ approaching zero: "c" closes up on "b," while "a" gets smaller, and at $\theta = 0$ we have $a = 0$. Hence

$$\sin 0° = a/c = 0/c = 0.$$

To understand the source of the negative values of sine and the meaning of negative values of θ, we would need to define the trigonometric functions in a more general way. We can perhaps see that this might be possible by considering point A of Fig. A.12 as the center of a circle and letting the side "b" rotate, as a radius vector, completely around a full circle.

A.8 CALCULUS

We shall here do no more than indicate to the reader, by means of Zeno's (495–435 B.C.) story of Achilles and the tortoise that a special mathematics is required to deal with the infinite. The ordinary arithmetic and algebra with which most people are familiar obviously will not cope with the infinitesimal distances referred to in Zeno's argument. This mathematics is the calculus, which is basic to any further and advanced studies in electricity and radiation physics.

Allowing that space and time are infinitely divisible, Zeno proposed that if Achilles were to run 10 times as fast as a tortoise but give the tortoise a 1000-yard head start he could never catch it. Why? Because by the time Achilles had run 1000 yards the tortoise would still be 100 yards ahead; by the time he had run this 100 yards the tortoise would still be 10 yards ahead; and so on forever. Achilles would get nearer and nearer to the tortoise but never quite to it.

This argument is one of the celebrated paradoxes of Zeno. It can be resolved, as we stated earlier, by employing mathematics invented in the seventeenth century, known as the *differential and integral calculus*.

Readers wishing to teach themselves, or refresh their knowledge of calculus, are referred to the book by Kleppner and Ramsay, listed below.

SUGGESTED READING

CRANE, H. R., *Programmed Math Reviews,* New York: Appleton-Century-Crofts, 1966. This is a set of five programmed reviews on angles and triangles, trigonometry, vectors, powers of ten, and algebra. Each set is composed of about 8 pages embracing some 50 frames each. A frame consists essentially of a statement followed by a question the reader must answer before proceeding. The answers to each frame are available for immediate confirmation of the correct response. These individual reviews would be excellent for one who desired a quick refresher in elementary mathematical techniques.

KEMP, L. A. W., *Mathematics for Radiographers,* Oxford: Blackwell Scientific Publications, 1964 (second edition). This book, which is exactly what its title states and hence fulfills the essential mathematical needs of the radiography student, can be highly recommended. This book would certainly be a valuable asset to any x-ray technician's professional library.

KLEPPNER, D., and N. RAMSAY, *Quick Calculus,* New York: John Wiley, 1965. As the subtitle of this book states, it is a short manual of self-instruction in the calculus. It is not a textbook in the traditional sense, but rather a type of "programmed learning" manual through which the reader works step by step. The book's emphasis on techniques and application, rather than rigorous theories, makes it particularly suitable for the technician who is interested in the calculus from the point of view of its application in electricity and radiation physics.

WEAST, R. C., S. M. SELBY, and C. D. HODGMAN (editors), *Mathematical Tables* (from the *Handbook of Chemistry and Physics*), Cleveland, Ohio: The Chemical Rubber Co., 1965 (forty-sixth edition). Any edition, in fact, of these tables fully provides all the numbers required when one works with trigonometric and logarithmic functions. Brief instruction on the use of logarithms is also provided, as are various differentials and integrals for those interested in pursuing the calculus.

The Metric System and English Equivalents

General system of multiples

Multiple	Prefix	Symbol
10^9	giga	G
10^6	mega	M
10^3	kilo	k
10^2	hecto	h
10	deka	da
10^{-1}	deci	d
10^{-2}	centi	c
10^{-3}	milli	m
10^{-6}	micro	μ
10^{-9}	nano	n

Length

Metric to English

1 angstrom = 1 Å = 10^{-8} cm (centimeter)
$= 10^{-10}$ m (meter)
1 micron = 1 μ = 10^{-3} mm (millimeter)
$= 10^{-6}$ m
1 cm = 0.3937 in. (inch)
1 m = 3.281 ft (foot)

English to metric

1 in. = 2.540 cm
1 ft = 30.48 cm

Volume

Metric to English

1 cm³ = 0.0610 cu. in. (or in.³)
1 liter = 0.2642 U.S. gal (gallon)
1 liter = 0.220 Imperial gal

English to metric

1 cu. in. = 16.387 cm³
1 U.S. gal = 3.785 liters
1 Imp. gal = 4.546 liters

Weight

Metric (gravitational to absolute units)

1 gram force = 980 dynes
1 kg-force = 9.8 newtons

English (avoirdupois) to metric (gravitational)

1 oz = 28.35 grams force
1 lb = 16 oz = 0.4536 kg-force

Temperature

Metric to English: degrees
   Fahrenheit = °F = (°C × $\frac{9}{5}$) + 32
English to metric: degrees
   Celsius = °C = (°F − 32) × $\frac{5}{9}$
Celsius to Kelvin (Celsius absolute):
   °K = °C + 273.2

Alphabetical List of the Elements

Element	Symbol	Atomic number Z	Element	Symbol	Atomic number Z
Actinium	Ac	89	Erbium	Er	68
Aluminum	Al	13	Europium	Eu	63
Americium	Am	95	Fermium	Fm	100
Antimony	Sb	51	Fluorine	F	9
Argon	A	18	Francium	Fr	87
Arsenic	As	33	Gadolinium	Gd	64
Astatine	At	85	Gallium	Ga	31
Barium	Ba	56	Germanium	Ge	32
Berkelium	Bk	97	Gold	Au	79
Beryllium	Be	4	Hafnium	Hf	72
Bismuth	Bi	83	Helium	He	2
Boron	B	5	Holmium	Ho	67
Bromine	Br	35	Hydrogen	H	1
Cadmium	Cd	48	Indium	In	49
Calcium	Ca	20	Iodine	I	53
Californium	Cf	98	Iridium	Ir	77
Carbon	C	6	Iron	Fe	26
Cerium	Ce	58	Krypton	Kr	36
Cesium	Cs	55	Kurchatovium	Ku	104
Chlorine	Cl	17	Lanthanum	La	57
Chromium	Cr	24	Lawrencium	Lw	103
Cobalt	Co	27	Lead	Pb	82
Copper	Cu	29	Lithium	Li	3
Curium	Cm	96	Lutetium	Lu	71
Dysprosium	Dy	66	Magnesium	Mg	12
Einsteinium	Es	99	Manganese	Mn	25

Element	Symbol	Atomic number Z	Element	Symbol	Atomic number Z
Mendelevium	Md	101	Ruthenium	Ru	44
Mercury	Hg	80	Samarium	Sm	62
Molybdenum	Mo	42	Scandium	Sc	21
Neodymium	Nd	60	Selenium	Se	34
Neon	Ne	10	Silicon	Si	14
Neptunium	Np	93	Silver	Ag	47
Nickel	Ni	28	Sodium	Na	11
Niobium	Nb	41	Strontium	Sr	38
Nitrogen	N	7	Sulfur	S	16
Nobelium	No	102	Tantalum	Ta	73
Osmium	Os	76	Technetium	Tc	43
Oxygen	O	8	Tellurium	Te	52
Palladium	Pd	46	Terbium	Tb	65
Phosphorus	P	15	Thallium	Tl	81
Platinum	Pt	78	Thorium	Th	90
Plutonium	Pu	94	Thulium	Tm	69
Polonium	Po	84	Tin	Sn	50
Potassium	K	19	Titanium	Ti	22
Praseodymium	Pr	59	Tungsten	W	74
Promethium	Pm	61	Uranium	U	92
Protactinium	Pa	91	Vanadium	V	23
Radium	Ra	88	Xenon	Xe	54
Radon	Rn	86	Ytterbium	Yb	70
Rhenium	Re	75	Yttrium	Y	39
Rhodium	Rh	45	Zinc	Zn	30
Rubidium	Rb	37	Zirconium	Zr	40

Answers to Selected Questions

Chapter 1

4. $E = hf$
6. Inner shell
9. Curie
14. 2.5 grams
15. 1 millicurie
16. $_{15}P^{31} + {_0}n^1 \rightarrow {_{15}}P^{32}$

Chapter 2

5. b) 5.4×10^3 newtons, attraction
6. a) 5.4×10^3 newtons, repulsion
    b) Force $\frac{1}{4}$ as large
9. 100 watts
10. a) $V_{AB} = -2000$ volts   b) Point B
11. Perpendicular to equipotential line
12. a) 7.0×10^4 eV   b) 7.0×10^4 eV
13. 2 cm
16. Leather-soled shoes
19. 6.8×10^{-3} coul

Chapter 3

1. 6.25×10^{18} electrons
2. 2×10^{-2} coul

3. Silver, copper, aluminum, tungsten, salt water, oil, glass

4. Low to high

10. a) Voltmeter has infinite resistance, ammeter has zero resistance

    b) Zero internal resistance   i) 8 ohms

    c) Zero resistance   j) 1 amp

    d) Clockwise   k) 8 volts

    e) 24 volts   l) a

    f) 2 ohms   m) +12 volts

    g) 2 amp   n) Zero

    h) 8 volts   o) Current would increase

    p) More current through R_3 than R_2

    q) Connect points e and a with good conducting wire

    r) Current rises, overheating wires, leading to fire hazard

    s) No change   t) Decrease

    u) Current would become twice as large; i.e., 4 amp

    v) Current would go to zero   x) Yes

    w) Nothing   y) No

Chapter 4

5. a) Clockwise

    b) North end of compass would point toward reader

    c) Oersted

6. a) Vacuum core   c) Ferromagnetic

    b) Paramagnetic

7. Transformers, relays, rotor

12. Toward magnet

13. Counterclockwise in coil

Chapter 5

2. a) Yes, from Y to X

    b) No

    c) Yes, from X to Y

3. a) Down right-hand wire   e) Increase

    b) Lenz's law   f) Double

    c) South   g) No change

    d) Much smaller

4. Increase the ratio of the secondary windings to primary windings; introduce a ferromagnetic core; increase current in primary.

5. a) Coil X is the primary; coil Y is the secondary

    b) Counterclockwise

    c) Counterclockwise

6. a) Generator   b) DC   c) From right to left

7. 60 cycles/sec
11. Induction motor
12. H.T. transformer
14. a) Increase   b) Increase   c) Faraday's law, Lenz's law
15. d) 3, 120° apart

Chapter 6

2. a) 0.067 sec
3. No; 15 amp RMS is required
7. a) Resistor   b) Inductor
9. Slightly less inductance with a diamagnetic core
10. No
11. a) 5.0 ohms   b) 12 ohms
12. Becomes less bright
13. a) $P = IV \cos \theta$ b) Watt   c) $P = I^2R$
14. Current and voltage in phase and in RMS values; circuit impedance entirely resistive, that is, reactance is zero.
15. a) RMS
    b) Capacitor has zero power consumption, inductor has zero power consumption, resistor has 1.5 kW power consumption.
    c) 1.5 kW
    d) Larger
17. a) 50 kV   b) 50 amp   c) 5 kW   d) Ideal transformer
19. 60 current pulses
20. Half wave
21. b) Silicon
22. a) Half wave   c) One
23. b) mAs meter
24. a) Yes; yes

Chapter 7

1. Filament may be damaged by electron emission from anode.
2. Higher peak values of current in half-wave than in full-wave for same mA, resulting in greater heating during the conducting half cycle.
10. 0.66%
14. X-rays and electrons, respectively

Chapter 8

3. Primary is at about mains voltage, secondary is connected to H.T. transformer output

9. In self-rectified x-ray machine, current flows only in one direction through the mA meter, even without its own rectification circuit.

11. b) Yes, if the exposure starts and stops when the voltage is close to, or at, its peak value. Five "spots" and two "half spots" could result. "Half spots" would be less dark.

13. About 50% of expected radiographic density (unless x-ray machine is equipped with circuits which automatically ensure correct mAs despite a valve-tube failure).

Chapter 9

3. Diffraction, polarization

4. Compton effect

5. Infrared, visible light, ultraviolet, diagnostic x-rays, gamma rays

6. 12.4 keV

10. a) A, glass envelope; B, cathode; C, target and anode; D, lead screen; E, crystal; F, radiation detector.

15. a) No, different λ_{min}
    b) Yes, same characteristic radiation

16. a) 90 keV   b) 90 keV   c) 27 keV to about 36 keV

17. b) 240 kV

18. $\lambda_{min} = \dfrac{(6.63 \times 10^{-34} \text{ joule-sec}) (3 \times 10^8 \text{ m/sec}) (10^{10} \text{ Å/m})}{(\text{kV})(10^3)(1.60 \times 10^{-19} \text{ coul})} = \left(\dfrac{12.4}{\text{kV}}\right) \text{Å}$

Chapter 10

3. b) Water, bone, copper, lead

8. a) A, pair production; B, photoelectric attenuation; C, Compton effect
   b) Photoelectric effect, on the assumption that "importance" refers to the amount of energy transferred to the patient.
   c) $\tau_{PE} \propto \lambda^3$, $\tau_{PE} \propto Z^3$.

10. $\Delta\lambda = 0.0243(1 - \cos\theta)$

Chapter 11

2. kV, mA, time, distance, filtration

3. 20 R

4. Reading larger when patient is in place, due to back scatter

5. 420 mR

6. Fluoroscopy, larger mAs
8. Low-energy photons
9. Increase filtration
11. Photographic effect, ionization, luminescence, heating effect, biological effect, change in conductivity
12. Calorimetry
14. a) Free-air chamber, Victoreen condenser chamber, Cutie Pie, Geiger counter
18. No
20. $\frac{1}{2}$
23. a) 300 R   b) Erythema
24. 0.1 rem/wk (based on 5 rem/yr after age 18)

Abbreviations of Units and Other Symbols

Abbreviations of Units

Å	angstrom unit
amp or A	ampere
cm	centimeter
eV	electron volt
gm	gram
HU	heat unit
j	joule
keV	kilo electron volt
kV	kilovolt
m	meter
mA	milliampere
mAs or mA-s	milliampere-second
MeV	million electron volts or mega electron volt
N	newton
°	degree
Ω	ohm
R	roentgen
sec or s	second
volt or V	volt
W	watt

Symbols

a	acceleration
A	atomic mass number; also activity of a radioactive material
B	magnetic field
C	capacitance
c	speed of light (in vacuum)
D	dose (that is, absorbed dose); also distance
Δ	Delta, meaning "a change in" or "a little bit of"
E	electric field; also energy
e	charge of a single electron; also base of natural logarithms
F	force
f	frequency
g	acceleration of gravity
h	Planck's constant
I	DC current; also RMS AC current
i	instantaneous current
I_{RMS} or I_{eff} or I: RMS AC current	
L	inductance
l	length
λ	decay constant; also wavelength
m	mass
p	momentum
P	power
Q or q	charge
R or X	exposure
R	resistance
RBE	relative biological effectiveness
s	distance
T	period; also half-life
t	time
V	DC potential (or potential difference); also RMS AC voltage
v	velocity; also instantaneous voltage
V_{RMS} or V_{eff} or V: RMS AC voltage	
W	work function or work (or energy)
X_C	capacitive reactance
X_L	inductive reactance
Z	impedance; also atomic number
$\perp$	Perpendicular; that is, $A \perp B$ means that if two quantities A and B, being vectors (that is, having both magnitude and direction), are multiplied, only their mutually perpendicular components should be multiplied.

Index

A B C D E 6 9 8